Fourth International Visual Field Symposium

Documenta Ophthalmologica Proceedings Series volume 26

Editor H. E. Henkes

Dr W. Junk bv Publishers The Hague – Boston – London 1981

Fourth International Visual Field Symposium
Bristol, April 13-16, 1980

Edited by E. L. Greve and G. Verriest

Dr W. Junk bv Publishers The Hague – Boston – London 1981

Distributors:

for the United States and Canada

Kluwer Boston, Inc.
190 Old Derby Street
Hingham, MA 02043
USA

for all other countries

Kluwer Academic Publishers Group
Distribution Center
P.O. Box 322
3300 AH Dordrecht
The Netherlands

ISBN-13: 978-94-009-8646-6 e-ISBN-13: 978-94-009-8644-2
DOI: 10.1007/978-94-009-8644-2

Cover design: Max Velthuijs

Softcover reprint of the hardcover 1st edition 1981

Dr. W. Junk bv Publishers, P.O. Box 13713, 2501 ES The Hague, The Netherlands.

INTRODUCTION

The 4th International Visual Field Symposium of the International Perimetric Society, was held on the 13–16 April 1980 in Bristol, England, at the occasion of the 6th Congress of the European Society of Ophthalmology. The main themes of the symposium were comparison of classical perimetry with visual evoked response, comparison of classical perimetry with special psychophysical methods, and optic nerve pathology. Understandably many papers dealt with computer assisted perimetry. This rapidly developing subgroup of perimetry may radically change the future of our method of examination. New instruments were introduced, new and exciting software was proposed and the results of comparative investigations reported.

There have been many confusing statements in the literature on the relative value of perimetry and the registration of visual evoked responses. Several reports attempted to bring some clarity in this issue. There is reason for further comparative research.

A number of papers dealt with special psychophysical methods, i.e. methods not using the simply monocular differential threshold.

The old critical fusion frequency received new attention. Fundusperimetry was used for testing spatial summation. Acuity perimetry, binocular perimetry etc. showed that there exist many possibilities for examining visual function.

At present it is not clear to us what exactly the place of these methods is in our diagnostic armament. However it is quite clear that some of them are promising and may lead to a further differentiation of perimetric methods.

An excellent invited report on colour perimetry was given by Hedin and Verriest. It demonstrated that this method has special merits and should be used more often in selected cases. Several other papers supported this concept.

New instruments and strategies that do not require computer assistance were presented, most of them dealing with the detection phase of perimetry.

Foulds presented his expert experience on optic nerve disease in a clear and informative invited lecture, which is warmly recommended to the reader. The defects in optic nerve disease were examined by several authors using a variety of test procedures, which may improve our detection rate. Apart from the optic nerve diseases several other diseases were presented in various papers. They concerned glaucoma, chiasmal lesions in pregnancy, cerebrovascular accident and others.

A report on mass-screening was given which presented figures similar to previous reports. Mass visual field screening is possible especially with computer assisted perimeters and may yield approximately 2% visual field defects.

There has always been a need for scoring of visual fields. Two papers deal with this subject. Esterman's system has been used in the USA for some time. The IPS will in the near future attack this urgent problem and hopefully come up with a system that incorporates not only area but also intensity of defects. Here, too, computer assistance may provide new possibilities.

Bristol and its surrounding countryside provided an excellent background for this 4th symposium of the IPS. Vincent Marmion and his family in a joint effort spent much time and energy in the local organization of the symposium. Alan Friedmann and Ronald Pitts Crick assisted in the organization. They can be proud of the result. Marmion's excellent secretary, Mrs. Maureen Pitman, and her colleague, Mrs. Joan Parker, were never visibly tired of organizing every single detail. They deserve our admiration and gratitude. Without them it would not have been the same.

As ever Mrs. Els Mutsaerts from the IPS secretariat in Amsterdam did much of the 'behind the curtain' work. Not only did she assist in the compilation of the scientific programme but also she played a major role in the realization of the proceedings. It has become almost a habit to thank Mr. Wil Peters of Dr. W. Junk bv, Publishers. After this, our sixth joint effort, we are still going strong!

THE EDITORS

CONTENTS

Part three: Special psychophysical methods

Part four: Colour perimetry

Part five: Instruments and strategies

Part six: Optic nerve

Part seven: Visual field defects in various diseases

Part eight: Varia

AUTOMATIC PERIMETER WITH GRAPHIC DISPLAY

HARUTAKE MATSUO, GEN KIKUCHI, SUSUMU HAMAZAKI,
JUNJI HAMAZAKI, EIJI SUZUKI & MAKOTO YAMADA

(Tokyo, Japan)

ABSTRACT

An improved type of automatic perimeter was devised based on the semi-automatic campimeter reported by Hamazaki *et al.* on the occasion of the 1978 symposium of the IPS [3]. The new perimeter is easier to manipulate and the entire examination process is computerized, with simultaneous T.V. monitor display and printout of the final result. Stimulus intensity and examination patterns are readily changeable according to the purpose of the examinations. Specific points of interest, arrangement of the stimulus points and stimulus intensity are all easily altered using the typewriter keyboard. In addition the perimeter is relatively cheap.

INTRODUCTION

An improved version of a semi-automatic campimeter was developed. The basic principle of the perimeter is the same as that of the former semi-automatic campimeter [3], reported in 1978, and is composed of a personal computer system combined with a television display. The versatile functions of the new perimeter permits various applications with suitable program using. Manipulation of the perimeter is simple and examinations short.

METHOD

1. The computerized automatic perimeter system is shown in Fig. 1.
   [1] *For patient*
      (1) C R T (Cathode Ray Tube) display
      (2) Response button
      (3) Button to proceed
   [2] *For examiner*
      (4) Personal computer
      (5) Monitor T.V.
      (6) Audio-cassette tape recorder
      (7) Videoplotter

The procedure begins with input of the desired program, which is stored in a tape recorder cassette, followed by input of biodata using the typewriter keyboard.

Doc. Ophthal. Proc. Series, Vol. 26, ed. by E. L. Greve & G. Verriest

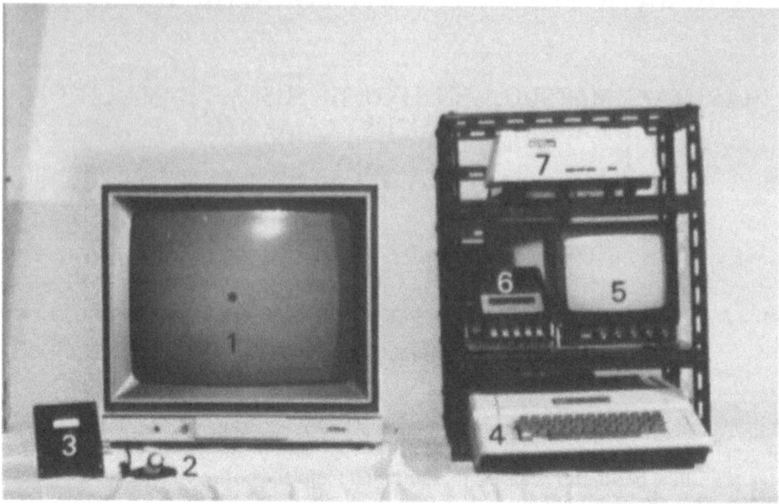

Fig. 1. Automatic perimeter system: 1. CRT display; 2. Response button; 3. Button to proceed; 4. Personal computer; 5. Monitor T.V.; 6. Audio-cassette tape recorder; 7. Videoplotter.

2. Examination conditions

[1] *Central fixation point and stimulus time*

The central fixation point is about 20 minutes in diameter. It is marked with a 1.0 cm round red filter, attached to the center of the screen and stands out clearly from the stimulus points. The fixation point light flashes twice at an interval of 0.5 seconds following which a mulitple-stimuli-pattern is displayed on the screen for 0.3 seconds. The fixation point, stimulus points and the beep from the computer are synchronized. Consequently the patient hears different rhythms and intervals of beeping sounds which draws attention to the fixation point and thus prevents unnecessary eye movements.

[2] *Adaptation*

The background luminance is adjusted by visual photometry to photopic conditions of 0.16 cd/m^2 adaptation level. The patient adaptation time is five minutes.

[3] *Luminance*

The size of one stimulus point is approximately nine minutes in diameter. The luminance is divided into five steps: 0, 1, 2, 3, 4, from low to high. Normal data determine lowest luminance threshold. The highest luminance is provided by the highest voltage of the computer. The stimulus luminance is increased gradually towards the periphery in order to maintain the plateau of the threshold within an area of 25°. This was determined by the results of studies of normal subjects. If the patient fails to recognize the highest luminance (4), 'x' is marked by the computer.

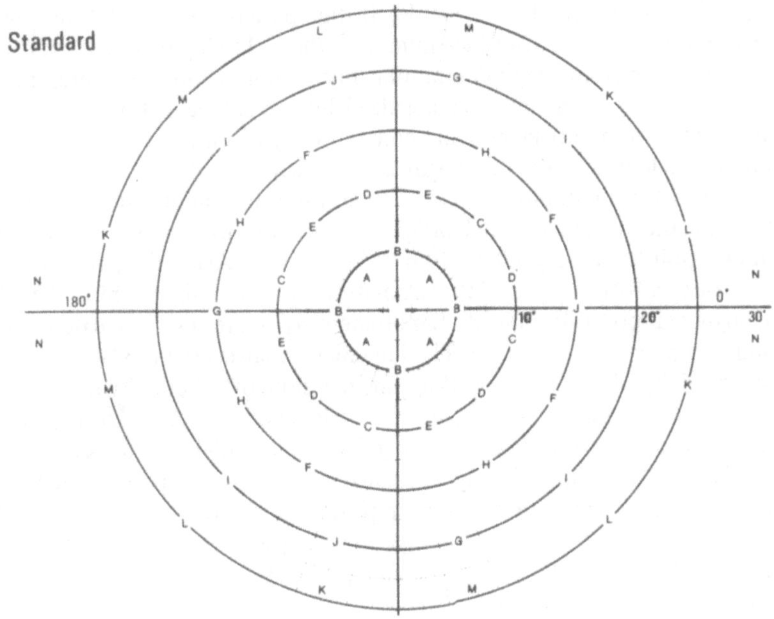

Fig. 2. Fifteen five stimulus points of standard program.

[4] *Patterns*

Fourteen types of multiple-stimuli-patterns are used. Each pattern has three or four stimulus points. There are 51 stimulus points within the 25° circle, and four more stimulus points are added to the 30° circle. Each of these four is situated at a site of five degrees above and below the horizontal meridian, in the hope of detection of nasal step (Fig. 2). The macula threshold appears three degrees apart from the center on the right side, and the patient is told to gaze at this point. Quick search of the lowest stimulus luminance recognized by the patient shortens the examination time. Four stimulus points are displayed on the central area, at a location of five degrees from the center, and if the patient is able to discern at least one of them, the examination can proceed from that luminance level.

3. Proceeding and interpretation

Patterns from A to N are displayed on the screen consecutively. Arrangement of the stimulus point is made as asymmetrical as possible on the same circle line. The patient pushes response button in accordance with the number of stimuli recognized, then pushes the proceed button for the next examination. On the examiner's side, when the patient responds correctly, the same examination is repeated for confirmation, then the next examination is performed. If the patient fails to respond correctly, all possible loss-factor permutations are displayed. Based on data of this examination, the computer calculates and judges which stimulus have been recognized on the basis of statistical probability. For example, if the patient answered three instead four in a four-stimuli-pattern examination, the following procedures are automatically carried out by the computer. Each stimulus point is represented by a, b, c, d. If 'a' point is not recognized by the subject, all possible permutations with one point lacking are consecutively displayed on the screen. The computer calculates the unrecognized site with false-unrecognized-stimuli. In a case of a four-stimuli-pattern, first all the four stimulus points are examined, then the aforementioned all possible permutations are surveyed, thus all stimulus points are examined four times evenly. After this, the computer carries out statistical probability calculations on the basis of which the falsely unrecognized point is judged. Simultaneously, a re-test is carried out by examinations 1, 2, 3, 4 (Fig. 3). The judging standards are preprogrammed and memorized by the computer, thus the decision of whether which stimulus point is truly or falsely recognized or not is made out. After examination of one luminance section examination of the next higher luminance section is performed, avoiding already recognized patterns. If patient response is unreliable, the examination can be repeated at anytime. Examination time for normal subjects, regardless of age, does not exceed five minutes per eye. Final results are displayed on the monitor T.V. and is printed out simultaneously by the videoplotter.

4. Other programs

In addition to the aforementioned program, other programs based on the principle of the Armaly-Drance technique are available.

[1] *Examination on the circle 15° from the center*

In order to check the Bjerrum area, 24 stimulus points are displayed on the circle 15° from the center. The distance between each point is 15°. The intensity of the luminance is the same as in the first program. Examination time, even if the patient has visual field disturbances does not exceed seven minutes.

[2] *Testing of the meridian*

Twenty four meridians from 0° to 345° at 15° intervals are set and 10 stimulus points are arranged along each meridian from the center to the 25° site at 2.5° intervals, these make a total number of 240 stimulus points. If the examiner wishes to examine one particular meridian, 10 stimulus points can be displayed. Examination time is less than four minutes. The intensity of the luminance of [1] and [2] is gradually raised to the maximum level automatically. Other programs aim at screening of two circles, at sites 10° and 20° from the center, with 24 stimulus points, using 1- and 4-luminance. This method is useful to shorten the examination time, e.g. is hemianopsia screening.

5. Clinical case

A diagnosis of open angle glaucoma had been made in this 51 year-old Japanese female 10 years ago. Fig. 4 shows the result of automatic perimeter

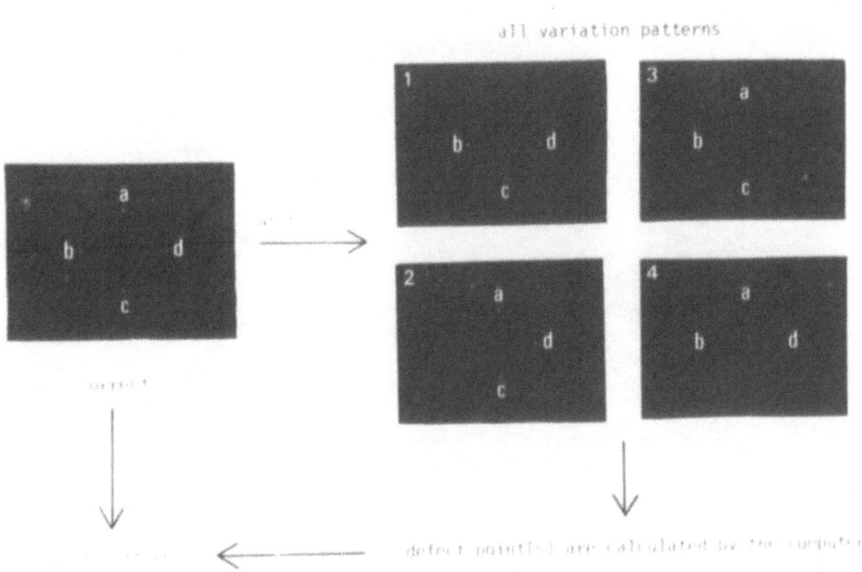

Fig. 3. Method of finding defect point(s).

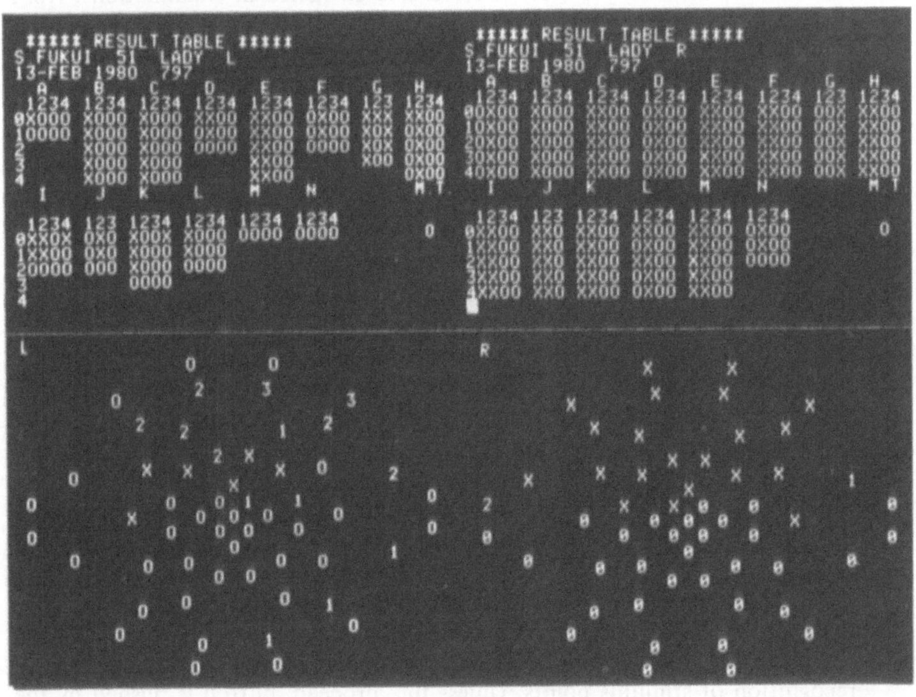

Fig. 4. Results of the automatic perimeter.

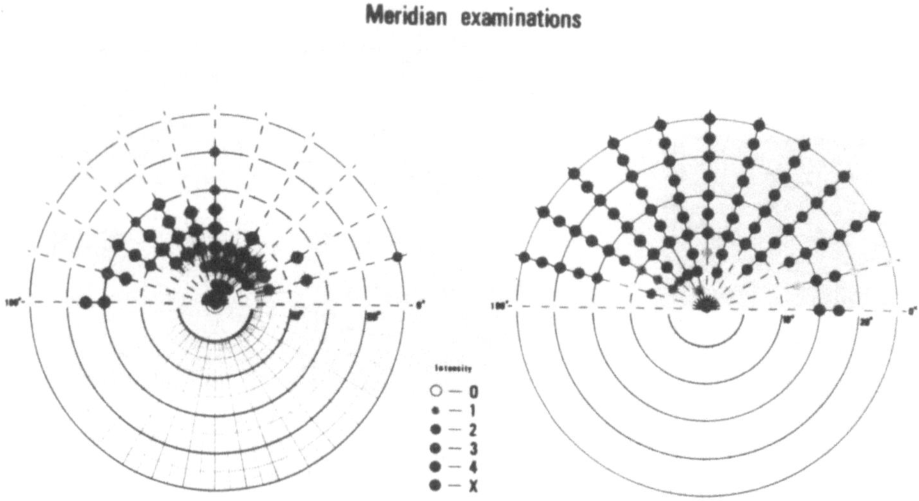

Fig. 5. Results of 13 meridian examinations (from 0° to 180°).

measurement. Both eyes were subjected to 13 meridian examinations, from 0° to 180° with a luminance of 0 to 4 (Fig. 5). The result of this examination was compared with the results of Goldmann Perimeter, Friedmann Visual Field Analyser, OCTOPUS, Perimetron and Tübinger Perimeter. The authors reached the conclusion that the automatic perimeter is valuable for screening purposes and also for quantitative measurement of visual changes.

DISCUSSION

Recently, various automatic perimeters have been developed for quantitative measurement of the visual field, such as OCTOPUS, Perimetron, Autofield and Fieldmaster among others. However, these instruments are rather expensive, space consuming and complicated. There are also problems with sensitively and permissible patient response time. In our automatic perimeter, in order to maintain the fixation point, the beeping sound and fixation point lamp are synchronized. The 0.3 seconds stimulating time is shorter than the former semi-automatic campimeter which lasted 0.5 seconds. Subsequently, the patient can easily observe the fixed point by means of the rhythms and flashing lamp. Due to adaptation of the application of multiple stimuli pattern method, the patient has to indicate the number of recognized points no time limit and it is not necessary to mention the site of direction of recognized stimuli. Consequently, the automatic perimeter is able to lessen errors in recognition of stimulus points. Unless the 'proceed' button is pushed by the patient, the procedure does not continue, so if the patient gets tired, he can rest anytime at will.

Results of a comparative study of the Goldmann Perimeter and the automatic perimeter revealed that the latter is suitable for daily clinical use. Also, shortening of the examination time is important.

CONCLUSION

An automatic perimeter with CRT display and a personal computer system was devised. The perimeter measures the visual field under stable conditions regardless of examiners' experience of the examiner, or the patient's response. As the system accepts a variety of programs, quantitative measurement of the visual field is simplified, efficient and precise.

REFERENCES

1. Fankhauser, F., J. Spahr & H. Bebie. Three years of experience with the OCTOPUS automatic perimeter. Docum. Ophthal. Proc. Series 14:7–15(1977).
2. Greve, E. L., M. T. H. J. N. Groothuyse & P. Bakker. Simulated automatic perimetry. Docum. Ophthal. Proc. Series 14:23–29(1977).
3. Hamazaki, S., J. Hamazaki, G. Kikuchi & H. Matsuo. Semi-automatic campimeter with graphic display. Docum. Ophthal. Proc. Series 19:311–317(1978).
4. Heijl, A. & C. E. T. Krakau. An automatic static perimeter, design and pilot study. Acta Ophthal. 53:293–310(1975).
5. Kelter, J. L., *et al.* Suprathreshold static perimetry. Arch. Ophthal. 97:260–272 (1979).
6. Shinzato, E., R. Suzuki & F. Furno. The central visual field changes in glaucoma using Goldmann Perimeter and Friedmann Visual Field Analyser. Docum. Ophthal. Proc. Series 14:93–101(1977).
7. Zingirian, M., V. Tagliasco & E. Gandolfo. Automatic perimetry:Minicomputers or microprocessors? Docum. Ophthal. Proc. Series 19:327–331(1978).

Authors' address:
Dept. of Ophthalmology
Tokyo Medical College Hospital
6-7-1 Nishishinjuku, Shinjuku-ku
Tokyo 160
Japan

STATISTICAL PROGRAM FOR THE ANALYSIS OF PERIMETRIC DATA

H. BEBIE & F. FANKHAUSER

(Berne, Switzerland)

ABSTRACT

Statistical test procedures may be used for determining whether the results of a static perimetric examination differ significantly from normal visual field values, or for the detection of significant trends in a series of such examinations. The advantages of such statistical evaluations by means of the Octopus automatic perimeter host computer, which has direct access to the visual field data bank, are described.

INTRODUCTION

The two main goals of clinical perimetric examinations are, on the one hand, the differentiation between normal and pathological behaviour and on the other, the determination of progression, regression or stationary behaviour with respect to time.

In clinical practice, such decisions are based half on intuitive, half on rational grounds. Decisions must be reached which may have far-reaching consequences, even though these are very often based on insufficient data. Such decisions are better made on statistical grounds, with the aid of a computer. Data processing is, however, only compatible with time restrictions imposed by clinical practice, when performed by a computer with adequate capacity, which furthermore has immediate access to the perimetric examination results. In addition, an elaborate, goal-oriented statistical interpretation program is a necessary prerequisite.

Such a program possesses the following advantages compared to the usual clinical-intuitive decisions: (a) Stability and clear definition of criteria. (b) Systematic use of all available data. (c) Careful avoidance of overestimating the importance of unusual data, which on a purely random basis are possibly more frequent than is generally assumed. (d) Knowledge of the percentage of cases in which the test is positive on the basis of random differences, even though there is no progression in actual fact (false positives).

THE DELTA PROGRAM

At the time of writing, a test version of a statistical program for the automatic perimeter Octopus has been developed [1]. The program makes use of examination results stored on floppy discs and performs a series of statistical tests upon this data. After a thorough evaluation of the data base, the program decides whether or not this is sufficient for the assumption of (a) deviation of an individual visual field from the norm, or (b) a trend in a series of examinations performed on different occasions. Furthermore, compressed data, which are aimed at a reduced characterization of the visual field, are produced. Statistical tests are, however, subject to the limits of each statistical method whose goal is the separation of two overlapping populations (normal vs. pathological). An increase in the sensitivity of detection of pathological deviations (low level of significance) by necessity leads to contamination of true deviations by random deviations (i.e. the specificity is lowered) and vice versa.

An optimal adjustment of test criteria, which includes interfering factors such as spatially synchronised long term fluctuations, 'learning effects' and others, is possible only by means of a feedback process between the program and a series of clinical evaluations. Such an evaluation has been performed using Octopus program 31 by Gloor *et al.* [2, 3, 4] and Gloor & Schmied [5], as a result of which a first adjustment of criteria was possible.

Refinement of this program Delta, as well as its generalization to include other Octopus examination programs, is at present in progress.

REFERENCES

1. Bebie, H. & F. Fankhauser. Ein statistisches Programm zur Beurteilung von Gesichtsfeldern. Klin. Mbl. Augenheilk. 177: 417–422 (1980).
2. Gloor, B., U. Schmied & A. Fässler. Glaukomgesichtsfelder – Analyse von Octopus – Verlaufsbeobachtungen mit einem statistischen Programm. Klin. Mbl. Augenheilk. 177: 423–436 (1980).
3. Gloor, B. P., U. Schmied & A. Fässler. Changes of glaucomatous field defects. Analysis of OCTOPUS fields with programme Delta. Doc. Ophthal. Proc. Series, Vol. 26, pp. 11–16 (1981).
4. Gloor, B. P., U. Schmied & A. Fässler. Changes of glaucomatous field defects. Degree of accuracy of measurements with the automatic perimeter Octopus (1980, in print).
5. Gloor, B. & U. Schmied. Erfahrungen bei Verlaufsuntersuchungen von glaukomatösen Gesichtsfeldern mit dem automatischen Perimeter Octopus. Klin. Mbl. Augenheilk. 176: 545–546 (1980).

Author's address:
F. Fankhauser
University Eye Clinic
CH-3000 Berne
Switzerland

CHANGES OF GLAUCOMATOUS FIELD DEFECTS
Analysis of OCTOPUS fields with programme Delta

B. P. GLOOR, U. SCHMIED & A. FÄSSLER

(Basel, Switzerland)

ABSTRACT

With the trial version of an analytical programme Delta, developed by Bebie and Fankhauser [1], the change in the 30°-visual field (OCTOPUS programme no. 31) of 125 eyes of 66 patients with chronic simple glaucoma or ocular hypertension, pseudoexfoliation glaucoma and pigmentary glaucoma included, were analysed. The mean age of the patients was 61.2±11.3 years, the intervals between the examinations were 59 to 473 days.

In the subsequent examinations the *size of the disturbed area*, the *total loss* and the loss *per examination per mean number of disturbed points* diminished. The verbal statement, evaluating 126 intervals, concluded 19 times on 'increased loss', 28 times on 'decreased loss'. As the examined sample consisted of patients in which the glaucoma was under observation since long time and in which no dramatic changes in the glaucomatous situation did occur, these changes, evaluated as 'improvements', are no factual ameliorations, but *learning effects* and *fluctuations*. By evaluating changes from the first to the second examination and comparing them to those occurring from the second to the third examination in 13 eyes, it became obvious, that the so-called improvements are considerable in size from the first to the second, but no longer from the second to the third examination. This *learning effect* runs up to 2 dB.

INTRODUCTION

Two qualities are essential for an insturment used for examination of visual fields of glaucoma patients:

1. capability to detect field defects as completely and fast as possible;
2. capability to detect changes in the visual field in reliable and reproducible manner.

The first requirement is essential for making the diagnosis, the second determines our therapeutical decisions.

With detection capability of the programme 21, together with the programme 31 of the OCTOPUS proved to be highly superior to manual Goldmann perimetry, as shown by Li *et al.* [4] and by Schmied [5].

But how are we performing, if we have to make up our mind, if an OCTOPUS field shows true changes or only fluctuations? How difficult this decision may be, is illustrated in Fig. 1. The sequence of 6 visual field examinations from November 1977 to March 1980 (OCTOPUS programme 31) of a 59-year-old mathematician with chronic simple glaucoma, myopia and developing

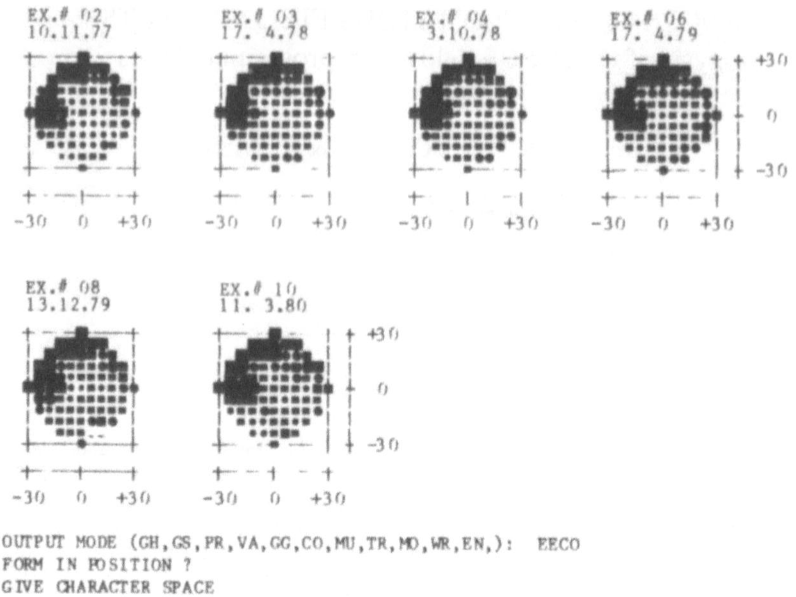

Fig. 1. 59-year-old patient with chronic simple glaucoma, myopia and beginning cataract. Sequence of six visual field examinations (OCTOPUS programme 31) from 1977 to 1980. Many changes from first to fifth examination, sometimes up, sometimes down, but obvious deterioration between the first and sixth examination. Source: Gloor, Schmied & Fässler [2, 3].

cataract is shown. Changes occurring from the 1st to the 5th examination alternate from improvement to deterioration several times, only between 1st and 6th examination a deterioration becomes obvious.

Becoming aware of these difficulties on one hand, taking into consideration on the other hand, that the OCTOPUS breaks up the visual field in a mass of numbers, really logarithmic units (dB), the claim for an analytical programme making use of all these numbers is the next logical step. We were fortunate to get the opportunity to use a trial and experimental version of such an analytical programme, developed by Bebie and Fankhauser [1].

METHODS

With this analytical programme Delta the change in the 30° visual field (OCTOPUS programme 31) of 120 eyes of 66 patients with chronic simple glaucoma or ocular hypertension, pseudoexfoliation glaucoma and pigmentary glaucoma included, were analysed. The mean age of the patients was 61.2±11.3 years, the 146 intervals between the examinations taken into account were 59 to 473 days (203±72 days). 13 eyes which had by chance 3 examinations are evaluated in more detail.

RESULTS

The Results are summarized in the following tables. Table 1a and 1b show, that from one examination to the next a diminution of the size of the

Table 1a. Development of glaucomatous visual field defects. OCTOPUS programmes 31 and Delta (122 eyes).
Disturbed area and total loss per examination per mean number of disturbed points.

	Distribution	S_M*	N
1. Disturbed area (%)			
A: 1. Examination	32.3 ± 33.6	3.1	120
B: Following examinations	29.4 ± 32.7	3.0	122
2. Total loss per examination per mean number of disturbed points			
A: 1. Examination	5.8 ± 5.7 dB	0.5	120
Minimum	0.0 dB		
Maximum	20.1 dB		
B: Following examinations	5.1 ± 5.0 dB	0.5	122
Minimum	0.0 dB		
Maximum	21.2 dB		

* Standard error of the mean.

Table 1b. Development of glaucomatous visual field defects. OCTOPUS programmes 31 and Delta (122 eyes).
Changes of total loss and changes in the single points.

	Distribution	S_M*	N
Change of total loss	−21.5 ± 78.5 dB	7.1	120
– All eyes with increased total loss	+31.8 ± 45.6 dB	5.9	60
– All eyes with decreased total loss	−68.8 ± 76.6 dB	9.9	60
Points			
– Normal in A, disturbed in B	4.7 ± 6.1		
– Disturbed in A, normal in B	6.4 ± 8.5		

* Standard error of the mean.

disturbed area, of the total loss per examination per mean number of disturbed points (TL . . . /DP) and of the total loss takes place. The *diminution* of the depth of the damage in the single point of 0.7 dB is statistically significant (these statistics are explained in Gloor *et al.* [2]).

Table 2 lists the verbal statements made by the two statistical tests, the one evaluating the change of total loss, the other the differences in an area of relatively disturbed points. Of special interest is the high number of 28 intervals, after which a decreased loss had to be assumed. Please also note that the second test is never in disagreement with the first test. There was no correlation between increase or decrease of loss and regulation of intraocular pressure. As there was no evidence of dramatic changes in the pressure situation in our sample of patients with glaucoma, observed since long time, we had no reason to believe that this 'improvement' is real. When the difference of disturbed area, total loss and TL . . . /DP from a first to a second observation was compared to the difference between second and third observation in 13 eyes, which by chance had more than two examinations, the difference of the size of disturbed area diminished from the first to the second interval from 6.1% to 2.6%, the difference of the total loss from

Table 2. Development of glaucomatous visual field defects. OCTOPUS programmes 31 and Delta.
Verbal statements of the two statistical tests of programme Delta.

OCTOPUS test 1:	Number	T-test of differences: NEE	Increased total loss	Decreased total loss
'No change'	1			
'Not enough evidence to assume change of total loss'	51 (7)	12	7 (1)	8 (2)
'Change within normal range of fluctuations'	28 (2)			
'*Increased* total loss may be assumed'	19 (3)		17 (3)	
'*Decreased* total loss may be assumed'	28 (8)	2 (1)		21 (7)

Intervals 127
Normal visual fields 19
N eyes 125
In ( ): tension not regulated (20)

Table 3. Development of glaucomatous visual field defects. OCTOPUS programmes 31 and Delta.
Three consecutive examinations of 13 eyes.

	1. Examination		2. Examination		3. Examination	
	Distribution	S_M	Distribution	S_M	Distribution	S_M
Disturbed area (%) $\bar{x}$	37.8 ± 38.2	10.6	31.6 ± 34.0	9.4	29.1 ± 34.4	9.6
Change of total loss $\bar{x}$			−46.3 ± 71.7 dB	19.2	+12.9 ± 59.4 dB	15.9
Change of total loss per examination per mean number of disturbed points $\bar{x}$			−2.4 ± 8.3 dB	2.2	−0.16 ± 3.6 dB	0.96

−46.3±71.7 dB to +12.9±59.4 dB ('−' means improvement, '+' means deterioration). Corresponding to that, the difference of TL . . . /DP diminished from −2.4±8.3 to −0.16±3.6 dB. The same tendency shows up in Fig. 1 and Tables 2 and 3.

As a first approach we would suggest, that the size of this so-called improvement really determines the size of the learning effect which is 0–2 dB per point. The considerable standard deviation in the determination of change of TL . . . /DP is inherent to the sensitivity of static perimetry to deviation of fixations, especially when a relatively wide grid of 6° is used. But this deviation may also point out, that reports on regression of field defects have to be evaluated with great care.

These difficulties, characteristic for static perimetry, can only be surmounted, if more time is invested in the examination of visual fields, even if an automatic perimeter such as the OCTOPUS is used. How much is added in accuracy by examining patients twice in short intervals, will be reported at the meeting of the Glaucoma Society in Brighton [3].

To conclude: The fascinating thing about the OCTOPUS perimetry is, that we have for the first time easy access to numbers and that we can characterize the visual field in terms of *disturbed area*, *total loss* and *loss per examination per mean number of disturbed points* immediately after an OCTOPUS examination. We are approximating the standards to differentiate between fluctuations and true changes. Some modifications seem necessary, as well as in the manner of application of the existing programmes as also of the programmes themselves.

REFERENCES

1. Bebie, H. & F. Fankhauser. Ein statistisches Programm zur Beurteilung von Gesichtsfeldern. Klinische Monatsblätter für Augenheilkunde 177, 4, 417–422 (1980).
2. Gloor, B., U. Schmied & A. Fässler. Glaukomgesichtsfelder – Analyse von OCTOPUS – Verlaufsbeobachtungen mit einem statistischen Programm. Klinische Monatsblätter für Augenheilkunde 177, 4, 423–436 (1980a).
3. Gloor, B., U. Schmied & A. Fässler. Changes of glaucomatous field defects – degree of accuracy of measurements with the automatic perimeter OCTOPUS. Presented at the First Symposium of the European Glaucoma Society, Brighton, 18th–20th April 1980. Int. Ophthal. 3, 1 (1980b).
4. Li, S. G., G. L. Spaeth, H. A. Scimeca & N. J. Schatz. Clinical experiences with the use of an automated perimeter (OCTOPUS) in the diagnosis and management of patients with glaucoma and neurologic diseases. Opthalmology 86, 7, 1302–1312 (1979).
5. Schmied, U. Automatic (OCTOPUS) and manual (GOLDMANN) perimetry in glaucoma. Graefes Arch. klin. exp. Ophthal. 213, 239–244 (1980).

This paper will be published in extenso in 'Klinische Monatsblätter für Augenheilkunde', in German.

Author's address:
Prof. B. Gloor
Universitäts-Augenklinik
Mittlere Strasse 91
CH-4056 Basel
Switzerland

THE PERITEST

ERIK L. GREVE

(Amsterdam, The Netherlands)

ABSTRACT

A more elaborate description of this instrument has been given in *Documenta Ophthalmologica Proceedings Series*, Vol. 22, pp. 71–74 (1980).

This perimeter (Fig. 1) has been constructed for automatic and non-automatic detection of visual field defects. Some technical data are presented in the table. The stimulus distribution is shown in Fig. 2.

The Peritest aims at completing a detectionphase within five minutes. At missed positions the intensity of defects can be further examined.

Table. Peritest technical data.

type:	hemispherical perimeter; radius 30 cm.
background L:	1 cd/m².
stimulus:	
L-source:	light emitting diodes (L.E.D.).
L-steps:	0.2 log. units.
L-range:	3.0 log. units.
colour:	peak at 575 nm.
size:	30′.
duration:	0.2 S.
presentation type:	Static, multiple and single.
positions:	fixed, no problems with reproducibility.
distribution:	see Fig. 2; a total number of 214 positions can be examined of which 157 are inside the 25° parallel and 57 in the periphery.

Author's address:
Eye Clinic of the University of Amsterdam
Wilhelmina Gasthuis
Eerste Helmersstraat 104
1054 EG Amsterdam
The Netherlands

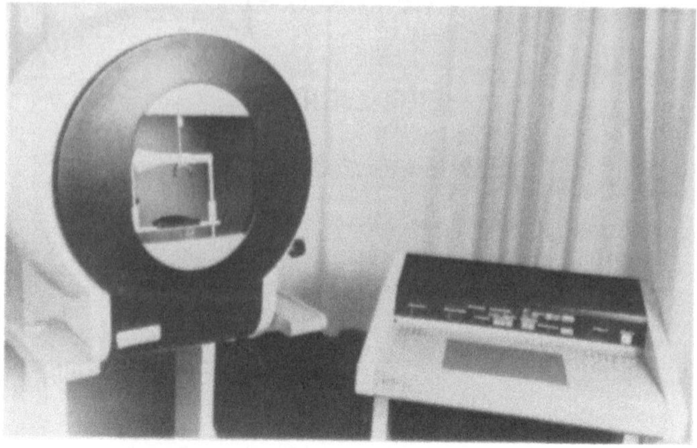

Fig. 1. Peritest.

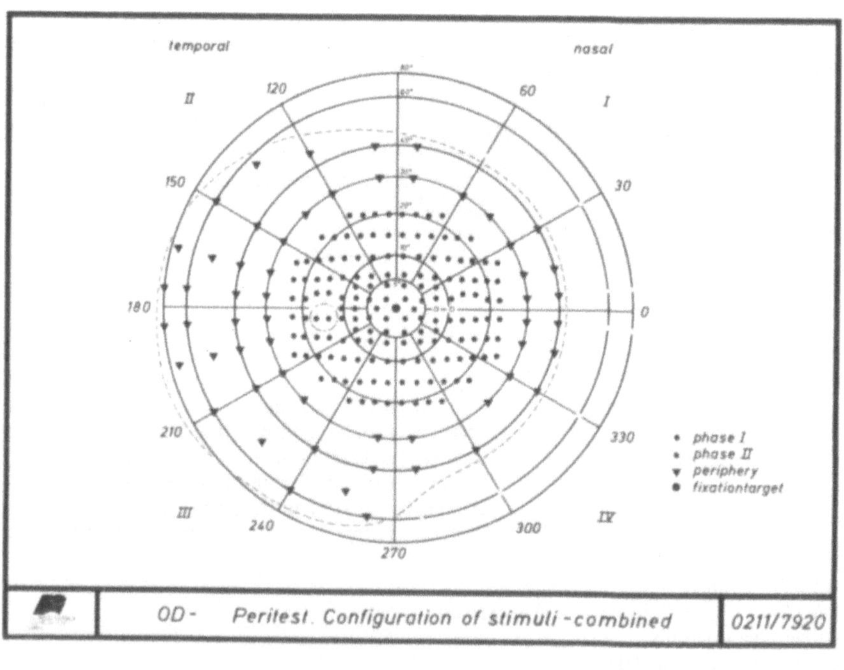

Fig. 2. Stimulus distribution of the Peritest.

DETECTABILITY OF EARLY GLAUCOMATOUS FIELD DEFECTS

A controlled comparison of Goldmann versus Octopus perimetry

G. K. KRIEGLSTEIN, W. SCHREMS, E. GRAMER & W. LEYDHECKER

(Würzburg, F.R.G.)

ABSTRACT

In a controlled study a group of 122 glaucomatous eyes with a high incidence of early visual field defects were examined with the Goldmann kinetic perimeter and the Octopus computerized perimeter. Discrepancies between both examinations were clarified by the use of a high resolution program of the Octopus placed into the disputed location of the field. In 55 of the 122 eyes field defects could be established by the kinetic procedure. The computerized perimeter verified early glaucomatous field defects in 87 of the 122 eyes. In 28 of the 32 eyes of nonconformity the field defect could be reproduced by the high resolution program. The results suggest that about every third glaucomatous defect is missed by kinetic perimetry and a sufficient degree of reproducibility of the examination in glaucomatous field defects is achieved by the computerized technique only.

INTRODUCTION

Anyone who knows the pitfalls of manual perimetry from his own clinical practice will appreciate the advantages of computerized perimetry [3]. The conceptual superiority of a static computerized perimetry with a repetitive bracketing for threshold determination is clearly preferable to traditional kinetic perimetry [1, 2]. Early glaucomatous visual field defects represent an ideal test group for the comparison of both methods. The aim of the present study was therefore to investigate the detection probability of glaucomatous defects comparing the Goldmann kinetic perimeter and the Octopus perimeter.

METHODS

The present study comprised 122 glaucomatous eyes of 84 subjects. The selection criteria for these patients should ensure a high incidence of glaucomatous field defects and were as follows:

a) known early glaucomatous visual field defects
b) glaucomatous disc findings
c) long-term history of considerably raised intraocular pressure

Patients with vision less than 0.5, anterior segment pathology, cataract formation or visual field changes other than glaucomatous were excluded from this study. In a randomized order the visual field was tested by observer I experienced for many years in kinetic périmetry utilizing the Goldmann instrument and by observer II using the Octopus perimeter (stimulus size 3, program 31) in a strictly masked fashion. Prior to the test the best near vision correction was obtained for both instruments. A minimum of 1 hr interval for resting was allowed between the repeated visual field examinations. In the case of a qualitative difference between both techniques the questionable defect was verified or rejected by means of the high resolution program 61 in the disputed location of the field. The definition of a pathological central kinetic field was orientated on isopter defects of a certain size and scotomas within an isopter all within 30° excentricity. For the static computerized field a threshold differential of 10 dB was defined to be the starting point of a true field defect.

RESULTS

In the 122 glaucomatous eyes investigated 55 pathological kinetic fields (45.1%) were obtained. The Octopus fields using program 31 exhibited in 87 eyes (68.0%) glaucomatous defects (Fig. 1). Consequently, a qualitative contradiction between both methods happened in 32 eyes (22.9%). Rechecking these eyes with program 61 the initial Octopus finding (minimum threshold differential of 10 dB) could be confirmed in 28 eyes. In the remaining 4 eyes the threshold differential was less than 10 dB but not within the fluctuation range. Fig. 2 shows a frequency distribution of pathologically decreased thresholds as determined with the program 31 stimuli pattern. There was no field pathological with the Goldmann perimeter which could be confirmed as normal by the Octopus, whereas Goldmann normal and Octopus glaucomatous occurred in the 28 double checked discrepancies. The reproducibility of the Octopus findings was elucidated by calculating the correlation between the threshold differentials (depth of the scotomas) obtained in program 31 and 61. There was a highly significant correlation coefficient of 0.90 with a regression line close to best line fit ($y = 1.01\,x - 1.27$; Fig. 3). Out of the 55 eyes exhibiting field defects in the kinetic as well as in the computerized

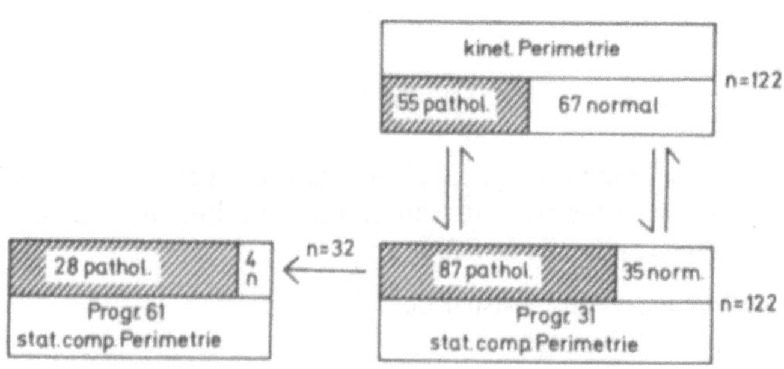

Fig. 1. Distribution of normal and pathological fields of 122 glaucomatous eyes using Goldmann kinetic perimetry and Octopus computerized perimetry program 31. In case of a qualitative discrepancy an additional Octopus field utilizing program 61 was performed.

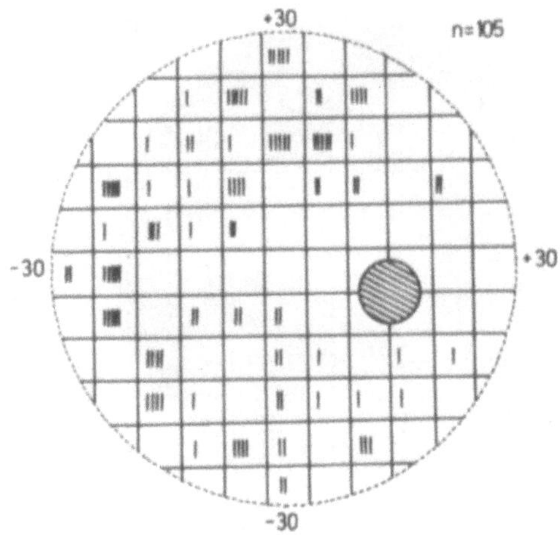

Fig. 2. Frequency distribution of 105 scotomas verified by Octopus perimetry in the central visual field.

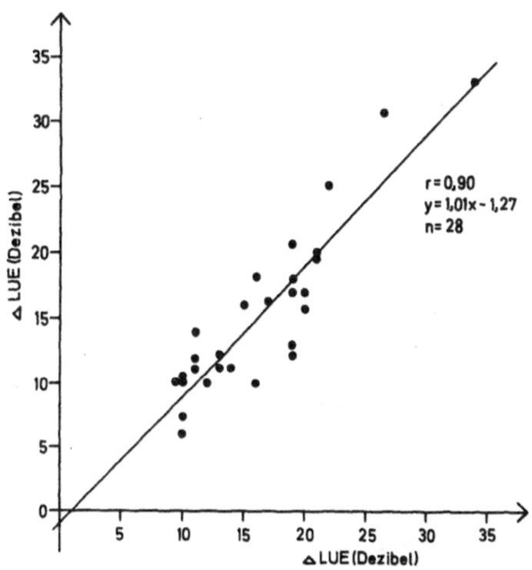

Fig. 3. Regression line between the threshold differentials of scotomas observed with the Octopus using program 31 (abscissa) and program 61 (ordinate). The threshold differentials (depth of the scotomas) could be confirmed with a highly significant correlation.

field quantitative differences occurred in 31 eyes (visual field defect different in Octopus and Goldmann with respect to size, shape and depth). Actually, comparable fields with both techniques were obtained only in 63 of 122 eyes.

An example of a rather advanced glaucomatous defect overlooked with kinetic perimetry is given in Fig. 4. Quantitative differences between a glaucomatous visual field obtained by kinetic technique and static computerized technique are shown in Fig. 5.

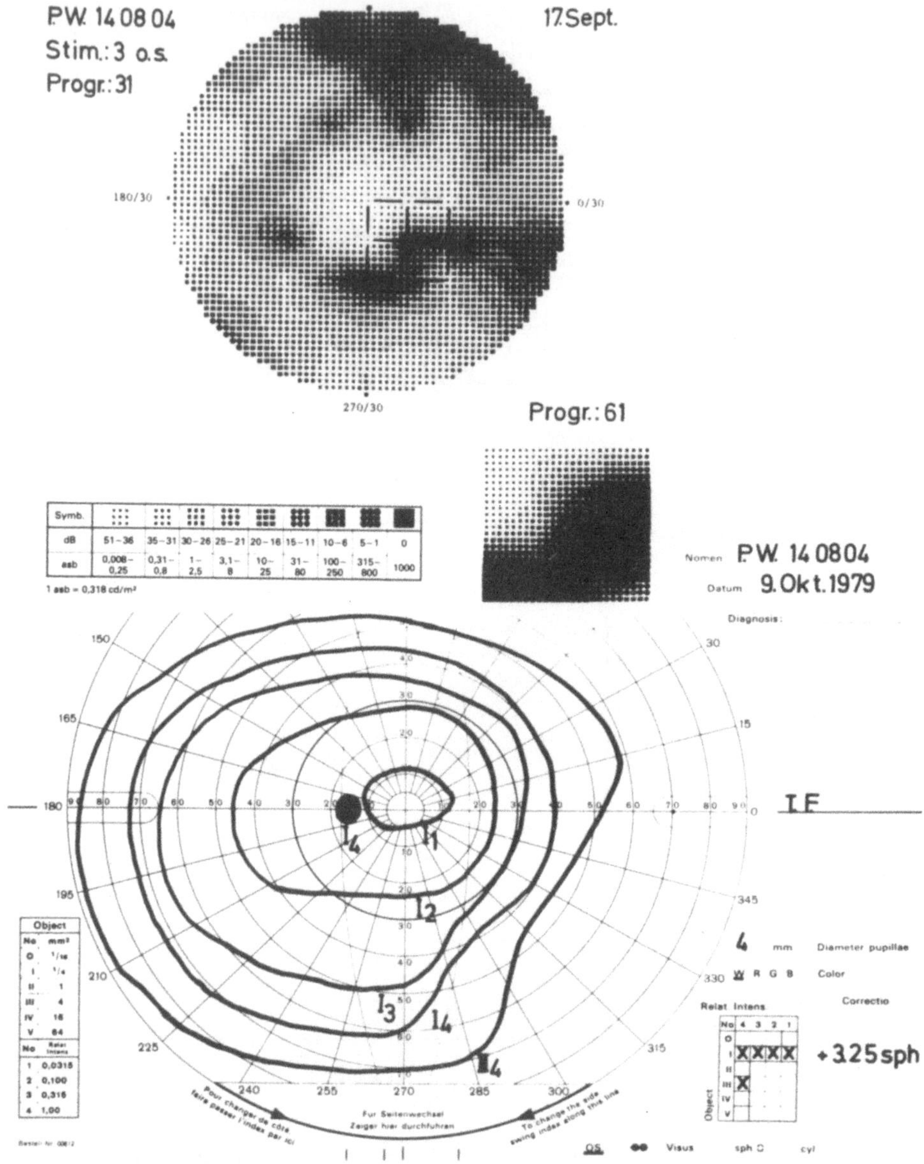

Fig. 4. Visual field of the left eye of a glaucoma patient with definite field loss observed with the Octopus (upper part) and only insignificant changes in the manual, kinetic field (lower part).

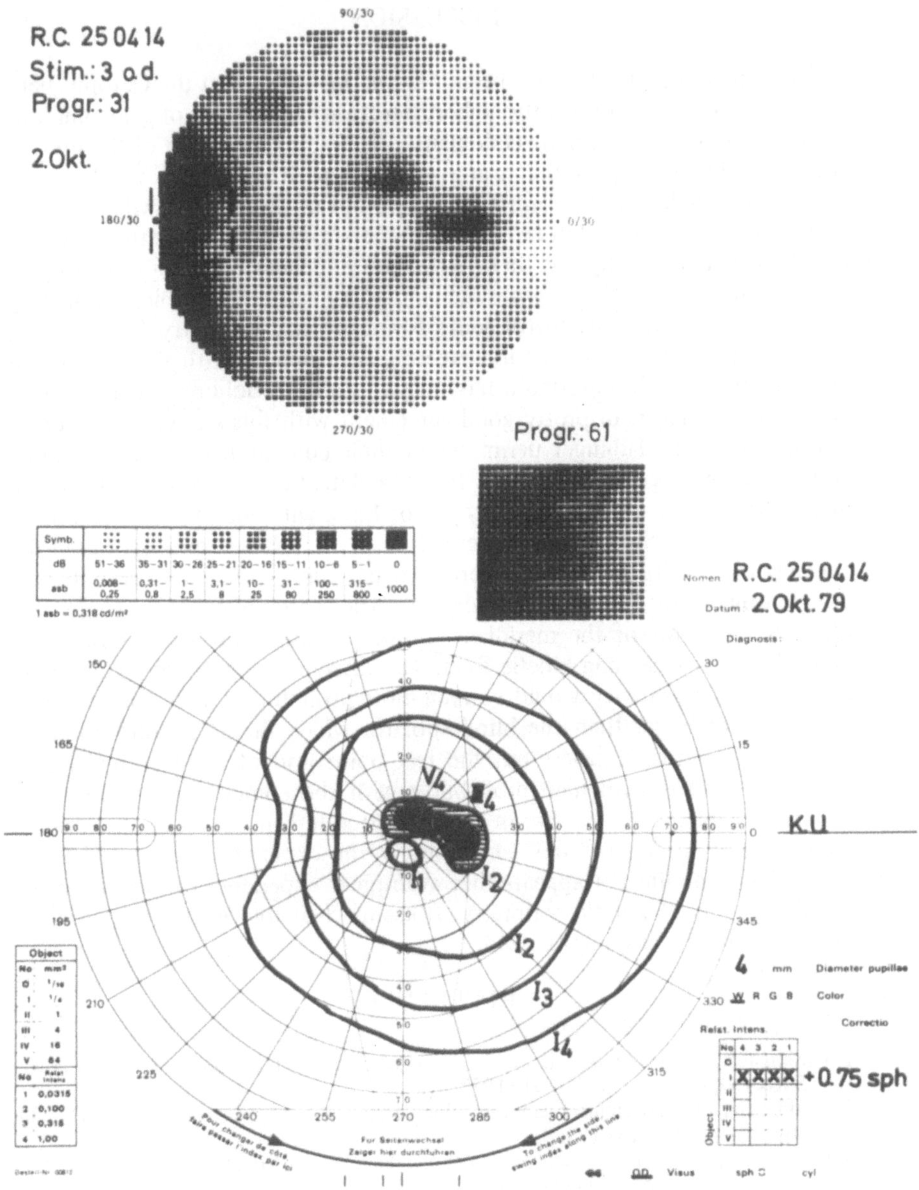

Fig. 5. Visual field of the right eye of a glaucoma patient with field loss verified by Octopus (upper part) and Goldmann (lower part) perimetry. There is an quantitive difference. The Octopus showed a paracentral scotoma close to the blind spot, whereas the Goldmann field shows an arcuate scotoma.

DISCUSSION

It was apparent from the very beginning of this study that the Octopus perimeter will show a significantly higher detection probability of glaucomatous field defects than the kinetic Goldmann perimeter. In the light of the present study one has to expect that using a kinetic perimeter every third glaucomatous field defect will be missed and two out of three which will be picked up will be misinterpreted in terms of size, shape and depth. Since the incidence of a field defect usually has therapeutic consequences it is important to pick up as many as possible, as reproducible and as early as possible. Comparing Goldmann and Octopus instruments for glaucoma perimetry Schmied [4] described a higher sensitivity in detecting field defects with the Octopus in 80% of the eyes. He reported a false-negative rate of Goldmann perimetry of about 30% which is in pretty good agreement with this study. Spaeth *et al.* [5] included the Tübinger perimeter in their comparative study of manual against Octopus perimetry. They found a detection probability of glaucomatous field defects using the Octopus of 82%, with the Tübinger perimeter of 60% and with the Goldmann perimeter of 53%. It is surprising that in the above study the Tübinger static perimeter is closer to the Goldmann than to the Octopus in its detection probabilities. The reason may be due to the fact that the selection of the meridians for the Tübinger profiles is orientated according to a foregoing kinetic field. The discrepancy between manual and computerized perimetry would be even more pronounced if we consider only scotomas not larger than the blind spot for which the detection by kinetic strategies is almost hopeless but the test point grid of the Octopus would catch the defects with high probability with the combination of two programmes. Facing the fact that in the present study and in the studies quoted above manual perimetry was performed by an experienced perimetrist of a large glaucoma clinic, it appears that even great experience cannot overcome the limitations of kinetic perimetry. It seems clear that glaucoma perimetry of tomorrow will be computerized.

REFERENCES

1. Fankhauser, F., J. Spahr & H. Bebie. Some aspects of the automation of perimetry. Survey Ophthal. 22, 131–141 (1977).
2. Fankhauser, F. Problems related to the design of automatic perimeters. Docum. Ophthal. 47, 89–138 (1979).
3. Gramer, E., G. K. Krieglstein & W. Leydhecker. Die Automatisation der Perimetrie. Zeitschr. prakt. Augenheilk. 1, 5–26 (1980).
4. Schmied, U. Automatic (Octopus) and manual (Goldmann) perimetry in glaucoma: first experiences. First International Meeting on Automated Perimetry, System Octopus. Interzeag AG, Schlieren, Switzerland (1979).
5. Spaeth, G. L., G. Li Suzanne & H. A. Scimeca. Clinical experiences with the use of Octopus automated perimeter in the detection of visual field loss in early glaucoma. First International Meeting on Automated Perimetry, System Octopus. Interzeag AG, Schlieren, Switzerland (1979).

Author's address:
Dr. G. K. Krieglstein
Univ. Augenklinik, Josef-Schneider-Str. 11
D-8700 Würzburg, F.R.G.

VISUAL FIELD IN DIABETIC RETINOPATHY (DR)

J.-H. GREITE, H.-P. ZUMBANSEN & R. ADAMCZYK

(Munich, F.R.G.)

ABSTRACT

By examination with the automated perimetry system OCTOPUS in Diabetic Retinopathy (DR) characteristic changes in the visual field show up in form of flecked, partially confluent relative scotomas. They can be correlated to areas of capillary non-perfusion. The average decrease of light sensitivity in the different stages of DR was ascertained. It ranges between 1.4 dB in the stage I and 6.7 dB in the stage IV. It is remarkable, that even in beginning DR the loss of retinal function is greater in the middle periphery than in the central area. This becomes more distinct in advanced stages of DR and especially in the proliferative form.

INTRODUCTION

At the first International Meeting on Automated Perimetry System Octopus in Zürich 1979 we showed that already in early stages of Diabetic Retinopathy (DR) characteristic visual defects can be detected with the automated perimeter Octopus [3]. The typical findings are relative scotomas, partly confluent and of different intensities and dimensions. They appear in the halftone display of the Octopus as a flecked or patchwork pattern, which reminds one of the damage done by moths.

We demonstrated that there is a close correlation between these scotomas and areas of capillary nonperfusion seen in the fluorescein angiograms (Fig. 1 and 2). So an accumulation of these scotomas is often found in the 40 to 60 degree zone of the visual field, which is as we well know, the preferred location of the development of capillary closure and consecutive neovascularisation, according to the findings of Taylor and Dobree [4]. It should be emphasized that these typical visual field defects occur before reduction of visual acuity, so we can say that the function of the peripheral retina in DR is much earlier affected than assumed hitherto because with traditional Goldmann perimetry these visual field defects were hidden. As well as these qualitative findings quantitative statements are of interest.

METHODS

For this purpose we systematically examined 107 eyes of 67 patients with different stages of DR. The stages of DR were defined as shown in Table 1.

All eyes were examined with the programmes 21, 31 and 41. For the numerical and statistical evaluation only the values of the programmes 31

Doc. Ophthal. Proc. Series, Vol. 26, ed. by E. L. Greve & G Verriest

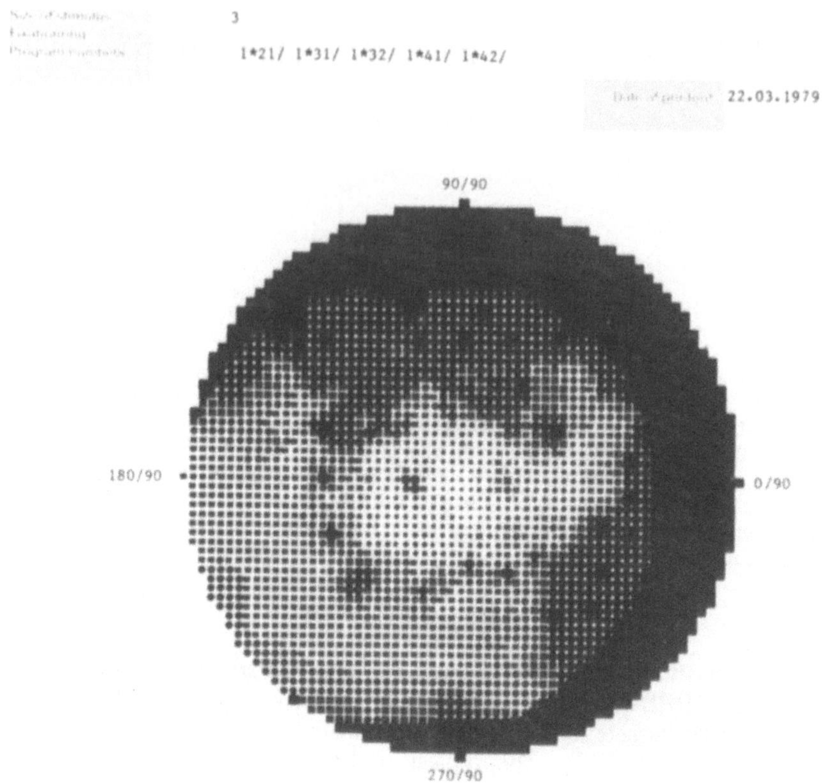

Fig. 1. Typical visual field in DR stage IV. Most of the scotomas are located in the middle periphery. The paracentral scotoma (opposite to the blind spot) corresponds to the area of capillary nonperfusion seen in Fig. 2.

Table 1. Definition of the stages in DR and number of examined eyes.

Stage of DR	Clinical appearance	No. of eyes
I	D.R. only seen in FLA	17
II	Microaneurysms only	23
III	Microaneurysms, haemorages and hard exudates	34
IV	Proliferative D.R.	33

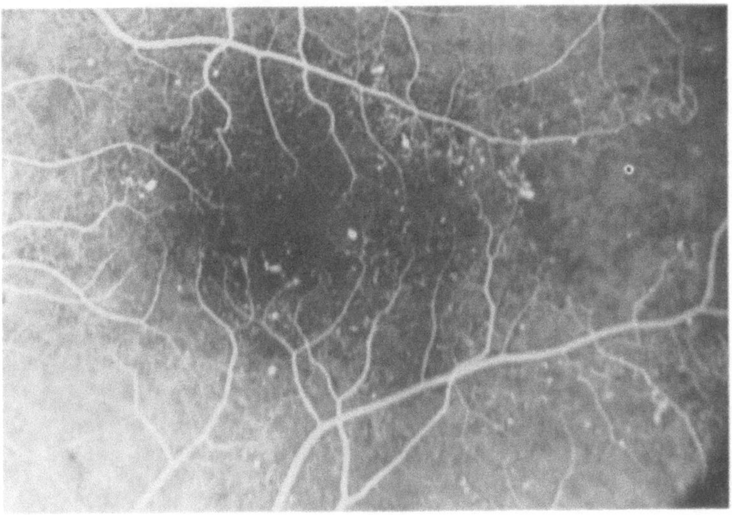

Fig. 2. Fluorescein angiogram of the case seen in Fig. 1. Notice the area of capillary nonperfusion, which is responsible for the paracentral relative scotom.

and 41 were used. The values of the blind spots were excluded. The findings were compared to the data of the normal average light sensitivities, which are published in the second edition of the Octopus Visual Field Atlas [3].

RESULTS

Typical individual findings of visual field defects in the different stages of DR are demonstrated in Figs. 3–6. In the profile section displays the normal curves are overprojected. The dotted areas show the actual decrease of light sensitivity.

With regard to the variation of the scotomas in DR it is only practicable and reasonable to bring into relation the summarized values of light sensitivity of all measurement points [2].

In Fig. 7 the findings of this study are summarized. It shows the average decrease of the light sensitivity in the different stages of DR in absolute dB-values. It ranges between 1.4 dB in stage I and 6.7 dB in stage IV. This seems to be low at first sight. However, considering a difference table of an individual case, one finds that the deviation from the normal values in separate measurement points can be very high. The decrease of average light sensitivity with increasing DR is obvious. Whether or not there is a linearity in this dependence we proved by analysis of regression. We found a significance of 95%. It is striking that the standard deviation is relatively high and increasing in the advanced stages of DR. This is intelligible because in the defined stages the individual extent of the morphological criterias show great variation. So a statistical comparison of the mean values of the different visual field areas may not be allowed. Nevertheless we can see tendencies. These are printed out in Table 2, in which the findings of the different visual

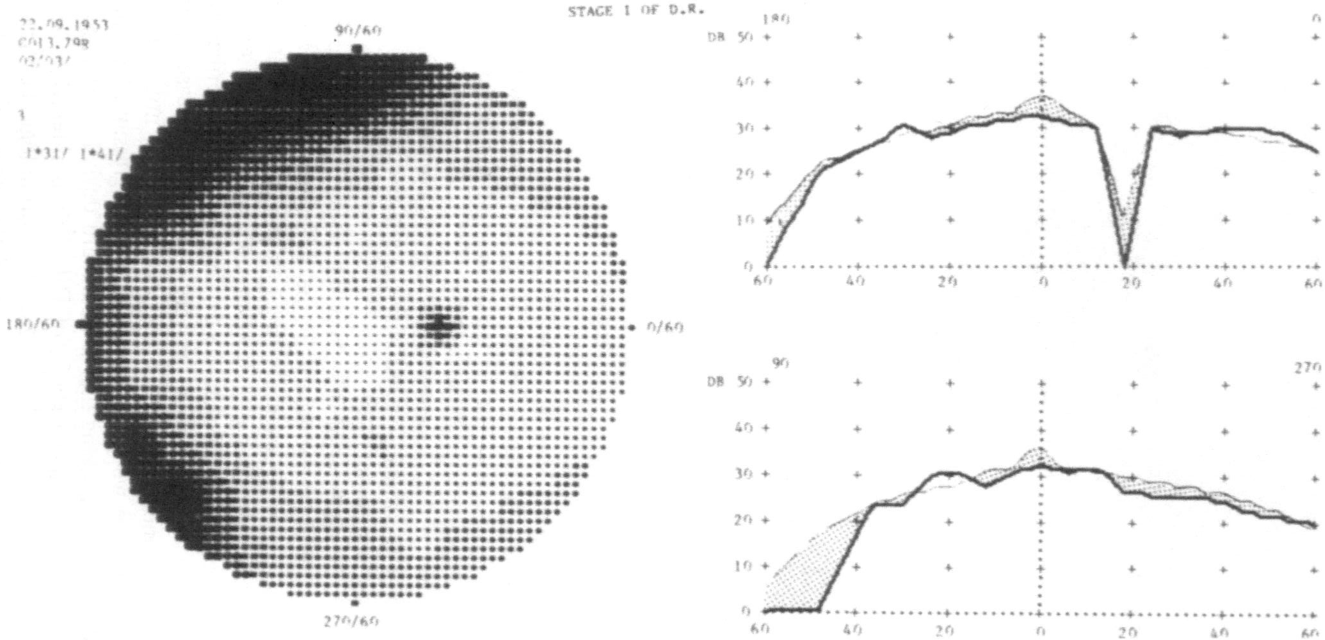

Fig. 3. Halftone and profile display of a case with DR stage I. In the profile display the average light sensitivity of this age group is over-projected, so that the dotted field show the decrease of light sensitivity.

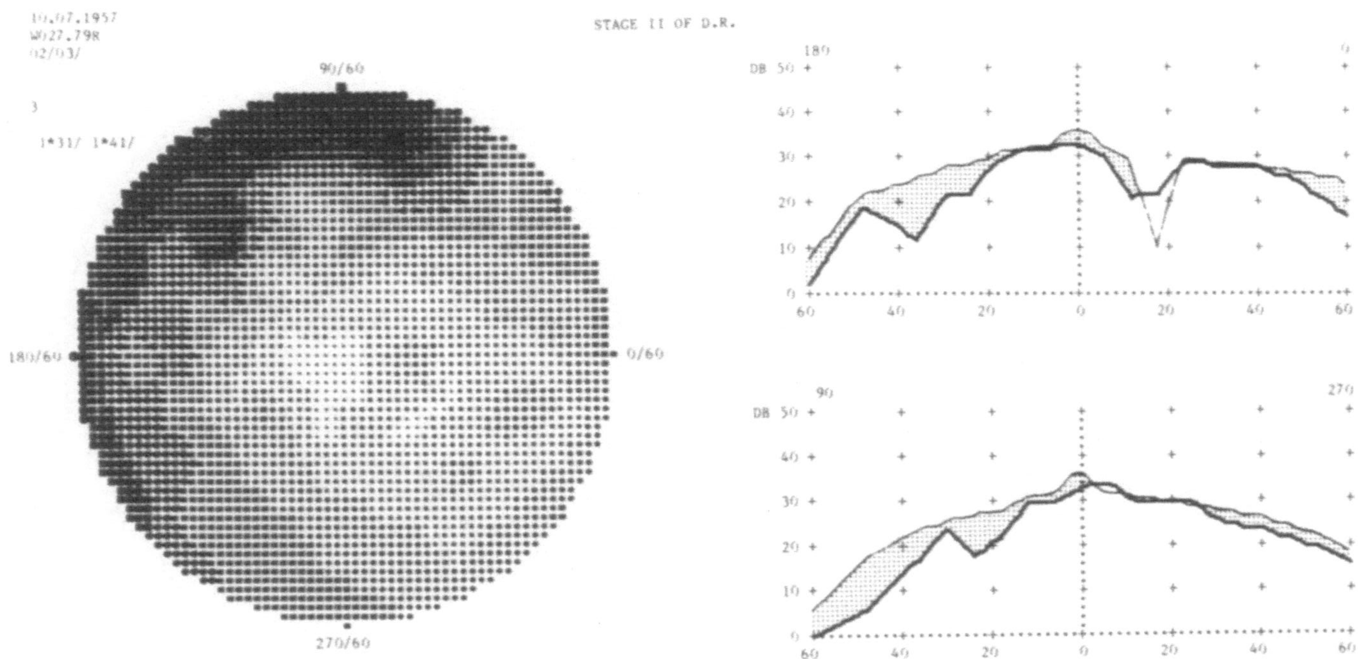

Fig. 4. Example of a case with DR stage II (see legend of Fig. 3).

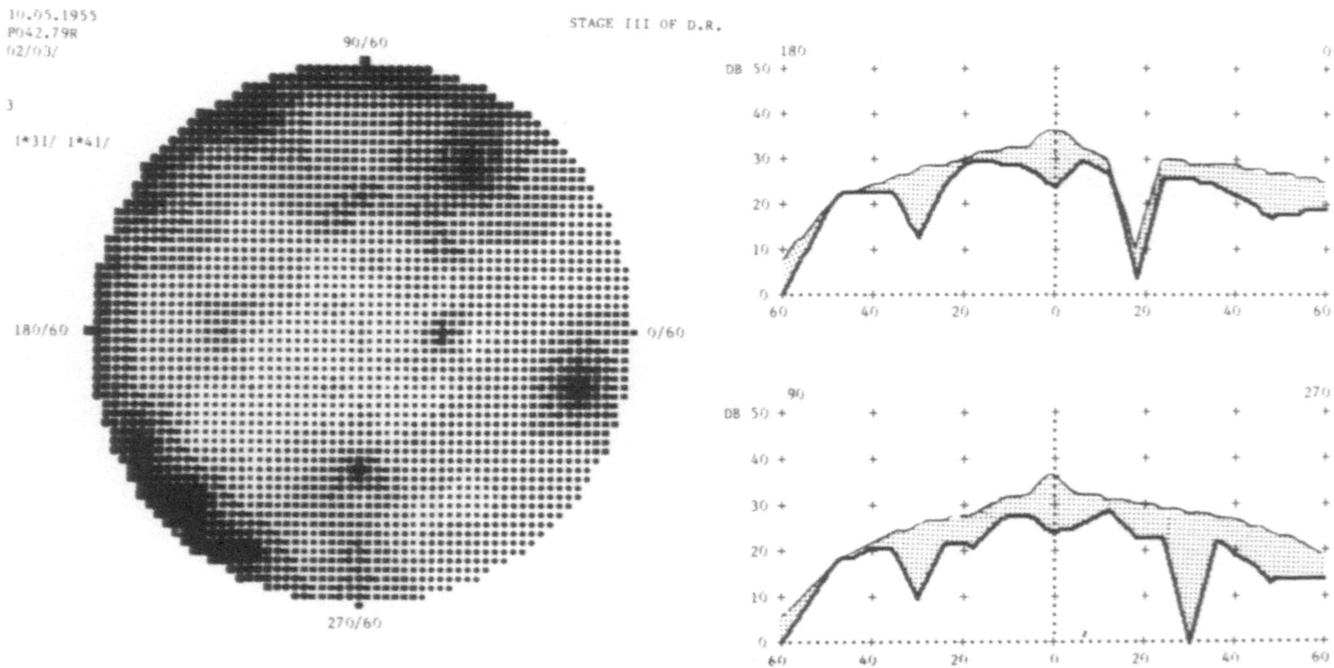

Fig. 5. Example of a case with DR stage III (see legend of Fig. 3).

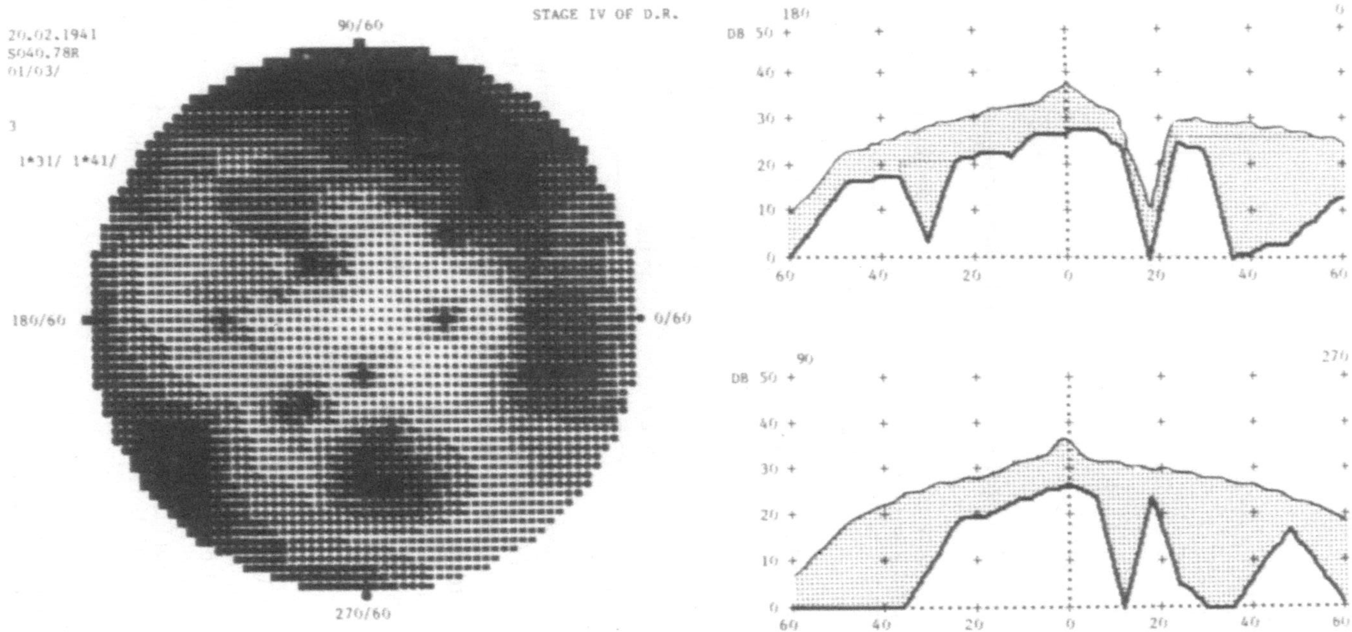

Fig. 6. Example of a case with DR stage IV (see legend of Fig. 3).

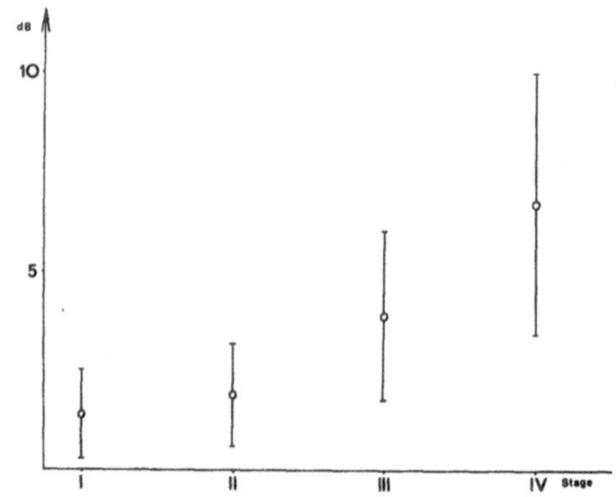

Fig. 7. Decrease of average light sensitivity in the different stages of DR.

Table 2. Decrease of average light sensitivity in the different stages in the different areas of the visual field.

Stage of DR	Areas of visual field 0°–30° (Progr. 31)	30°–60° (Progr. 41)	0°–60° (Comb. 31/41)
I	4.5%	7.5%	5.6%
II	5.7%	10.7%	7.7%
III	13.0%	21.2%	16.5%
IV	22.4%	37.0%	28.0%

field areas are shown. It is remarkable that even in beginning DR the loss of retinal function is greater in the middle periphery than in the central area, which becomes more distinct in advanced stages of DR and especially in the proliferative form.

In current and further investigations, establishing better comparable collectives, we try to find out if these findings can be statistically confirmed.

REFERENCES

1. Fankhauser, F. & H. Bebie. Personal communication.
2. Greite, J.-H. Octopus-Perimetry in Diabetic Retinopathy Proceedings of the I. Intern. Meeting on Automated Perimetry System OCTOPUS, published by Interzeag AG Schlieren, Switzerland, 107–116 (1979).
3. OCTOPUS Visual Field Atlas. 2nd ed. Interzeag AG Schlieren, Switzerland (1978).
4. Taylor, E. & J. H. Dobree. Proliferative diabetic retinopathy. Brit. J. Ophthal. 54:11 (1970).

Author's address:
Priv. Doz. Dr. J.-H. Greite
Augenklinik der Universität
Mathildenstr. 8
D-8000 München 2
F.R.G.

DETECTION AND DEFINITION OF SCOTOMATA OF THE CENTRAL VISUAL FIELD BY COMPUTER METHODS

J. FLAMMER, G. NAGEL, A. GLOWAZKI,
H. R. MOSER & F. FANKHAUSER

(Berne, Switzerland)

ABSTRACT

The early detection of visual loss has long been a major goal in perimetry. Shallow scotomata of small diameter can only be detected by high resolution measurements combined with appropriate attenuation of the threshold fluctuations. Detectability of such scotomata by different Octopus programs, varying in these two basic strategies, is shown.

PROBLEM

The task of separating true local loss of contrast sensitivity from threshold fluctuations is the more demanding the shallower a scotoma, the smaller its diameter and the larger the local measurement error (the measurement error, as defined here, includes all factors contributing to threshold instability) [5]. Detectability can only be improved by high spatial resolution (i.e. a high scanning density) and averaging procedures. Both steps may drastically increase examination duration [4] unless the visual field area to be examined is appropriately reduced. When such time restrictions are taken into account this leads to the well known dilemma: we may either (1) analyse large visual field areas, in which case detectability will be limited, or (2) we may analyse small field areas, whereby high resolution scanning together with averaging procedures greatly increase detectability within the area examined. In this latter case, large field areas remain unexplored. Depending on the clinical problem we may be forced to choose either (1) or (2). It is the intention of this report to demonstrate the effects of Octopus programs differing in the basic strategies (1) or (2) upon the perimetric result. Since it was not the intention to perform a systematic analysis of the pathological class examined, only a few typical results will be displayed and commented.

MATERIALS AND METHODS

9 patients (total 18 eyes) suffering from multiple sclerosis and having undergone at least one episode of retrobulbar neuritis, were analysed using Octopus programs 33, 34, 61 and F8. These patients had a visual acuity of 0.6 or better but the latency of the VEP was increased. 115 ms was taken as the limiting

normal value. Target size 3 (diam.: 0.43°) was chosen. Otherwise, the basic procedure for Octopus perimetry was adhered to [4]. Octopus programs 33, 34 and 61 have been described previously (Octopus user's manual). Programs 33 and 34 scan a visual field area of r = 30°. The spatial resolution of these programs, when combined, is 4.2°. The luminance intervals of the repetitive bracketing procedure are 4 . . . 2 . . . 1 dB [6].

Program 61 performs 3 threshold determinations at 25 test locations with a separation of 3°. At each test location the local average value together with the local r.m.s. fluctuations is calculated. The global r.m.s. fluctuations are computed as well. The bracketing strategy operates with luminance intervals of 2 . . . 1 . . 1/2 dB. This results in a reduction of the measurement error by about 20% [3].

The F8 program used here is one of a family of programs including programs F1, F2, F4 and F8. Program F8 permits distribution of a maximum of 11 test locations at an arbitrary resolution along a 'profile' or 'section' which may be oriented arbitrarily across the visual field (minimum interstimulus distance: 0.2°). 8 determinations per test location are peformed. The luminance steps are 2 . . 1 . . 1/2 dB. Graphical printouts of the examination results may be produced together with numerical tables which display the contrast sensitivities, their means and local normal values. The local as well as the global r.m.s. fluctuations are printed out.

The graphical displays were produced by the host computer of the Octopus and printed out by its terminal (Fig. 1 and 4a) and via data transfer to a large scale IBM computer, model 3033, and plotted by a calcomp graphics system 1039.

RESULTS

Analysis by programs 33 and 34

Two categories of results were obtained: (1) normal visual fields (Fig. 1a). No deviations, when compared with normal standards (Visual Field Atlas, 2nd edition) could be detected. (2) Suspicious visual fields were recorded (Fig. 1b and 1c) displaying variable degrees of deviations from standard values. However it was not known whether such deviations were purely fortuitous or whether these deviations ought to be accepted as real and if so, at which level of confidence. Statistical program Delta [1, 2] was not applied to these results because the part of program Delta, discriminating normal and pathological states (in contrast to the part of the program assessing progression or not) had not yet reached optimum performance at the time when these experiments were performed.

Analysis by program 61

4 eyes belonging to category 2 were analysed by 4 programs 61 coupled together, covering a visual field area of 27 degrees². Examinations performed upon an arbitrarily selected eye are displayed in 3-dimensional views (Fig. 3). The basic properties of such displays are shown in Figure 2. For a better

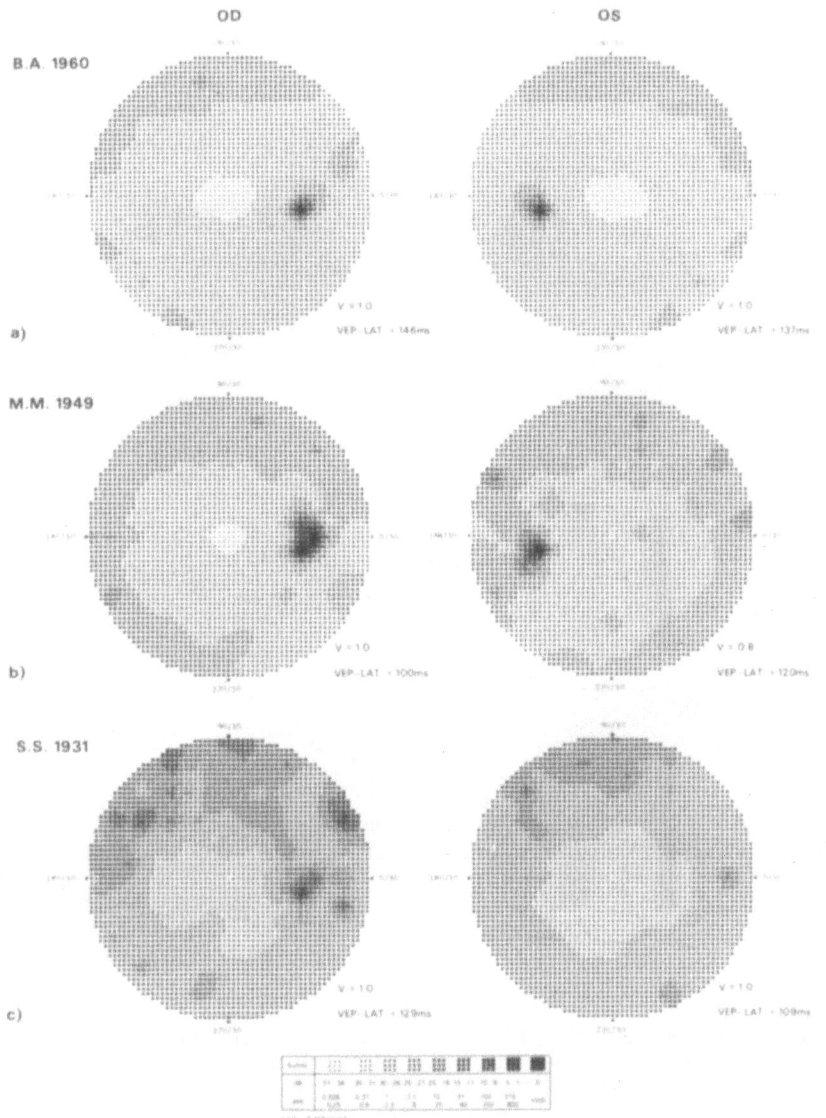

Fig. 1. Visual fields of patients with history of retrobulbar neuritis. Grey scale displays. programs 33 + 34 (mixed mode). Visual acuity and VEP latency are indicated in each graph.

1a. Normal visual fields of subject B.A.: OD and OS.

1b and 1c. Suspicious visual fields. Variable degrees of real or apparent pathology.

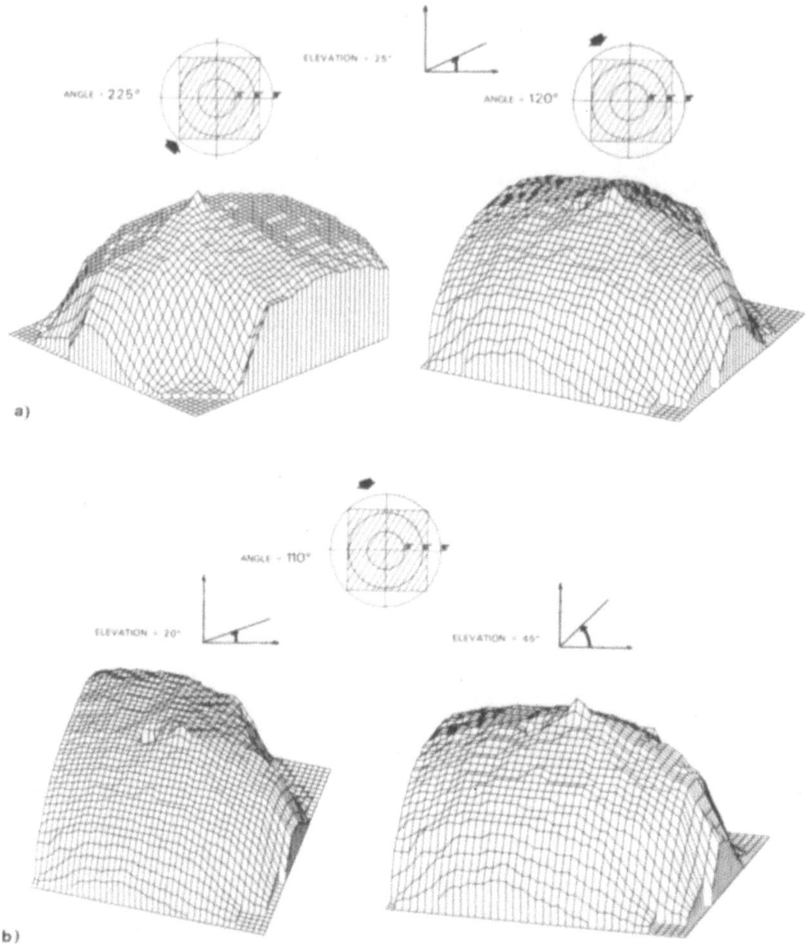

Fig. 2. 3-dimensional display of sections of normal visual fields. Fig. 2a: 3-dimensional contrast sensitivity distribution from various sides (angle of rotation: see insert). Fig. 2b: displays at various degrees of elevation (insert).

understanding of the contrast sensitivity relief such displays may be viewed from various sides (i.e. they may be rotated around their axes) or they may be looked at from various angles of elevation. In figure 3, three-dimensional aspects of the 27 degrees^2 area analysed (centre coordinate, x: −16; y: −13) are shown. The contrast sensitivity reliefs of the first, second and third determination, together with the mean value and the standard normal value are shown. The graphs are shown at two different angles of rotation. The results differ markedly from the norm and considerable differences between the 3 single determinations are noted, which are due to measurement error. The mean value represents a good approximation to the truth but without further

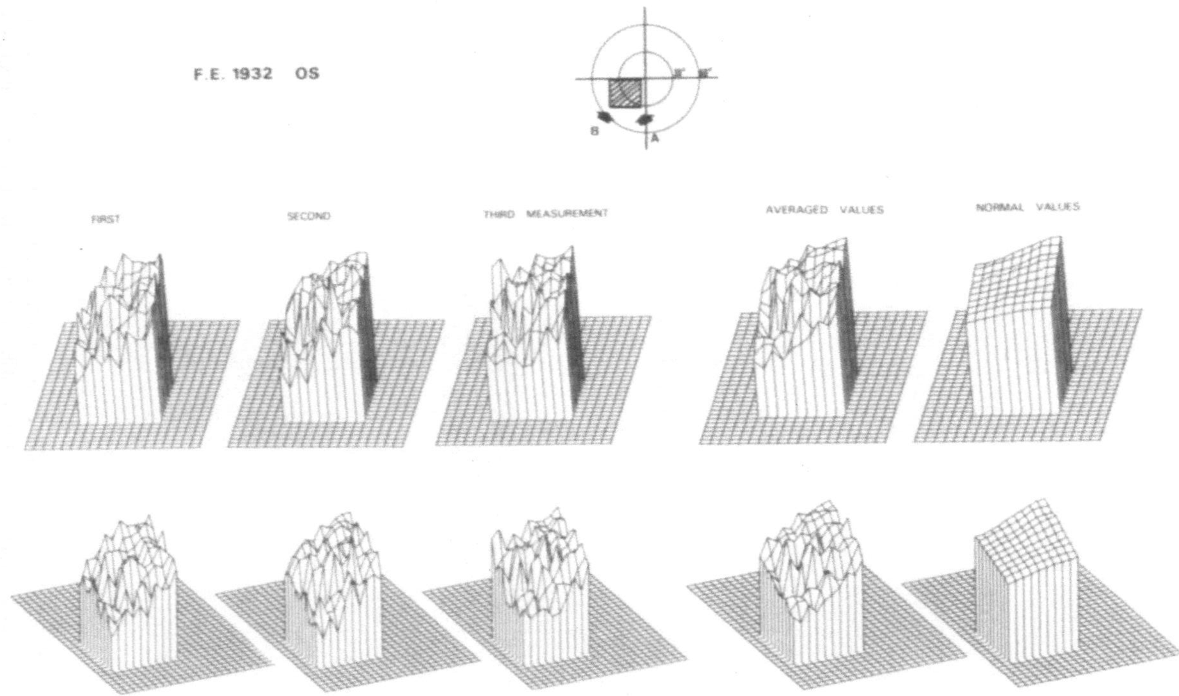

Fig. 3. From left to right: display of single measurements and mean values of Octopus programs 61 (see text). First, second and third measurement and mean values of subject F.E. (visual acuity = 0.6, VEP.LAT = 153 ms) are shown. Right: normal values. Top and bottom row differ in angle of rotation of 3-dimensional display.

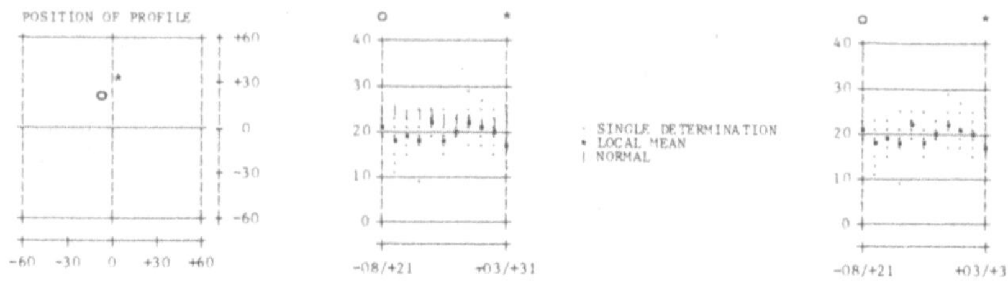

Date of printout: 17.03.1980

Number of questions: 491

Number of repetitions: 34

STRATEGY : UP-DOWN (NORMAL)
LENGTH OF PROFILE (DEG) : 14.9
NUMBER OF TEST LOCATIONS : 11
RESOLUTION (DEG) : 01.5
NUMBER OF REPETITIONS : 08
R.M.S. FLUCTUATION (DB) : 03.8

NN	X	Y	V1	V2	V3	V4	V5	V6	V7	V8	MEAN +-	S.D.	NORM
0	- 8.0	21.0	21	23	19	21	21	21	23	23	21.5 +-	1.4	25
1	- 6.9	22.0	19	23	23	19	11	15	13	21	18.0 +-	4.5	25
2	- 5.8	23.0	21	21	21	15	17	23	15	23	19.5 +-	3.3	24
3	- 4.7	24.0	19	17	19	21	21	9	17	25	18.5 +-	4.6	24
4	- 3.6	25.0	21	19	23	23	25	23	23	19	22.0 +-	2.1	24
5	- 2.5	26.0	19	19	25	21	17	15	15	19	18.8 +-	3.3	23
6	- 1.4	27.0	19	23	19	21	21	19	19	23	20.5 +-	1.8	23
7	- 0.3	28.0	29	21	21	17	25	21	23	23	22.5 +-	3.5	23
8	0.8	29.0	27	17	21	21	21	25	19	17	21.0 +-	3.5	22
9	1.9	30.0	21	25	17	15	19	21	21	23	20.3 +-	3.2	22
10	3.0	31.0	26	18	12	16	24	20	20	4	17.5 +-	7.0	23

a)

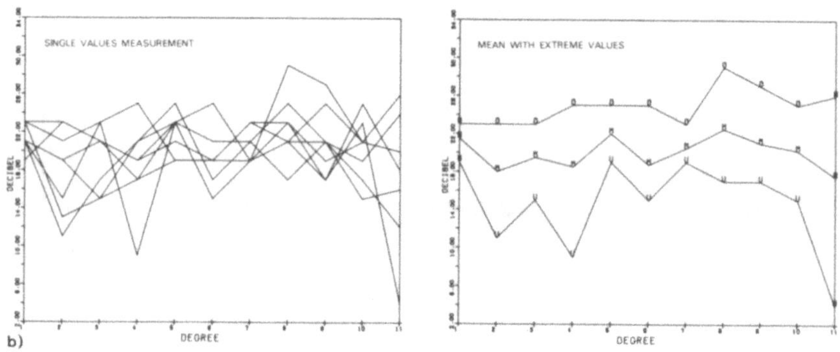

b)

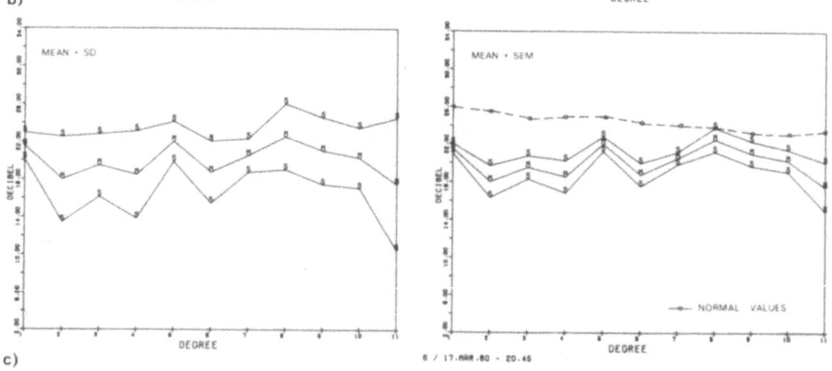

c)

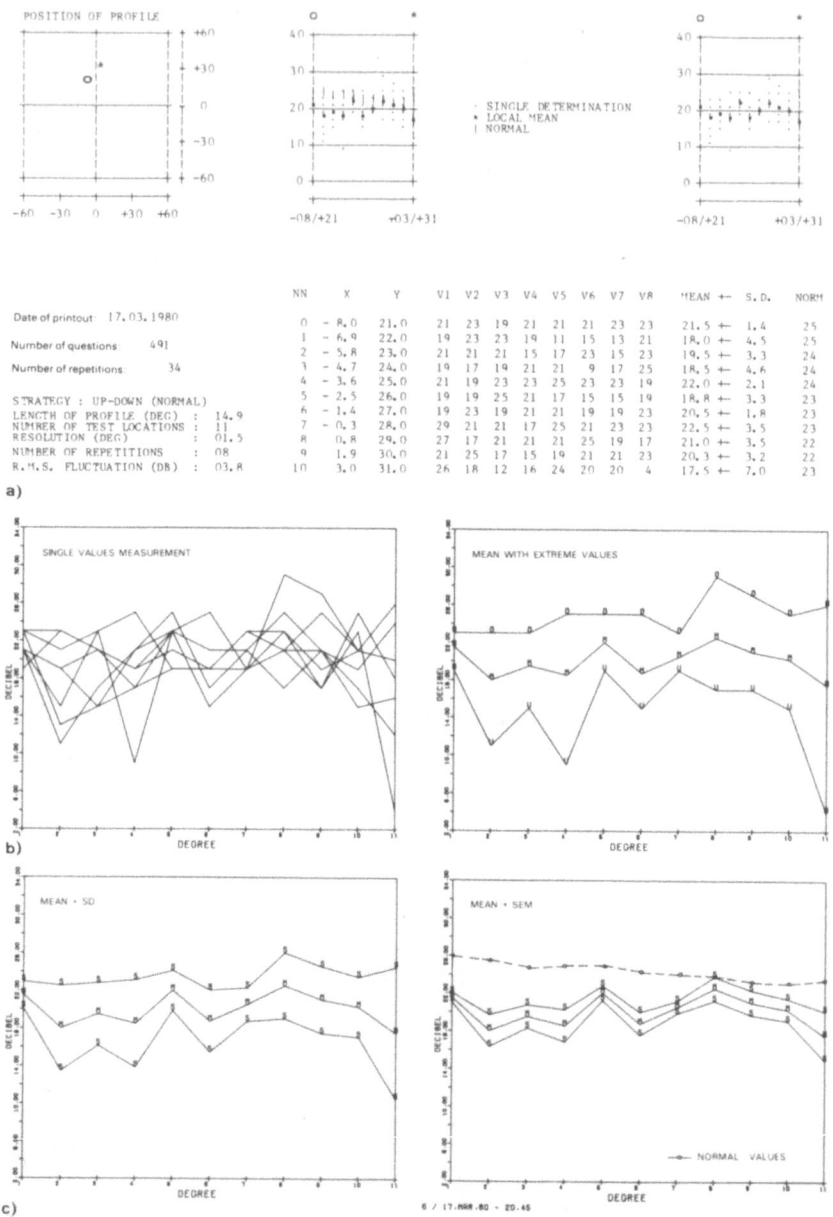

Fig. 4. Subject W.M., OD. Program F8. Profile positioned in visual field is shown in top figure, left. Fig. 4a: top left: position of profile in visual field. Top right: display of 8 individual values + mean at each test location. Top centre: same, but standard values are added (lengths of vertical lines = 1 stand. dev.). Bottom: figure table (see text). Fig. 4b: Curves represent same values as Fig. 4a. Left: single values. Right: mean values + extreme values. Fig. 4c: left: Mean values and standard deviations of single values. Right: normal mean values (dashed line), mean values and standard errors of the standard deviations.

statistical scrutiny, the evaluation of the local contrast sensitivity losses is incomplete. For a statistical evaluation a new data base was considered necessary.

Analysis by program F8

OD of subject W.M. belonging to category 2 was examined. A profile measuring 14.9° was analysed. The various Octopus printouts (graphs and numerical table) are shown in Figure 4a. For a better visualisation and evaluation the graphical results were again displayed by the large scale computer system in figures 4b and 4c. Figure 4b shows the single values (left) together with the mean and the extreme values (right). Figure 4c shows the mean values together with the standard deviations (left) and the means together with the standard errors of the means. This graph includes in addition the normal contrast sensitivity curve (right). F8 allows us to arrive at the conclusion that the mean contrast sensitivity curve recorded is situated, at most test locations, below the normal contrast sensitivity curve (Figure 4c, right). Whether this behaviour may be considered as a true pathological loss was not further explored. However it is apparent that the single values disturbed by the measurement error are highly contradictory (Fig. 4b, left) whereas the means of 8 determinations together with their standard deviations allow a much more valid evaluation of the true contrast sensitivity distribution (Fig. 4c).

An evaluation was carried out on both eyes of subject F.E. (Fig. 5). A profile was adjusted from x: −6° to x: +4° at y: 0° (i.e. across the fixation point). Figure 5b displays the means and the standard errors of the means of OD and OS. It emerges very clearly that the single value determinations (Fig. 5a) are highly contradictory and represent a poor approximation to the truth. One scotoma appears quite consistently on both eyes but its depth and extent are relatively uncertain. A smaller scotoma is apparent from some of the single determinations. From others it is not (Fig. 5a). In contrast, the mean values display very clearly two scotomata of comparable diameter but of different depths. The reliability in declaration of these scotomata emerges from the fact that the ratio of the loss of contrast sensitivity to the standard error of the mean is large in both eyes. Two homonymous relative scotomata may therefore be accepted as real. These results were considered definitive for these investigations and no statistical manipulations were carried out which might have revealed further details.

CONCLUSIONS

Provided spatial resolution is high and noise attenuation is good enough, it is possible to diagnose shallow relative scotomata having a small diameter with a high degree of fidelity and accuracy. This has been achieved with Octopus program F8. Without such measures these defects would probably have passed undetected. Although these scotomata appear to have the shape of a funnel, a geometrical assumption of this kind is not warranted. In order to classify the scotomata geometrically, a much higher degree of resolution, still

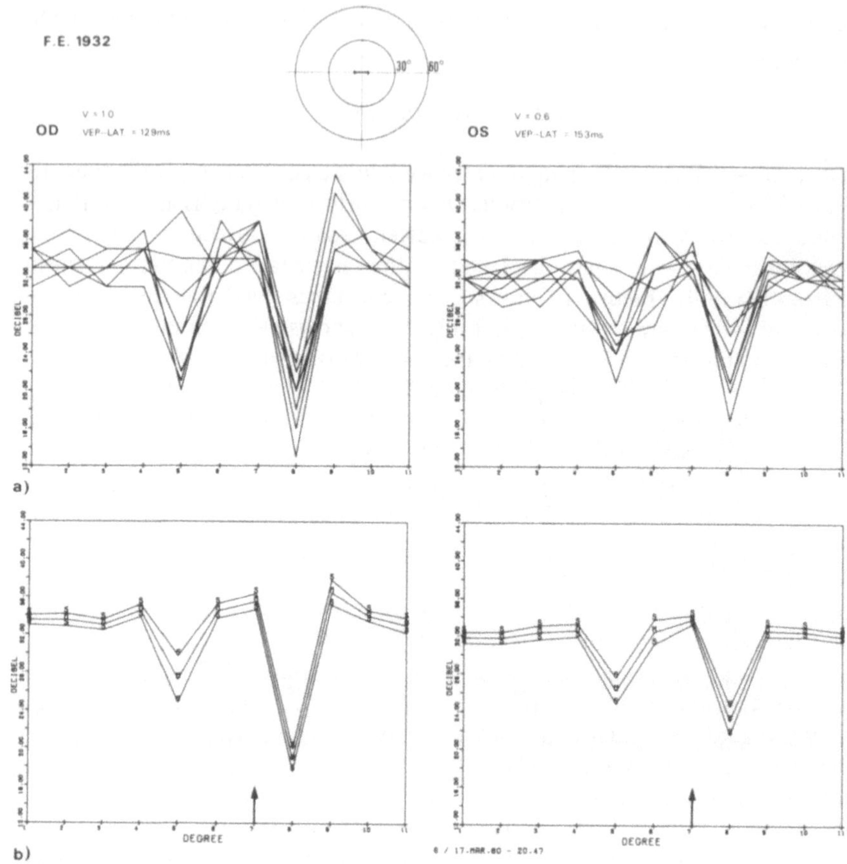

Fig. 5. Subject F.E. OD and OS. F8 program. Fig. 5a: single values of OD (left) and OS (right). Fig. 5b: mean values and standard errors of the mean, OD (left); OS (right). Arrow indicates the fixation point.

combined with higher noise attenuation, would be necessary. The contrast sensitivity profiles obtained when using program F8 and target size, diameter 0.43° (Goldmann standard 3), displays steep borders. This indicates good spatial resolution of contrast sensitivity by target 3, as expected. The reduction of target size to diameters 2, 1 or 0 would only make sense when attempting to detect scotomata having a diameter of 1/2° or less. However, the problems related to the detection of scotomata of this size may be considerable [5].

ACKNOWLEDGEMENTS

We would like to thank Prof. H. Bebie and Mr. F. Jenni for technical advice, Prof. H. P. Ludin for the V.E.P. measurements and Miss E. Ulrich and Miss E. Widmer for typing the manuscript.

REFERENCES

1. Bebie, H & Fankhauser, F. Statistical programs for the analysis of perimetric data. Doc. Ophthal. Proc. Sereis, Vol. 26 (this volume).
2. Bebie, H. & Fankhauser, F. Ein statistisches Programm zur Beurteilung von Gesichtsfeldern. Klin. Mbl.Augenheilk. 177, 417–422 (1980).
3. Bebie, H., Fankhauser, F. & Spahr, J. Static perimetry: Strategies. Acta Ophthal. 54: 325–338 (1976).
4. Fankhauser, F. Problems related to the design of automatic perimeters. Doc. Ophthal. 47: 89–138 (1979).
5. Fankhauser, F. & Bebie, H. Threshold fluctuations, interpolations and spatial resolution in perimetry. Doc. Ophthal. Proc. Series 19: 295–309 (1979).
6. Spahr, J. Optimization of the presentation pattern in automated static perimetry. Vision Res. 15: 1275–1281 (1975).
7. Operator's Manual. Interzeag, Schlieren, Switzerland.
8. Visual Field Atlas, 2nd edition. Interzeag, Schlieren, Switzerland.

Author's address:
Dr. J. Flammer
Universitäts-Augenklinik
CH-3010 Bern
Switzerland

A CLINICAL COMPARISON OF THREE COMPUTERIZED AUTOMATIC PERIMETERS IN THE DETECTION OF GLAUCOMA DEFECTS

ANDERS HEIJL & STEPHEN M. DRANCE

(Malmö, Sweden/Vancouver, Canada)

ABSTRACT

The ability to detect glaucomatous field defects of 3 automatic computerized perimeters (COMPETER, OCTOPUS and PERIMETRON) was compared in a clinical study of 74 patients, some suffering from established glaucoma, with normals, and glaucoma suspects in whom the visual fields were completely normal. The reference fields were obtained by careful static and kinetic manual perimetry on the Tübingen perimeter. All the automatic instruments gave similar high rates of detection of field loss and low false positive results. Quality conventional manual perimetry is still necessary to back up automatic perimetric results but automatic perimeters can already take over a large proportion of routine perimetric screening.

INTRODUCTION

A number of semiautomatic and automatic perimeters have been introduced into Ophthalmology. Some of these have developed sophisticated computerized test logic which measures increment thresholds at selected predetermined points in the visual field. One instrument is capable of determining contrast thresholds by means of kinetic perimetry. Some of these perimeters have been clinically tested and their performance compared with conventional manual perimetry and the reported results have been encouraging (1, 3, 4, 5a, 5b, 5c, 6, 7, 8, 9a). No study has so far been published comparing the screening sensitivity and specificity of these computerized perimeters. It was the aim of this study to compare clinically the COMPETER, the OCTOPUS, and the PERIMETRON in screening for glaucoma defects. These three instruments were the only fully automatic machines commercially available when the study was carried out in the summer of 1979. One of the most important parts of the study was to develop criteria for each of the perimetric tests which would indicate an abnormality that would have to be more fully explored. It was not the purpose of the study to compare the ability of each perimeter and its program to detect and quantitate visual field defects in an unlimited time, but rather to compare the ability of these devices to detect field defects in a practical and limited period of time.

Doc. Ophthal. Proc. Series, Vol. 26, ed. by E. L. Greve & G. Verriest

METHOD

Seventy-four patients with established glaucomatous field defects or glaucoma suspects without field defects, and normal people were tested. The ages ranged from 21 to 84 years (average 60.8 years). Only eyes with small or medium-sized field defects were included. Extensive field defects were avoided. The patients were not selected according to their previous perimetric reliability. The COMPETER (5d), the OCTOPUS (9b) have been described in detail elsewhere. The PERIMETRON is a projection perimeter which employs both kinetic and static modes of testing using stimuli and background illuminations of the same sizes and intensities available on the Goldmann perimeter. The stimuli are presented in a non-randomized sequence such as a perimetrist would employ. Fixation is checked by an infrared monitor and can be overridden by a manual fixation through a telescope similar to that on the Goldmann perimeter.

Our choice of test programs was guided by 2 principles:

1. Screening should take a finite and practical amount of time which was considered to be 20 to 30 minutes per eye. Programs were selected for each instrument which would take approximately that time.
2. On the COMPETER the central pattern of test points tested by a fairly fast threshold measuring test logic (Test logic 1 described by Heijl [5f]) was chosen. In addition profiles of 2 meridians 15° above and below the nasal horizontal out to 30° from fixation were automatically tested. The OCTOPUS perimeter program '31' was used, which is a standard threshold measuring program consisting of 73 points within 30° from fixation with a 6° interstimulus distance (2). The PERIMETRON was used utilizing its Test program '10' which plots kinetically 2 to 4 isopters in the central and peripheral field and performs static spot-checking between the isopters. Spot-checking commences at the threshold level of the enveloping isopter and increment thresholds of all missed points are then established.

The criteria used to classify the automatic fields as abnormal were developed with experience and were chosen to maximize sensitivity with a reasonably good specificity. The details of the criteria used will be published elsewhere (5h).

Automatic perimetry was performed on each patient using all three computerized instruments during a single session lasting 2½ to 3 hours. The order of the automatic perimeters was randomly selected so that each machine had an equal number of first, second and third tests. The patients were allowed to rest for at least 15 minutes between the different instruments and operator interference during the testing was avoided as much as possible. Correction for ametropia and for near was always used when appropriate. Previous manual fields employing static and kinetic perimetry on the Tübingen perimeter were available in all glaucoma patients with field defects. Screeners employing a modification of Armaly's selective screening on the Goldmann perimeter or full Tübingen fields were available in all patients with full visual fields. All automatic fields were compared with the manual reference fields. When a discrepancy arose between any of the automatic fields and the manual fields the patients were retested with another careful kinetic and static evaluation on the Tübingen perimeter without the technician knowing the area of discrepancy. The technicians were then handed an envelope which showed the area of disagreement and that area was fully explored with static perimetry. COMPETER fields with poor fixation quotient (greater than 0.15) were disregarded and repeated. The final manual perimetry was the standard for reference and eyes with inconclusive results on this test were excluded.

RESULTS

The manual reference perimetry classified 42 fields as abnormal and 32 fields as normal. Using the criteria for establishing abnormal automatic fields the computerized perimeters yielded the following results.

Sensitivity

The COMPETER correctly identified 39 out of 42 abnormal fields with a sensitivity of 93%. The OCTOPUS identified 36 fields with an 86% sensitivity and the PERIMETRON correctly identified 38 of the 42 abnormal fields with a sensitivity of 90%.

Specificity

The COMPETER falsely classified 6 of 32 normal fields as abnormal which resulted in a specificity of 81%. The corresponding figures for the OCTOPUS were 4 abnormals of the 32 normal fields with a specificity of 87% while the PERIMETRON produced 6 false positives with specificity of 81%.

COMMENT

The results of a clinical study such as this depends on many factors including the types and sensitivity and severity of field defects of the population sample and their perimetric reliability. The quality of the manual reference perimetry, the criteria selected for the classification of automatic fields and the duration and difficulty of the tests used were other factors. In this study the composition of the population sample excluded large visual field defects and many of the field defects were small and would easily have been overlooked by the usually practiced manual perimetry. Most of the abnormal fields that were missed by the automatic perimeters were quite subtle. The selection of more extensive visual field defects would have given a better sensitivity and specificity. Had the study also been confined to perimetrically trained and reliable patients the figures for both the sensitivity and specificity would have been increased. The patients in this study were not selected in such a way and were considered to be representative of a population in a normal clinical setting.

One can only compare the performance of the automatic instruments with one another if the reference patients are evaluated by meticulous and painstaking manual perimetry, no matter how long that requires. We believe that this standard comes closest to a 'true' visual field. In view of the fact that our reference fields were in fact of this quality it is not surprising that the sensitivity figures obtained in this study are a little lower than those of some other studies of automatic perimeters in which the ordinary kinetic perimetry on the Goldmann perimeter used as a reference would miss many subtle scotomata. Some false positives in our study could represent early field loss that could not be confirmed even with the most careful scrutiny by the manual examination. There were indeed one or two instances in which several automatic machines indicated the same area of the field as defective but which could not be confirmed by manual perimetry. These were exceptions and did not affect our results to any significant degree. It was our opinion that at this time automatic perimetry can only be compared with the most careful manual perimetry as a reference. It is probably erroneous to conclude that automatic perimetry is more sensitive because more points automatically determined appear to be defective, as is reported in some recent studies in which the manual perimetry could be questioned (6, 7, 8). Both automatic and manual perimetry shows considerable variation which can also be demonstrated by repeating the automatic tests. Not all defective points found on the automatic perimeters are reproducible. The inclusion of tests on normal fields provide an estimate of the frequency of false positive results which must be part of any comparative study.

The choice of criteria for the classification of the automatic fields is all-important and presents a problem at this time. The more stringent the criteria the more field defects will be found but always at the expense of an increased number of false positives. It was our intention to optimize the criteria for each instrument and screening program towards a maximum sensitivity with a reasonable and acceptable rate of false positives. In order to allow a meaningful comparison between the three automatic instruments we avoided criteria which would give one instrument a much higher sensitivity than the other two if this resulted in a much lower specificity compared with the other two instruments. We therefore modified our earlier COMPETER criteria (5b, 5c) to make them less sensitive as they would have yielded a 98% sensitivity but at a considerably lower specificity than obtained with the other automatic perimeters. The OCTOPUS criteria presented some problems as our previous experience with the perimeter was rather limited. We applied the rules used by Schmied (8) but had to abandon this method when we found that it led to a 98% sensitivity but a specificity of only 25%. The criteria used in this study were found by trial and error and will be fully reported elsewhere. There were no previous data available for the PERIMETRON. We found that the majority of false positives from the PERIMETRON were due to small nasal steps. The specificity would in fact have risen to 94% if the nasal step criteria had been excluded but the sensitivity would have fallen to 71%.

The results of the study were probably unfavourably influenced by the fact that patients were subjected to three strenuous tests within a few hours. Prolonged automatic perimetry can lead to deterioration of patient performance (5e). Randomization of the sequence of automatic testing should minimize this in a comparative study. We found the test results from the three instruments equally useful. The PERIMETRON covered the full field and often indicated nasal steps more clearly than the other two machines but it can miss the full depth of localized visual field defects.

The method of presentation of the results on the PERIMETRON are most easily interpreted by ophthalmologists. The OCTOPUS program used covers the central fields up to 30° while the COMPETER covered the central 20°. Nasal wedge-shaped defects were often more clear in the OCTOPUS than in the COMPETER central pattern charts. The peripheral points in the OCTOPUS tests are often affected by lens artifacts which had to be disregarded in the study. The resolution of OCTOPUS Test program '31' is lower in the central visual field than the resolution of the other two instruments but the use of a complementary program '32' which increases the resolution at the cost of doubling the test time can be employed. The OCTOPUS as we employed it can therefore miss small paracentral defects including narrow arcuate scotomas curving between 5° and 10° from fixation towards the nasal parafoveal area. It seldom indicates the full depth of the physiological blind spot.

CONCLUSION

The objectivity and standardization of testing of the automatic perimetric programs are major advantages. All three perimeters tested proved very useful and gave similar results which in our opinion is superior to much of currently used standard kinetic visual fields plotted. The ophthamologist cannot solve all his perimetric problems at this time by purchasing an automatic perimeter. Conventional manual backup system with a competent technician is still necessary, particularly for quantitative perimetry. The automatic perimeters can relieve technicians from much tedious and time-consuming routine screening and it is our belief and hope that automatic perimetry will become a standard procedure within the next decade. Judiciously used computerized perimeters will prove to be of great benefit to ophthalmologists and their patients. They can already improve the quality of perimetry as currently practiced.

REFERENCES

1. Aulhorn, E. & W. Durst. Comparative investigation of automatic and manual perimetry in different visual field defects. Doc. Ophthalmol. Proc. Ser. 14: 17–22 (1977).
2. Bebie, H., F. Fankhauser & J. Spahr. Static perimetry: Strategies. Acta Ophthalmol. 54: 325–338 (1977).
3. Bynke, H., A. Heijl & C. Holmin. Automatic computerized perimetry in neuro-ophthalmology. Doc. Ophthalmol. Proc. Ser. 19: 319–325 (1979).
4. Dyster-Aas, K., A. Heijl & L. Lundqvist. Computerized visual screening in the management of patients with ocular hypertension. In press.

5a. Heijl, A. Automatic perimetry in glaucoma visual field screening. A clinical study. Albrecht von Graefes Arch. Klin. Exp. Ophthalmol. 200: 21–37 (1976)

5b. Heijl, A., S. M. Drance & G. R. Douglas. The value of an automatic perimeter (Competer) in detecting early glaucomatous visual field defects. Arch. Ophthalmol. Accepted for publication.

5c. Heijl, A. & S. M. Drance. Computerized profile perimetry in glaucoma. Arch. Ophthamol. Accepted for publication.

5d. Heijl, A. & C. E. T. Krakau. An automatic perimeter for glaucoma visual field screening and control. Construction and clinical cases. Albrecht von Graefes Arch. Klin. Exp. Ophthalmol. 197: 13–23 (1975).
5e. Heijl, A. Time changes of contrast thresholds during automatic perimetry. Acta Ophthalmol. 55: 696–708 (1977).
5f. Heijl, A. Computer test logics for automatic perimetry. Acta. Ophthalmol. 55: 837–853 (1977).
5g. Heijl, A. & C. E. T. Krakau. A note on fixation during perimetry. Acta Ophthalmol. 55: 854–861 (1977).
5h. Heijl, A. & S. M. Drance. A clinical comparison of three computerized automatic perimeters in the detection of glaucoma defects. In preparation.
6. Li, S. G., G. L. Spaeth, N. J. Schatz *et al.* Clinical experiences with the use of an automated perimeter (Octopus) in the management of patients with glaucoma and neurological disease. Ophthalmol. 85: 74 (1978).
7. Proll, M. Die Varianz der Befunderhebung bei der kinetischen und der computergesteuerten Perimetrie. Inaugural-Dissertation, Julius-Maximilians-Universität, Würzburg, Federal Republic of Germany (1979).
8. Schmied, U. Automatic (Octopus) and manual (Goldmann) perimetry in glaucoma. In: Proc. Int. meeting automated perimetry system Octopus. Interzeag. publ., Schlieren, Switzerland (1979).
9a. Spahr, J., F. Fankhauser, A. Jenni *et al.* Praktische Erfahrungen mit dem automatischen Perimeter Octopus. Klin. Mbl. Augenheilk. 172: 470–477 (1978).
9b. Spahr, J. Zur Automatisierung der Perimetrie. I: Die Anwendung eines computergesteuerten Perimeters. Albrecht von Graves Arch. Klin. Exp. Ophthalmol. 188: 323–338 (1973).

Supported in part by B.C. Health Care Research Foundation and in part by the Carmen and Bertil Regnér's Eye Research Fund and the Swedish Medical Research Grant #K78-17F-5303-01.

Authors' addresses:
Stephen M. Drance
Dept. of Ophthalmology
University of British Colombia
and Vancouver General Hospital
2550 Willow Street
Vancouver V5Z 3NG
Canada

Anders Heijl
Dept. of Ophthalmology
University of Lund
S-21401 Malmö
Sweden

CAPABILITIES AND LIMITATIONS OF AUTOMATED SUPRATHRESHOLD STATIC PERIMETRY

JOHN L. KELTNER & CHRIS A. JOHNSON

(Davis, Calif., U.S.A.)

ABSTRACT

Automated suprathreshold static perimetry is a technique for performing rapid, quantitative visual field testing to detect visual field defects. Over the past three and one-half years, we have had the opportunity to evaluate five commercially-available automated perimeters that utilize this technique. Our research has emphasized the development of optimal test procedures for automated suprathreshold static perimetry, and clinical comparison studies with manual perimetry to define the capabilities and limitations of the technique. To date, more than 2,500 eyes have been evaluated in these clinical comparison studies. Among the various commercial devices we have examined, there are many similarities and differences. This blend of common and unique components for each device has allowed us to determine many general principles of automated suprathreshold static perimetry. The present paper describes an overview of our investigations with regard to test conditions, principles of operation and performance capabilities in automated suprathreshold static perimetry. The ultimate role of automated suprathreshold static perimetry, in conjunction with automated static or kinetic testing, remains to be defined.

INTRODUCTION

Our investigations of automated suprathreshold static perimetry now encompass three and one-half years of study, five commercially-available automated devices and evaluation of more than 2,500 eyes (1–8). Similarities and differences among various approaches to automated suprathreshold static perimetry have become apparent through this work. It has also been possible to determine stimulus conditions, test procedures, validation techniques, capabilities and limitations of this technique, cost considerations, and possibilities for future development. The present paper describes an overview of our experiences with automated suprathreshold static perimetry and discusses some considerations for the development of the 'ideal' automated perimeter (5). This information is directed only to the specifications of automated suprathreshold static perimetry and does not apply to the more sophisticated test procedures of automated static or kinetic testing devices.

Doc. Ophthal. Proc. Series, Vol. 26, ed. by E. L. Greve & G. Verriest

STIMULUS CONDITIONS

1. Background luminance

There are presently no standards for background luminance in automated suprathreshold static devices. It is our opinion that a background luminance of 31.5 asb (10 cd/m²) should be employed until further research warrants an alternative value. These automated devices would then be in correspondence with the most widely used background luminance for manual perimetry. The uniformity of background luminance in most automated suprathreshold static perimeters is comparable to that of conventional manual perimeters, exhibiting good uniformity along the horizontal meridian and a modest luminance gradient along the vertical meridian.

2. Target size

Ideally, automated suprathreshold static perimeters should offer a variety of target sizes as provided on most manual perimeters. However, many of the available automated devices of this type are restricted to a single target size. In this instance, we recommend that a target size of 7–10 minutes of arc diameter be employed.

3. Target luminance

The most desirable stimulus for automated perimetry is a target that exhibits a sharp, symmetric intensity profile and maintains constant luminance, color temperature and spectral distribution, irrespective of its location. Thus, a projection system for target presentation is the preferred method of stimulus display. Our second alternative for target presentation consists of individual fiber optics elements. It is necessary to insure equal transmission characteristics of each fiber optics element, and to carefully position and calibrate them in the perimeter bowl, since directionality of the fiber optics elements can influence the effective luminance to the eye. However, fiber optics elements retain the advantage of using a common light source for all stimuli, and exhibit a sharp, symmetric luminance profile.

Our third choice consists of individual light emitting diodes (LEDs). In this instance, each target utilizes a separate light source, thereby increasing the difficulty of maintaining target uniformity and precise calibration. We have also found that luminance profiles of individual LEDs are often asymmetric and can exhibit considerable variation from one LED to another. We recommend that if LEDs are used, a good diffuser combined with a small aperture stop should be used for each individual target. We have also found that the luminance and spectral distribution of LEDs can exhibit considerable individual variation. It should also be noted that LEDs introduce the additional complications of color perimetry, since their spectral distribution is not neutral. It is our opinion that the use of LEDs for automated suprathreshold static perimeters should be approached with caution and must include extremely careful calibration procedures.

4. Target color

Because of the increased complexity and precision required for color perimetry, we feel that achromatic targets should be utilized for automated suprathreshold static perimetry. This technique is a relatively new form of visual field testing, and the introduction of complex test procedures and stimuli is probably not beneficial at this time.

5. Target presentation sequence

Most automated suprathreshold static perimeters utilize a target presentation sequence that is random or pseudo-random. We favour this type of approach because it minimizes the influence of expectancy, unstable fixation and other factors that are deleterious to the test results.

6. Target presentation rate

We find that rapid target presentation rates are sometimes hard for patients to follow, particularly in elderly populations. On the other hand, a presentation rate that is too slow often produces boredom or inattentiveness on the part of the patient. We recommend a target presentation rate of approximately 1 per second. However, this presentation interval should be somewhat sporadic or non-rhythmic. The use of a constant target presentation rate will sometimes cause patients to develop a 'rhythm of response' that produces spurious results.

7. Target duration

As with target presentation rate, stimulus duration that are too long or too short may produce difficulties in some patient populations. We therefore recommend a target duration of approximately 0.5 to 1 second for each stimulus presentation.

8. Target presentation pattern

A number of target presentation patterns are available on the various commercially-available automated suprathreshold static perimeters. These target distributions are generally based upon the clinical experience and opinions of expert consultants in the area of visual field testing. While this approach has validity, there is presently no quantitative, empirical basis for the various presentation patterns employed. The efficiency, accuracy and sensitivity of automated suprathreshold static perimetry are critically dependent upon the presentation pattern. We have no formal recommendation for target presentation patterns for automated suprathreshold static perimetry, but are curently in the process of defining an objective, quantitative method of deriving optimal target presentation patterns for this type of automated testing.

9. Fixation

An eye monitor to assess the accuracy of fixation is useful for many patients undergoing automated testing. The efficacy of a fixation monitor depends upon its sensitivity and reliability. It must be able to consistently detect significant eye movement but should not be so sensitive as to be repeatedly triggered by non-significant movements. An eye monitor sensitivity adjustment is helpful to select a reasonable criterion for detecting eye movements that may affect the test results, and to be able to select eye movement tolerance levels that are within the capabilities of each individual patient. Our experience indicates that unless an eye monitor is reliable and its sensitivity is adjustable, it may create more problems than it solves.

TEST PROCEDURES

1. Multiple luminance testing

In order to achieve high rates of detecting visual field defects with automated suprathreshold static perimetry, it is necessary to perform testing for at least two different target luminances. A high target luminance will provide an evaluation of the full visual field, but is likely to miss shallow or moderate scotomas. On the other hand, a low target luminance will be able to detect shallow-to-moderate visual field defects, but will not be appropriate for evaluating the far periphery. It is, therefore, necessary to perform testing for two or more target luminances to optimize test results.

2. Refractive correction

For testing the central 30° at low target luminances, an appropriate refractive correction for the target distance should be used. Unless this is done, a high incidence of false alarms will occur as a result of refraction scotomas.

3. Automatic retest

Another factor that is necessary to reduce false alarm rate is the performance of an automatic retest of all targets missed during the first presentation sequence. It is particularly important that this be done automatically to insure consistent test conditions from the initial testing to the retest. It is also useful to retest several spots that were detected on the initial presentation in order to keep the patient alert during the retest period.

VALIDATION STUDIES

1. Controlled clinical trials

We feel that controlled clinical trials should be performed with automated perimeters before they are released to eye care specialists. This includes the use of standardized manual perimetric techniques for comparison. In the past, some of the commercial automated perimeters have been marketed before proper validation studies were performed and appropriate deficiencies in the devices were corrected. This has understandably caused some concern over the validity of automated suprathreshold static testing.

2. Criteria for interpreting data

Once the results have been obtained, it is necessary to interpret the findings according to standard established criteria. One of the great advantages of automated testing is that each patient is subjected to a standardized, reproducible test procedure. These benefits are diminished if the results of the test procedure are interpreted in a non-systematic fashion.

CAPABILITIES AND LIMITATIONS

Our findings indicate that most automated suprathreshold static perimeters are capable of achieving detection rates of 90 per cent or better in comparison to manual perimetric testing, provided that proper stimulus and test conditions are employed. In contrast, false alarm rates can vary considerably. When factors such as appropriate refractive correction, automatic retest and standardized criteria for interpreting results are employed, false alarm rates can be below 5 per cent. In the absence of these factors, the false alarm rate can be as high as 25 per cent or more. Detection and false alarm rates for three automated suprathreshold static perimeters we have evaluated (the CFA-120, the Autofield-I and the Fieldmaster Model 101-PR) are presented in Table 1. Because of the greater simplicity and speed of automated suprathreshold static perimetry, some patients produce test results that are superior to those derived from manual techniques. Overall, these findings indicate that automated suprathreshold static perimetry can be an excellent technique for the detection of visual field defects.

The ability of automated suprathreshold static perimetry to provide detailed assessment of visual field defects and to follow the progression and/or regression of visual field loss appears to be somewhat limited. At the present time, only preliminary data are available on the efficacy of this technique for such purposes. From a theoretical standpoint, the lack of flexibility for test and stimulus conditions in these devices imposes a strict limitation upon detailed assessment of visual field loss.

Table 1. Detection and false alarm rates for the Autofield-I, CFA-120 and Fieldmaster model 101-PR as compared to manual kinetic perimetry

Device	# of eyes	# of defects	Detection rate	False alarm rate
Autofield-I	103	65	93.8%	24.2%
CFA-120	99	54	90.7%	17.9%
Fieldmaster model 101-PR	1,019	436	96.1%	4.7%

COST CONSIDERATIONS

In analyzing the efficacy of automated perimetry, cost must be a consideration. Automated suprathreshold static perimeters have done relatively well regarding cost containment. The simplicity of the testing technique has permitted the development of these moderately low cost devices. In our modern cost conscious health delivery system, this becomes a significant consideration.

FUTURE DEVELOPMENTS

Our experience suggests that the future development of automated suprathreshold static perimetry is dependent upon several important factors. These include: (1) a quantitative empirical basis for defining the distribution and number of target locations necessary for performing automated suprathreshold static perimetry; (2) the development of specialized test protocols to evaluate specific types of visual disorders; (3) an updated method of data representation for automated suprathreshold static perimetry. After having viewed thousands of visual field results from automated suprathreshold static perimetry, we still find them to be more difficult to interpret than the traditional data representation methods used in manual perimetry. The general problem of data representation for visual field information, irrespective of manual or automated testing, is a significant problem that requires further attention. (4) Perhaps the most significant development for automated suprathreshold static perimetry will be the establishment of well-defined standards. Clearly, as the field of automated perimetry advances from its infancy, the standards will need to be modified. However, it is desirable to achieve some consistency among automated devices before their pathways become too divergent. We feel that one of the greatest advantages afforded by automated perimetry is the capability of achieving widespread standardization of stimulus conditions and test procedures, a goal that should be easier to achieve for automated devices than for existing manual techniques. The role of automated static, kinetic and suprathreshold static testing procedures in the development of the 'ideal' automated perimeter remains to be seen. Factors such as cost, simplicity of operation, ease of data interpretation and reliability in detecting and following visual field loss will determine the type of device to gain acceptance by the practicing eye care specialists throughout the world.

SUMMARY

Automated suprathreshold static perimetry is now a reality, and has been shown to be an effective method of accurately detecting visual field defects. The capabilities and limitations of this technique for detailed assessment of visual field loss and following the progression and/or regression of visual field defects remains to be determined. Future developments many enhance the effectiveness of this form of automated visual field testing.

REFERENCES

1. Johnson, C. A. & J. L. Keltner. Comparison of manual and automated perimetry in 1,000 eyes. Computers in Ophthalmology, New York; IEEE Publishing Service, 178–181 (1979).
2. Johnson, C. A., J. L. Keltner & F. G. Balestrery. Suprathreshold static perimetry in glaucoma and other optic nerve disease. Ophthalmology 86: 172–1286 (1979).
3. Johnson, C. A. & J. L. Keltner. Automated suprathreshold static perimtetry. Amer. J. Ophthalmol., 89: 731–741 (1980a).
4. Johnson, C. A. & J. L. Keltner. Comparative evaluation of the Autofield-I, CFA-120 and Fieldmaster Model 101-PR automated perimeters. Ophthalmology, 87: 31–37 (1980b).
5. Keltner, J. L. & C. A. Johnson. Automated perimetry. Western Journal of Medicine 129: 543 (1979).
6. Keltner, J. L., C. A. Johnson & F. G. Balestrery. Suprathreshold static perimetry: Initial clinical trials with the Fieldmaster automated perimeter. Arch. Ophthalmol. 97: 260–272 (1979).
7. Keltner, J. L. Comments on automated perimetry. Ophthalmology 86: 1317–1319 (1980).
8. Keltner, J. L. & C. A. Johnson. Mass visual field screening in a driving population. Ophthalmology, 87: 39–44 (1980).

Supported in part by National Eye Institute Research Grant #EY-01841 (to JLK) and National Eye Institute Academic Investigator Award #EY-00095 (to CAJ)

Author's address:
John L. Keltner, M.D.
Department of Ophthalmology
University of California, Davis
Davis, CA 95616
U.S.A.

RELIABILITY OF VISUAL FIELD EXAMINATION IN CLINICAL ROUTINE

T. NEUHANN & J.-H. GREITE

(Munich, F.R.G.)

ABSTRACT

152 eyes of 86 patients with retinal diseases affecting the periphery as well as the center, and glaucoma visual defects were examined with the Fieldmaster 200 and Octopus. Manual kinetic perimetry with a Goldmann perimeter was used for comparison, to find out how reliable field defects are, detected by a single examination. Patients aged between 20 and 50 years have shown in about 94% reliable results.

In the age group 51–70 years still 90% gave good answers in visual field examination. Patients aged over 70 years gave only in 25% reliable answers in their examinations.

The reliability of defects in visual fields is not different between the Fieldmaster and the Goldmann perimeter, while the Octopus provides objective data for their evaluation.

INTRODUCTION

Due to the rapid development of automated perimetry, a variety of instruments is available today, creating new problems for the ophthalmologist by their differences in controls, programs, measuring units, stimulus variables, results display etc. (5, 10). What the practitioner is primarily interested in is how efficient such a perimetry is.

First experiences with new automated perimeters have recently been reported by numerous authors (1–4, 6, 9, 11, 12). We are fully aware that a direct comparison of fully automated, semi-automated and manual perimeters is virtually not permitted. Since, however the Goldmann perimeter is the most widely used instrument today, the practicability of any newly developed perimeter will be evaluated in comparison to it.

Thus, we do not intend to give you an evaluation of the quality of each one of these systems; what we have examined instead, is how reliable a single examination with either one of the above systems is in detecting visual field defects.

METHOD

The examinations were carried out on a Goldmann perimeter, the semi-automatic system Fieldmaster 200 and the fully automated perimetric system Octopus. The following table contains the principal differences among the three perimeters:

Table 1. Shows the principal differences among the three named perimeters (see also text).

Strategy	OCTOPUS static	FIELDMASTER static	GOLDMANN kinetic
Stimulus presentation	in random spatial order in a square grid of variable size	in random spatial order in a pre-fixed grid	by examiner
Stimulus size	variable	not variable	variable
Exposure time	fixed	variable	variable
Stimulus luminance	varied to determine threshold by repetitive bracketing	to be preset	to be preset
Surround field calibration	automatic	manual	manual
Setting of fix. contr.	by examiner	by patient	by examiner
Fix. contr.	by infrared TV-monitoring and visually	by infrared cell monitoring	visually
Result display	electronic data storage and three kinds of graphic display	semi-automatic	manual
System	fully automatic	semi-automatic	manual

While with the Octopus the threshold for every tested spot in the field is determined by means of a repetitive bracketing technique, the information provided by the Fieldmaster is, whether the threshold of the tested area in the field is above or below the preset luminance, for the fixed target size.

We have examined 152 eyes of 86 patients (Table 2). They were first examined on the Goldmann perimeter all by the same technician. On the following day, instruction and examination on the Octopus was performed by one of the authors (TN). Finally, instruction and testing was carried out on the Fieldmaster, model 200, also by one of the authors (TN).

For optimal program selection with the automated systems, different procedures were used for

group I: patients with retinal diseases, affecting the periphery as well as the center and for
group II: glaucoma patients.

In group I, the 90° field was tested using the Octopus program 21. Background luminance was calibrated automatically before each examination, target size was standard size 3. On the Fieldmaster, program 2 was chosen for the left eye, program 3 for the right eye; the background luminance was set at 31.5 asb, the stimulus luminance at 134 asb, both figures corresponding to the recommendations given by the manufacturer.

In the second group, the 30° field was tested on the Octopus using program 31. On the Fieldmaster, program 'central 30°' was chosen; background

Table 2. Shows the exact numbers of the examined patients and the age groups.

A G E (years)	G R O U P I central +peripher retinal diseases	G R O U P II glaucoma visual field defect	
20 - 50	28 patients 53 eyes	11 patients 19 eyes	39p 72e
51 - 70	13 patients 25 eyes	14 patients 24 eyes	27p 49e
over 70	6 patients 9 eyes	14 patients 22 eyes	20 p 31e
		total	86 patients 152 eyes

luminance was the same as above, the stimulus luminance, however, was set at 43 asb, also corresponding to the manufacturer's recommendations.

The patients tested were further subdivided into three age groups:

20–50 years
51–70 years
over 71 years

RESULTS

In the patients aged between 20 and 50 years, the results were almost identical with all three methods. Small paracentral relative defects, however, were only detected on the Octopus. Two patients, who had been examined for diffuse 'pressure' in both eyes, exhibiting a concentric field constriction had a significant percentage of false negative responses on the Octopus. This led to more detailed anamnestic exploration and finally made the diagnosis of a psychogenic visual disturbance possible. On the Goldmann perimeter and the Fieldmaster, the false negative nature of the responses had not been so clearly demonstrable.

The patients in the second group, i.e. 51 to 70 years, also presented a surprisingly high quality and coincidence of the findings with all three methods. False positive and false negative responses occurred only occasionally. Fixation was generally sufficient to allow for good information to be drawn from the examinations. Here, too, small paracentral relative scotomata were detected only by the Octopus, but could then be reproduced with the Goldmann perimeter and, by adjusting test luminance, with the Fieldmaster.

The third age group of those over 71 years, was not only the smallest, but also the most difficult to test. Diabetic and glaucomatous eye disease were predominant. Whereas in all 20 patients Goldmann perimetry was performed very sensibly, testing on the Octopus and on the Fieldmaster proved to be extremely difficult. The main sources of errors were the following:

– Premature replies: these occurred when the response to the previous stimulus coincided with the new stimulus.

- Insufficient fixation.
- Physical disabilities: this can result, for example in insufficient setting of the fixation target by the patient with the Fieldmaster, thus making proper fixation and reproducibility impossible.

False positive and false negative responses occurred frequently. The mean fluctuation, given in dB, by the Octopus was significantly higher than in the precedent age groups. Thus, the accumulation of these interfering factors with the automated perimetry often reduced its reliability to a minimum. This, however, is by no means to say that patients above the age of 70 cannot perform good perimetry: We also had excellent results with none or only few false negative or positive responses, low fluctuation rate and good reproducibility. It was the frequency of unreliable responses that was noticeable. The overall reliability results are presented in Fig. 1.

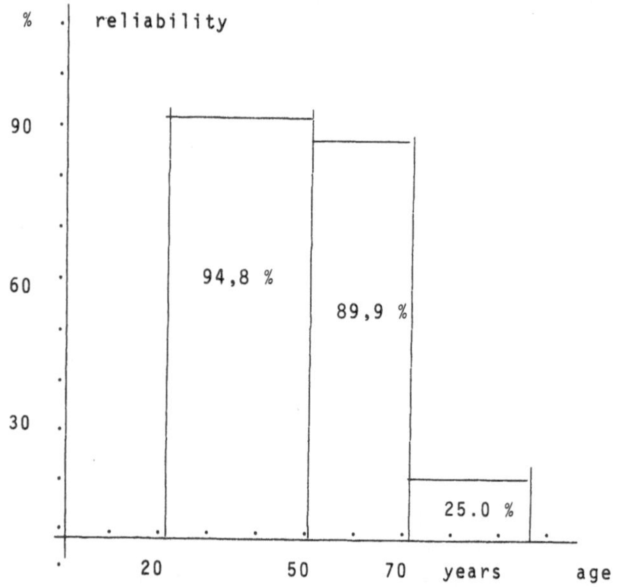

Fig. 1. Reliability in different age groups.

COMMENT

Focussing back on our question, how reliable are visual field defects detected by a single examination with each one of the three methods, it may be answered as follows:

Under optimal conditions, that is a well-observing, cooperative patient and a trained perimetrist, all three methods are of virtually identical reliability in detecting field defects, the Octopus being somewhat superior in detecting small paracentral relative scotomata under the conditions of this trial. When the preconditions are less favorable, a sensible manual Goldmann perimetry may well prove superior to automated systems. However, with the Fieldmaster or the Goldmann perimeter, the examiner must try to get a clue as to the reliability of the patients. The Octopus provides plenty of objective data for the evaluation how good or how bad the result is. Thus, with the Fieldmaster or the Goldmann perimeter the reliability must be judged subjectively for the examination, whereby false positive or false negative responses may easily be overlooked, while the Octopus offers objective data for its evaluation.

REFERENCES

1. Aulhorn, E. & W. Durst. Comparative investigation of automatic and manual perimetry in different visual field defects. Doc. Ophthal Proc. Series, Vol. 14: 17–27 (1977).
2. Bynke, H. & A. Heijl. Automated computerized perimetry in the detection of neurological visual field defects. A pilot study. Albrecht von Graefes Arch. Klin. exp. Ophthal. 206: 11–15 (1978).
3. Dannheim, F. Klinische Erfahrungen mit einem halbautomatischen Perimeter 'Fieldmaster'. Der Augenspiegel, Nr. 6, 270–280.
4. Fankhauser, F. Automated perimetry. In. Glaucoma. 204–211, 1978, K. Heilmann (Hrsg.), G. Thieme, Stuttgart.
5. Greve, E. L. Automatic and non-automatic perimetry. In: Proceedings of the 1st Int. meeting on automated perimetry, 81–88 (1979).
6. Kampik, A., O.-E. Lund & H.-J. Greite. Computer Perimeter OCTOPUS (nach Fankhauser). Klinischer Vergleich mit dem GOLDMANN-Perimeter. Klin. Mbl. Augenheilk. 175: 72–81 (1979).
7. Portney, G. L. & M. A. Krohm. The limitations of kinetic perimetry in early glaucoma detection. Trans. Amer. Acad. Ophthal. Otolaryngal. 85: 287–293 (1979).
8. Rönne, H. Über klinische Perimetrie. Arch. Augenheilk. 87: 137 (1921).
9. Schmied, U. Automatic (OCTOPUS) and manual (GOLDMANN) perimetry in glaucoma – first experiences. In: Proceedings of the 1st Int. meeting on automated perimetry, 53–59 (1979).
10. Spahr, J. Zur Automatisierung der Perimetrie. Die Anwendung eines computergesteuerten Perimeters. Graefes Arch. Ophthal. 188: 323–388 (1973).
11. Spahr, J., F. Fankhauser, F. Jenni & H. Bebie. Praktische Erfahrungen mit dem automatischen Perimeter OCTOPUS. Klin. Mbl. Augenheilk. 172: 470–477 (1978).
12. Spaeth, G. L., S. G. Li & H. A. Scimeca. Clinical experiences with the use of Octopus automated perimeter in the detection of visual field loss in early glaucoma. In: Proceedings of the 1st Int. meeting on automated perimetry, 40–52 (1979).

Author's address:
T. Neuhann
Mathildenstr. 8
University Eye Clinic
D-8000 Munich 2
F.R.G.

PSYCHOPHYSICAL AND ELECTROPHYSIOLOGICAL DETERMINANTS OF MOTION DETECTION

ROBERT P. SCOBEY

(Davis, Calif. U.S.A.)

ABSTRACT

Displacement thresholds for moving line targets were measured for man and for retinal ganglion cells of cat and monkey. Several studies are summarized and should be of interest for perimetry. A luminous line was stationary at one site and moved at constant velocity to a test site where it again remained stationary. The optimal stimulus parameters for kinetic perimetry were considered to be the range of target luminance, line length and duration of motion which produced minimum and consistent thresholds. For durations of motion below 0.5 seconds, displacement thresholds remained constant for both foveal and peripheral (18°) vision. Increases in stimulus luminance and line length produced a successive reduction in displacement thresholds in peripheral vision, whereas foveal displacement thresholds were essentially unaffected by these variables. Displacement thresholds were as small or smaller than acuity measures throughout the central 40° of visual field.

INTRODUCTION

Detection of motion is of practical interest in kinetic perimetry. Although the visual literature spans a period of over 100 years, the effect of some stimulus parameters on motion thresholds is unknown. Little is known about the neural mechanisms for detecting motion in the primate visual system. Furthermore, there are technical difficulties in motion studies which are not present in studies with static targets. Perhaps it is not surprising that the optimal parameters for motion are not yet established.

There are several stimulus paradigms used in motion studies (2). The displacement threshold is the smallest distance that a target can be detected as changing in position. Displacement thresholds have been obtained under nearly identical stimulus conditions for man using psychophysical techniques (5) and for retinal ganglion cells in monkey using electrophysiological techniques (7). In these and other studies, a stationary luminous target was seen against a constant background. It moved at constant velocity from the initial site to a test site where it again remained stationary. This stimulus paradigm has the theoretical advantage that the response to motion is not confounded with the response to onset and offsets of a flashing target. It has the practical advantage that the time delay between neural excitation and response does not change the motion thresholds because the subject does not respond until motion is completed. These advantages are the basis for our selection of displacement threshold as a measure of motion detection.

METHODS

The methods used for the psychophysical experiments on humans and the electrophysiological experiments on Rhesus monkey have been reported in detail (5, 7). A brief description is given here. A cathode ray tube (CRT) stimulator provided a 'white' line target that could be controlled with the aid of a minicomputer. In the psychophysical studies, the stimulus was seen against a uniform background of $10\,cd.m^{-2}$ at a distance of 1 m. Similar stimulus conditions were used for anesthetized animals. Optimal refraction was placed before the test eye.

Psychophysical displacement thresholds were obtained by a randomly interleaved double staircase with a variable step size. An average of 10 reversals at the minimum step size was used as a threshold value. The presentation order of the stimulus conditions was counterbalanced across 4 sessions and these 4 thresholds were averaged to give the data points in Figs. 1c, 2a, 2b. The line through the data points was drawn by eye to average the data of two subjects. Both subjects exhibited a corrected visual acuity of better than 20/20, had no ocular abnormalities and received extensive practice in the task before collection of the data.

The stimulus paradigm is illustrated in Figs. 1A, 1B. The stimulus line was stationary at the initial site until the subject pressed the start button on his control panel. Then the stimulus line moved at constant velocity to the test site and stopped. After the subject responded, the line returned to the initial site and waited for the subject to proceed.

Displacement thresholds were measured as a function of movement duration, line length and luminance of the target in the fovea and at 18° eccentricity in the nasal field (horizontal meridian). In order to isolate the effects of an individual parameter, it was necessary to select constant optimum values for other stimulus conditions while testing one parameter. A movement duration of 80 msec, a stimulus luminance of 1.0 log unit above the increment threshold, and a line length of 40 minutes of arc were used as standards. As a single stimulus parameter was varied, the other stimulus conditions were adjusted to these standard values.

RESULTS

Psychophysics

At each duration of movement, displacement thresholds at 18° eccentricity were higher than for fovea, although the overall shape of the functions for both visual field locations was highly similar (Fig. 1c). Notice that the displacement thresholds were essentially constant for motion durations between 0.005 and 0.5 sec. This is a two log unit range over which minimum (optimum)

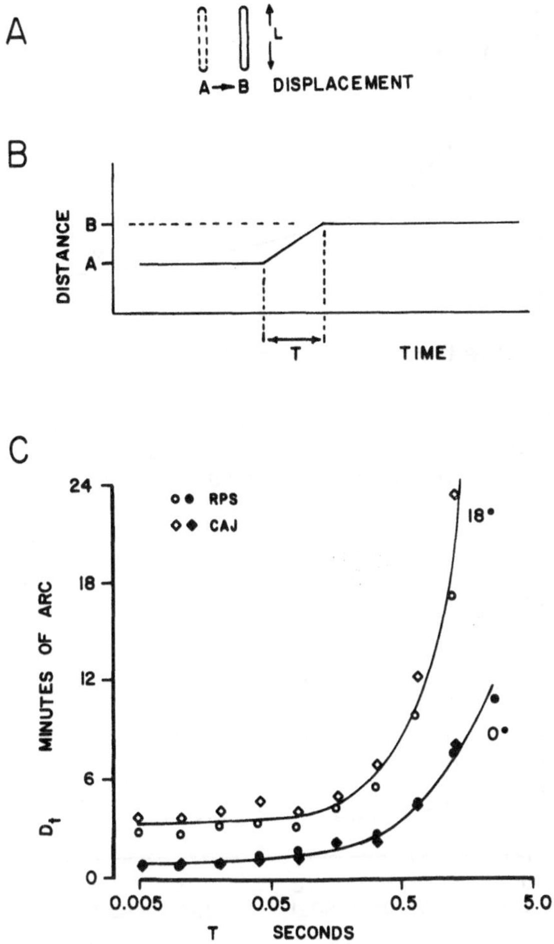

Fig. 1. Displacement threshold as a function of duration of motion.
A. The stimulus line is shown as seen by the subject. B. The position of the stimulus line is plotted as a function of time. C. Data for two subjects and two eccentricities are illustrated. Data (Fig. 1c, 2a, b) was replotted from the study of Johnson and Scobey (in press) to show the average of two subjects as the continuous line. Symbols for subjects in this figure are also used in Fig. 2.

motion thresholds can be obtained. It is likely that faster motion would give similar thresholds. Thus, for motion thresholds obtained in this manner, the optimum duration of motion is any duration less than 0.5 sec.

Displacement thresholds were obtained as a function of stimulus line length with the duration of motion and luminance held at the aforementioned standard values (Fig. 2a). In contrast to the results obtained for various durations of movement, the displacement threshold functions for line length exhibit rather significant differences between foveal and peripheral viewing. Foveal displacement thresholds were essentially independent of the length of the stimulus line. At 18° eccentricity, however, displacement thresholds exhibited a progressive decrease for longer stimulus lines up to approximately 30′,

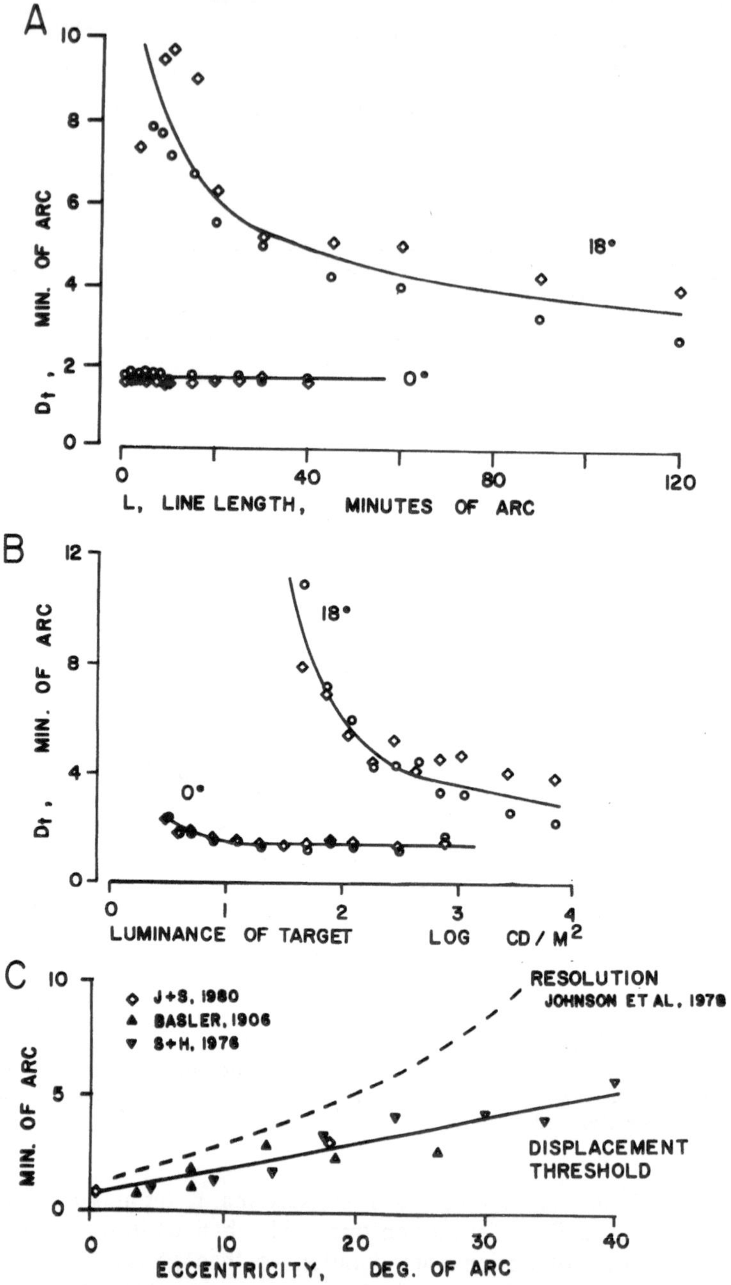

Fig. 2. Displacement threshold as a function of line length, luminance and eccentricity. A. The displacement threshold is plotted as a function of line length (L in Fig. 1). In foveal vision (0°), the displacement threshold is independent of line length. In peripheral vision (18°), the displacement threshold decreases markedly with line length. B. The displacement threshold is plotted as a function of luminance. C. Displacement threshold is plotted as a function of eccentricity in the visual field. Data for the displacement thresholds were taken from three studies, see text. For comparison, the normal resolution properties determined with stationary flashing spots is shown as the dotted line (Johnson, Keltner and Balestrery, 1978).

beyond which displacement threshold changes were rather minimal. Therefore, optimal line length for eccentricities up to 18° would be about 30′ or more.

Displacement thresholds were obtained as a function of stimulus luminance with the duration of motion and line length held at the standard values (Fig. 2b). A slight decrease in foveal displacement thresholds for increases in stimulus luminance of approximately 0.3 log units above the increment threshold was found. A more dramatic effect of stimulus luminance was found for four displacement thresholds at 18° visual field eccentricity. Changes in displacement threshold were minimal for stimulus luminance greater than 1.0 log unit above the increment threshold. Thus, over the central 18° of viewing, the value of luminance for optimal motion detection would be a target luminance about 1 to 2 log units above the increment threshold.

In Fig. 2c, displacement thresholds are plotted as a function of eccentricity in the visual field. Two data points are from this study while the others were measured by Basler (1) and Scobey and Horowitz (7). Although stimulus conditions were not identical in these studies, measurements are similar, indicating that the displacement threshold increases progressively with retinal eccentricity. The minimum angle of resolution for acuity of static targets has not been obtained under identical conditions as the motion studies. Nevertheless, we can compare cautiously motion and acuity thresholds. The dotted line represents resolution properties determined by the discrimination of circle and square targets (4). The tentative comparison suggest that motion thresholds are less than acuity thresholds.

Electrophysiology

When the size of receptive fields of single units in the visual system are determined with stationary flashing spots, it is found that the receptive field is always much larger than the displacement threshold. For example, displacement thresholds as small as 15″ in human foveal vision have been reported (8). Diffraction of light alone would produce larger receptive fields. Retinal ganglion cells respond to movements which are much smaller than the diameter of their receptive fields (6). An example will illustrate the mechanism for this exquisite sensitivity to motion.

In this experiment on a single retinal ganglion cell of monkey (unpublished data), a spot of light (3′) was positioned along the diameter of the receptive field and flashed with different luminance until a barely detectable increase in discharge rate was evoked. The reciprocal of threshold luminance was plotted on the ordinate of Fig. 3A to define the sensitivity profile of the receptive field. The nearly symmetric sensitivity profile had a maximum sensitivity to the onset of the flashed spot in the center of the receptive field.

Post-stimulus time histograms (20 iterations) were made following a small displacement (T = 4 msec) of the luminous spot from a site near the edge of the receptive field to a site of higher sensitivity. The spot was 2 log units above the minimum increment threshold. A 8.6′ displacement evoked a large response. Note that the spot of light moved to a more sensitive site in the receptive field (difference of about 0.6 log units). Smaller displacements

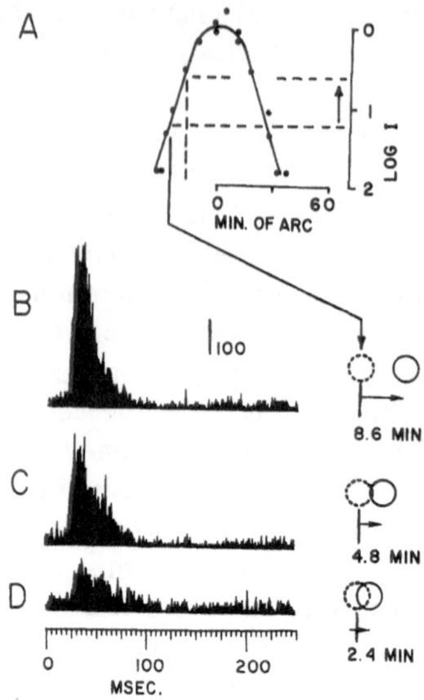

Fig. 3. Response of monkey retinal ganglion cell to small displacements within its receptive field center.
A. The sensitivity profile of a phasic on-center type unit from the peripheral retina of monkey (about 24° in the nasal retina) is plotted to define the location of the receptive field and illustrate the sensitivity to stationary flashing spots. The same small spot of light (3′) used for plotting the sensitivity profile was displaced in the receptive field center to evoke the histograms in Figs. 3B, C, D. The initial site for all three displacements is the same. The final position of the displacement for 3B (8.6′) is illustrated in A as dotted lines. The final site was about 0.6 log units more sensitive to stationary flashing light than the initial site. Smaller displacements caused correspondingly smaller responses.

moved the spot to less sensitive sites and a correspondingly less response was obtained (Figs. 3c, d). Displacement threshold was found to be the distance required to move the spot to a site that has a sensitivity increase equal to the increment threshold in that region of the receptive field (7).

Minimum displacement thresholds of on- and off-type retinal ganglion cells are similar in magnitude, but occur in different parts of the receptive field. A response to image displacement was found when a luminous spot moved to a site of lower sensitivity in off-type fields. Recent unpublished studies indicate that all retinal ganglion cells respond to small displacments. While quantitative differences have been identified between different types of cells, the major determining factor for motion sensitivity was the sensitivity gradient of the receptive field.

DISCUSSION

These findings indicate that reliable and small motion thresholds can be obtained with a stimulus line which is stationary at site 1 and moves to site 2 where it again remains stationary. Motion thresholds obtained in this manner obey a simple rule: to detect movement, a stimulus must travel a distance equal to the minimum displacement threshold (for the specific visual field location) within 0.5 sec or less.

The results for various line lengths reveal differences across the visual field. As previously reported by Graham (3), foveal displacement thesholds were essentially independent of line length. On the other hand, peripheral displacement thresholds exhibited a summation-type function; displacement thresholds decreased with line length up to about 30′, after which threshold reductions were more gradual.

Substantial changes in displacement thresholds were found as a function of line luminance in the periphery (18°), but not in the fovea. These findings correlate well with receptive field characteristics (Johnson and Scobey, in press). Changes in displacement threshold were minimal with luminance more than one log unit above increment threshold.

The displacement threshold paradigm provides a means to examine cellular response of single units under similar stimulus conditions as used in psychophysical studies. Likewise, theoretical predictions from electrophysiological experiments on subhuman primates are being used to design experiments for testing human visual fields. Thus, both models based on neural response and empirical data are available for choosing optimal parameters for motion studies.

It is not yet possible to state that the techniques described here have distinct advantage in detecting pathology from the use of conventional kinetic or static perimetry. Studies to date suggest that the displacement threshold paradigm can have significant increase in spatial resolution over the detection of a slowly moving spot as used in the Goldmann Perimeter. Optimum parameters for displacement threshold measures have a broad range of parameter values which yield optimum motion detection. Unfortunately, commercially available perimeters lack necessary stimulus control to implement these advantages in clinical perimetry.

REFERENCES

1. Basler, A. Über das Sehen von Bewegungen. Pflügers Arch. ges. Physiol. 115: 582–601 (1906).
2. Graham, C. H. Vision and visual perception. John Wiley and Sons, New York (1965).
3. Graham, C. H. Depth and movement. Am Psychol. 23: 18–23 (1968).
4. Johnson, C. A., J. L. Keltner & F. G. Balestrery. Effects of target size and eccentricity on visual detection and resolution. Vision Research 18: 1217–1222 (1978).
5. Johnson, C. A. & R. P. Scobey. Foveal and peripheral displacement thresholds as a function of stimulus luminance, line length and duration of movement. Vision Research, in press.
6. Scobey, R. P. & J. M. Horowitz. The detection of small image displacements by cat retinal ganglion cells. Vision Research 12: 2133–2143 (1972).
7. Scobey, R. P. & J. M. Horowitz. Detection of image displacement by phasic cells in the peripheral visual fields of the monkey. Vision Research 16: 15–24 (1976).
8. Westheimer, G. Spatial sense of the eye. (Proctor lecture). Invest. Ophthal. and Visual Sci. 18: 893–912 (1979).

Supported in part by National Eye Institute Research Grant EY-01495

Author's address:
Robert P. Scobey
Section of Neuroscience
School of Medicine
University of California
Davis, CA 95616
U.S.A.

PERIMETRY AND PATTERN – VECP IN CHIASMAL LESIONS

F. DANNHEIM, A. MÜLLER-JENSEN & S. ZSCHOCKE

(Hamburg, F.R.G.)

ABSTRACT

Pattern-evoked cortical potentials proved as a useful tool for the detection of chiasmal lesions in 27 patients, when hemifield stimulation was applied. Both the reduction of the amplitude and the latency delay correlated well with the degree of subjective perimetric changes evaluated by a highly sensitive technique.

INTRODUCTION

Objective perimetry with the aid of Visual Evoked Cortical Potentials (VECP) has successfully been employed in patients with demyelinating disease (1 and others). The diagnostic value of VECP in compressive lesions of the visual pathways has not been convincing (2, 3, 5, 6). In this report an attempt is made to evaluate the possibilities and limits of hemifield pattern-evoked potentials in chiasmal lesions in comparison with subjective perimetry.

MATERIAL AND METHODS

27 patients with reasonably good cooperation had been examined. A pituitary adenoma was surgically verified in 17 patients, suspected in 4. The others suffered from craniopharygeoma, epidermoid cyst, demyelinating disease, trauma and aneurysm of the carotide artery.

Visual fields have been taken with a TUEBINGEN perimeter, an OCTOPUS computer perimeter, or both. In the examination emphasis was placed on the evaluation of shallow paracentral defects which often are missed in clinical routine. The degree of changes has arbitrarily been divided into severe (Fig. 1a), moderate (Fig. 2a, above; Fig. 3a) or minimal (Fig. 2a, below).

Cortical potential analysis was performed by checkerboard reversal stimulation with an electronic triggered video device. The pattern was monocularly presented at 1 m distance subtending a visual angle of 30° x 25°. The size of each single square was 0.76°, the temporal frequency 2/sec. Stimulation of the whole field was followed by stimulation of the temporal or nasal hemifield. Occipital midline cortical potentials were recorded and graphically

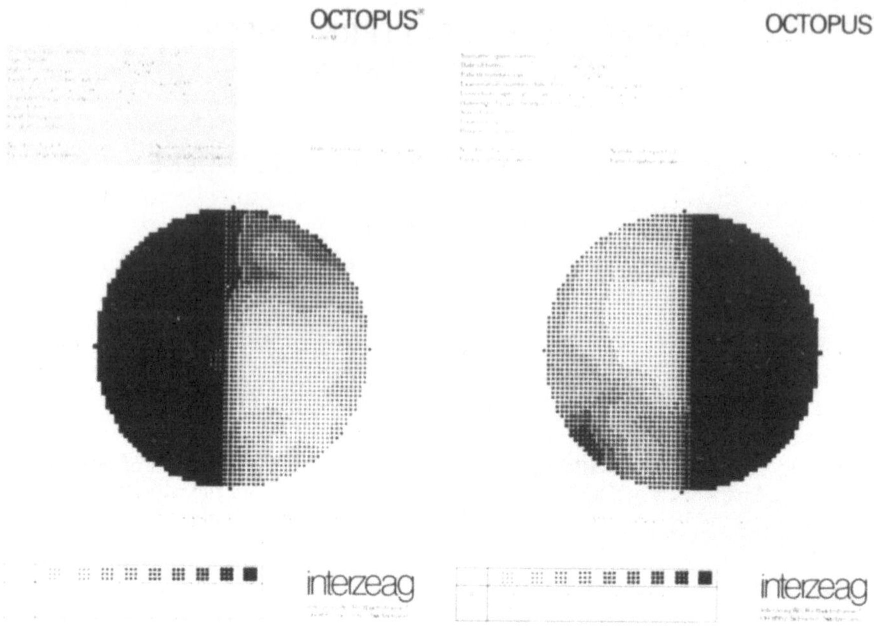

Fig. 1a. Severe bitemporal visual field defects due to a pituitary tumor, plotted with the OCTOPUS computer perimeter, program 32.

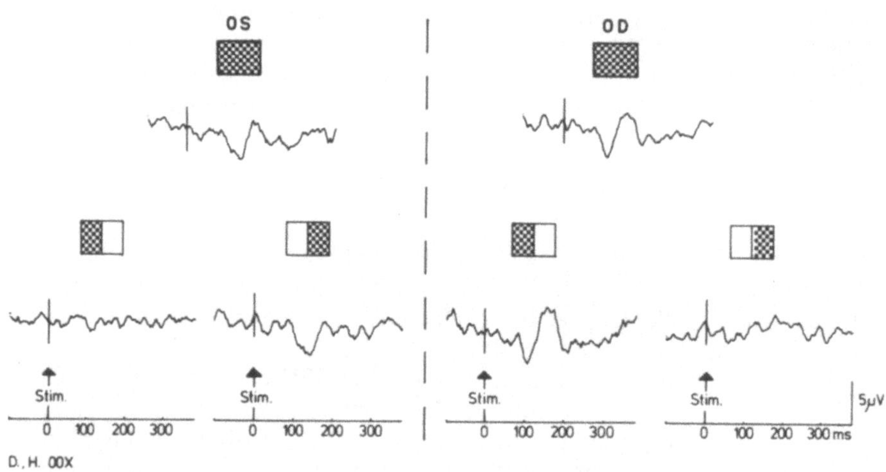

Fig. 1b. VECP with whole field stimulation (above): OD with normal wave form, OS with slight reduction of amplitude and delayed latency. Hemifield stimulation (below): No distinct response for both temporal hemifields (extreme right and left); wave form for nasal hemifield OD normal, OS moderately deformed and delayed.

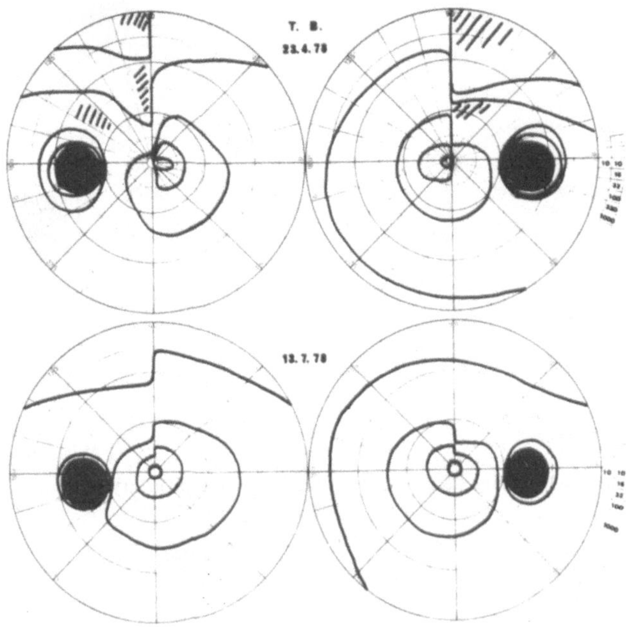

Fig. 2a. Moderate bitemporal field defects due to a pituitary adenoma (above), kinetically plotted with a TUEBINGEN perimeter (30°). OS with minimal alterations also in the nasal paracentral hemifield. Marked improvement to minimal bitemporal defects after removal of the tumor (below).

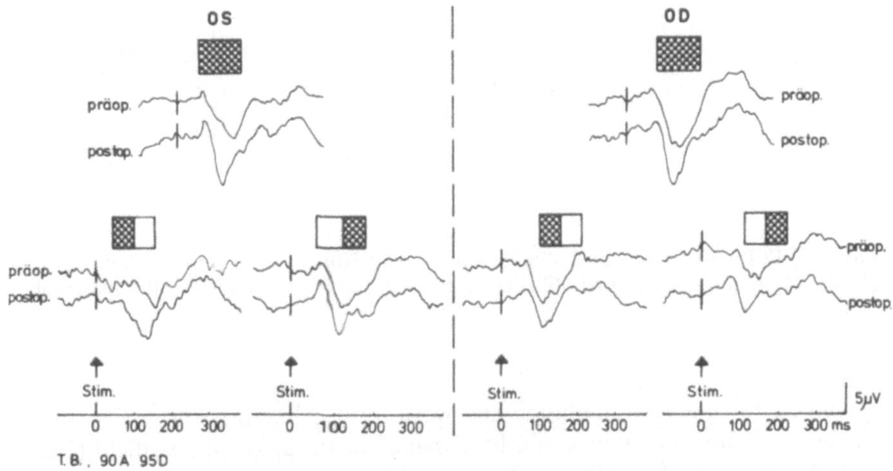

Fig. 2b. VECP with whole field stimulation (above): OD with some deformation and delay preoperatively (upper tracing) and normal wave form postoperatively (lower tracing); OS with marked deformation and delay preop. and normal wave form postop. Hemifield stimulation (below): Marked deformation and delay bitemporal and minimal changes in the nasal hemifields before operation. After surgery OD with normal wave form for both hemifields, OS with some deformation and delay for the temporal hemifield only.

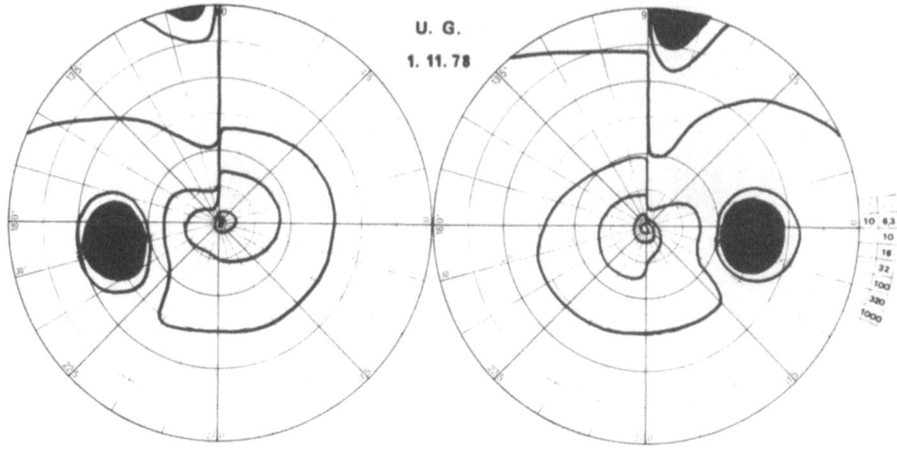

Fig. 3a. Moderate bitemporal defects before removal of a pituitary adenoma, plotted as in Fig. 2a).

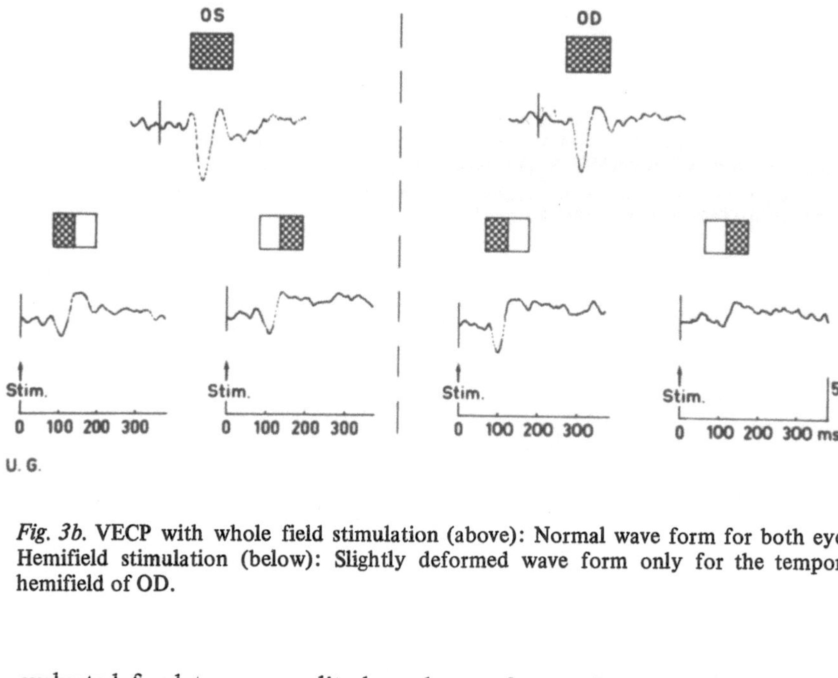

Fig. 3b. VECP with whole field stimulation (above): Normal wave form for both eyes. Hemifield stimulation (below): Slightly deformed wave form only for the temporal hemifield of OD.

evaluated for latency, amplitude and wave form. Alterations were classified as severe, if no potentials could be obtained in the affected hemifield (Fig. 1b). A reduction of amplitude of at least 1/3 as compared to the unaffected hemifield and a definite latency delay for the first negative component was graded as moderate change (Fig. 2b, preop.). Lesser degrees of asymmetries of the two hemifields were judged to be minimal (Fig. 2b, left eye postop.; Fig. 3b, right eye). All these recordings had not been available to the perimetrist in the subjective testing procedure.

RESULTS

From the 27 patients all had changes for subjective perimetry in one or both eyes due to a chiasmal lesion except for one patient with an enlarged sella and refraction scotomata in both eyes. Only 4 out of 26 patients were not found to be abnormal by VECP, all of which having minimal perimetric alterations. The one patient with refractional defects was correctly classified by VECP in showing the expected general reduction of potentials (4) without hemiopic asymmetries. The findings of VECP were never pathological, when subjective perimetry was undisturbed.

Such good results could only be obtained by hemifield stimulation: 21 of all 38 eyes with pathological VECP-findings would have been missed, if only the whole field had been stimulated. In these 21 eyes the degree of alterations for perimetry or VECP was about equally distributed in minimal, moderate and severe and the nasal hemifield was unaffected (Fig. 1, right eye; Fig. 2, left eye postop.; Fig. 3, right eye). To correlate the degree of alterations for the subjective and objective test all 54 eyes were evaluated separately. Two eyes of one patient entered twice due to a marked improvement following the removal of a pituitary adenoma (Fig. 2).

There is a good correlation (Fig. 4): In the majority the degree of alterations was the same. Less changes in VECP than expected from perimetry occurred in 12 eyes. The deviation of response was only 1 group except for one eye with a deviation of 2 groups (Fig. 3, left eye). More pronounced changes in VECP than expected was present in 11 eyes, which had moderate or severe findings for VECP and falling off the ideal correlation by 1 group.

PERIMETRY: \ VECP:	normal	minimal	moderate	severe	
normal	7				7
minimal	9	2	7		18
moderate	1	2	10	4	17
severe				14	14
	17	4	17	18	56

Fig. 4. Correlation of perimetric and VECP findings in 56 eyes of 27 patients with chiasmal lesions. Description of degree of alterations in the text. Optimal correlation along the diagonal, especially marked.

With a reduction in size of checkerboard squares as was performed in the last few patients of the series, a minimal alteration was found in one eye which had been missed with the standard set up.

The latency of the cortical response could be assessed with sufficient accuracy in 18 of 21 eyes with moderate or minimal changes (Fig. 5). All values except one fall outside the normal range of latency of ±2.5 sd. All values for the perimetrically unaffected hemifields except one lie in the upper half of the normal range.

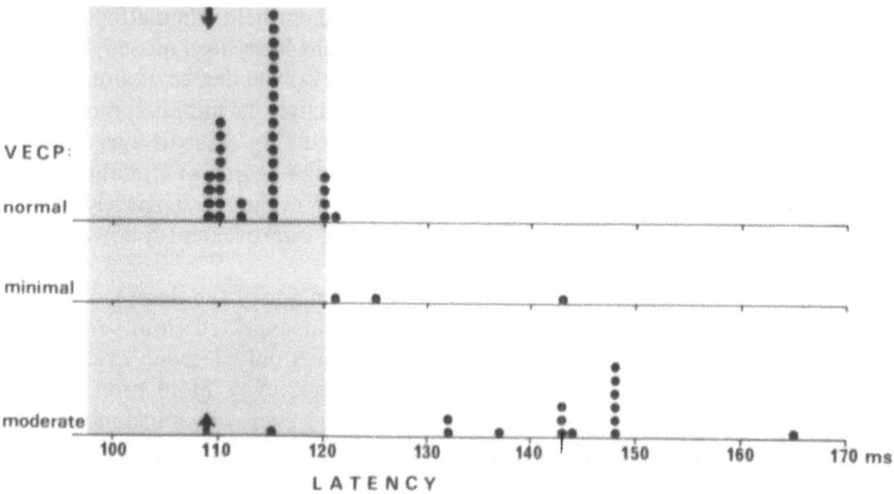

Fig. 5. Scattergram of values for latency of the first negative component of the VECP. Normal range (109 ms ± 2.5 sd) marked grey. Bottom line: 15 values of moderately affected hemifields, with one exception outside of the normal range. Middle line: 3 values of minimally affected hemifields outside of the normal range. Upper line: 35 values of unaffected hemifields, all except one in upper half of normal range.

COMMENT

The arrangement of this study differs from others in the relatively high number of cases not only with extensive, but also with moderate or minimal functional alterations (2, 3, 5, 6). The perimetric evaluation was performed with higher sensitivity; VECP were recorded with hemifield checkerboard stimulation of low temporal frequency.

The results disclose a better correlation of the two test procedures: Not only does the reduction of amplitude follow that correlation, but also the latency delay in the affected hemifields. Both features may improve following the removal of the compressive lesion. Stimulation of the whole field yielded a considerably higher rate of false negative findings. A reduction of visual acuity unrelated to the chiasmal lesion produces lower cortical potentials and thus limits the possibility for an accurate evaluation. A reduction of the size of checkerboard squares does also result in lower amplitudes. It may enhance the sensitivity of cortical responses in certain cases, however, and reduce the rate of false negatives even more.

ACKNOWLEDGEMENT

The author is indebted to the Claere Jung Foundation for the donation of an OCTOPUS computer perimeter.

REFERENCES

1. Halliday, A. M., W. I. McDonald & J. Mushin. Delayed visual evoked response in optic neuritis. Lancet 1: 982–985 (1972).
2. Halliday, A. M., E. Halliday, A. Kriss, W. I. McDonald & J. Mushin. The pattern-evoked potential in compression of the anterior visual pathways. Brain 99: 357–374 (1976).
3. Korol, S. Le syndrome chiasmatique – L'intérêt des potentiels évoqués visuels pour le diagnostic. Klin. Mbl. Augenheilk. 170: 314–320 (1977).
4. Millodot, M. & L. A. Riggs. Refraction determined electrophysiologically. Responses to alternation of visual contours. Arch. Ophthal. (Chic.) 84: 272–278 (1970).
5. Wildberger, H. G. H., G. H. M. van Lith, R. Wijngaarde & G. T. M. Mak. Visually evoked cortical potentials in the evaluation of homonymous and bitemporal visual field defects. Brit. J. Ophthal. 60: 273–278 (1976).
6. Wildberger, H. G. H., G. H. M. van Lith, R. Wijngaarde & G. T. M. Mak. Differential diagnostic aspects between optic neuritis and chiasm tumors. Ophthalmologica (Basel) 174: 106–110 (1977).

Senior author's address:
Priv.-Doz. Dr. Fritz Dannheim
Universitäts-Augenklinik
Martinistr. 52
D 2000 Hamburg 20

ACKNOWLEDGEMENT

[illegible] Foundation [illegible]

REFERENCES

[illegible]

[illegible]

[illegible]

[illegible]

VISUAL FIELD (VF) VERSUS VISUAL EVOKED CORTICAL POTENTIAL (VECP) IN MULTIPLE SCLEROSIS PATIENTS

J. T. W. VAN DALEN, H. SPEKREYSE & E. L. GREVE

(*Amsterdam, The Netherlands*)

ABSTRACT

29 Patients with multiple sclerosis were examined by means of static perimetry and visual evoked cortical response. In 16 eyes with a normal VECP an abnormal visual field was detected, while in 2 eyes with a normal visual field an abnormal VECP was found. Static perimetry appears to be at least as sensitive as VECP.

INTRODUCTION

During the last few years several examinations have been added to our diagnostic schemes in multiple sclerosis patients. For instance color vision tests (1) and grating sensitivity tests (2), are very sensitive in demonstrating demyelination in patients with multiple sclerosis. Therefore we felt the need for a comparison of visual field (VF) and visual evoked cortical potential (VECP) examinations in multiple sclerosis patients. A comprehensive review of our results will be published elsewhere.

METHODS

Subjects. 29 Subjects (19 women and 10 men) with well documented multiple sclerosis (3) were examined. All patients had a complete ophthalmological and neurological examination. Seven patients (8 eyes) had a history of at least one attack of optic neuritis; 22 patients never experienced any visual symptoms suggesting involvement of visual pathways (the so-called asymptomatic group).

Visual field examination. The fields were assessed by means of:

– Friedmann visual field analysis
– Kinetic perimetry
– Static perimetry.

Visual evoked cortical potential. The visual evoked cortical potentials were obtained by checkerboard stimulation on a TV-screen. The checksize was 20′

Doc. Ophthal. Proc. Series, Vol. 26, ed. by E. L. Greve & G. Verriest

and 55′. The pattern reversal frequency was 2 Hz and 10 Hz. The VECP latency was considered to be abnormal when the latency of the major positive peak was more than 126 msec. (For further details see 4 and 5). VF and VECP were determined on the same day.

RESULTS

Examination results per patient. 22 Patients showed a delayed VECP (in one or both eyes). Twenty-one of these 22 patients showed an abnormal visual field (in one or both eyes). Seven patients had a normal VECP. From these patients 5 had an abnormal visual field.

Examination results per eye. In 32 eyes (out of 58 eyes: 55%) an abnormal VECP was found and in 46 eyes (79%) an abnormal VF, i.e.:

- In 10 eyes a normal VF and VECP were found,
- In 30 eyes an abnormal VF and VECP were found,
- In 2 eyes with a normal VF an abnormal VECP was found, but on the other hand
- In 16 eyes with a normal VECP an abnormal VF was detected!

N.B. In the series of 8 eyes with a history of optic neuritis an abnormal VF and VECP was found in 6 eyes, while there was a discrepancy between the VF and the VECP in the remaining 2 eyes.

The above mentioned data suggest that VF assessment in multiple sclerosis patients is at least as informative as determination of VECP.

Visual field defects. The visual fields in our patients show interesting, characteristic defects. Of 46 eyes in which a defect was found, in 6 eyes only a central defect was detected, while 28 eyes showed a central defect *and* a defect in the intermediate visual field and 12 eyes showed a defect in the intermediate visual field only. (The intermediate visual field in this context means between 10° and 30° of eccentricity.)

In these 12 eyes a delayed VECP was found in 5 eyes. In Fig. 1a-b and Fig. 2a-b characteristic field defects in two of our multiple sclerosis patients have been shown. We often noticed relative patchy small scotomata 10°–20° off center. These intermediate area defects assessed by static perimetry turned out to be much more pronounced than could be suspected on the basis of a Friedmann visual field analysis. Often Friedmann visual field analysis did not detect any significant abnormalities in these regions, where static perimetry was extremely helpful. Kinetic perimetry did not provide any information in the asymptomatic group.

DISCUSSION AND CONCLUSION

In our asymptomatic group (50 eyes) in 26 eyes (52%) an abnormal VECP was found. This is consistent with previous studies that demonstrated a VECP

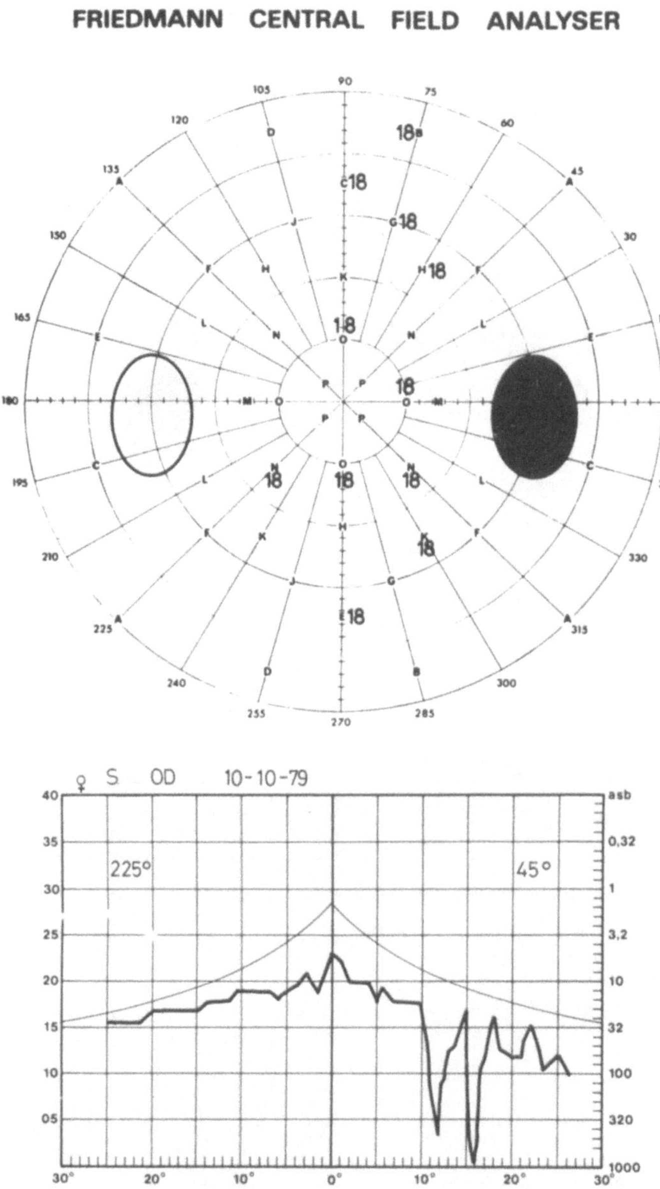

Fig. 1

A. Approximately normal Friedmann visual field analysis of the right, asymptomatic eye of a 39-year-old female patient.

B. Static perimetry (45°–225°) of the right eye shows remarkably deep defects 10°–20° off center. These defects are much more pronounced in the static profile than could be suspected on the basis of a Friedmann visual field analysis. The VECP of the right eye was delayed.

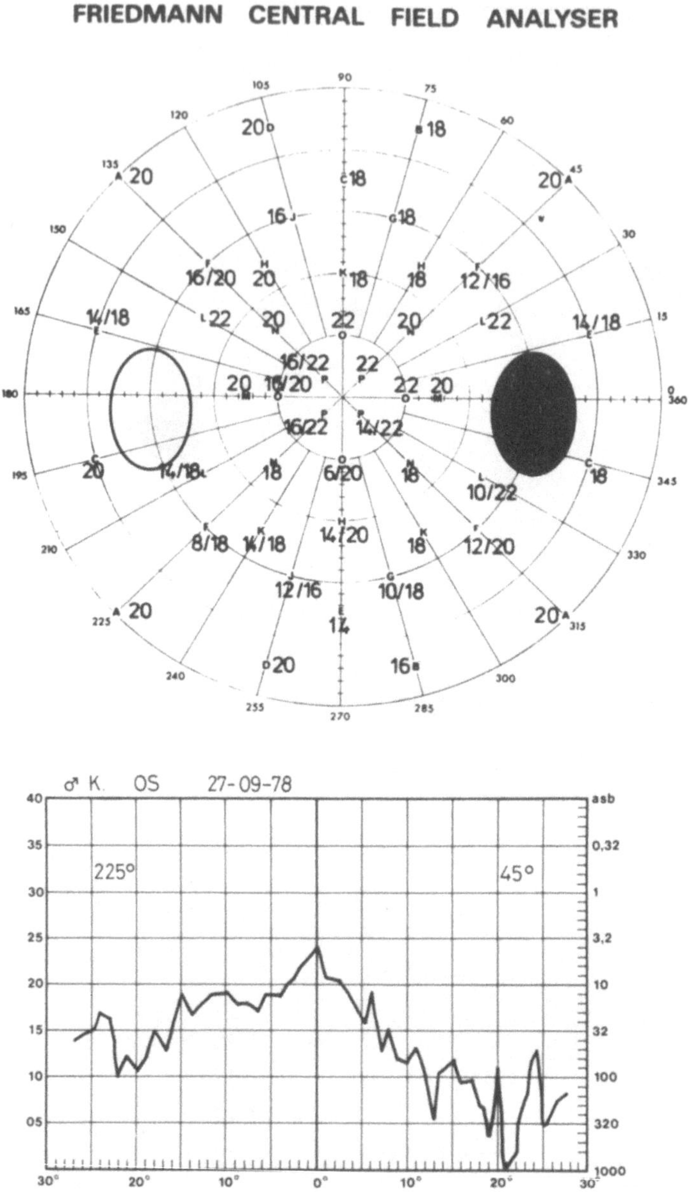

Fig.2

A. Friedmann visual field analysis of the asymptomatic right eye in a 22-year-old male patient. There are many small defects with extremely strong scattering. The other, also asymptomatic, eye showed the same pattern.

B. Static perimetry (45° –225°) of the right eye shows marked defects in the peripheral parts of the visual fields. Scattering is less pronounced. The VECP of the right and left eye were normal.

delay in nearly 100% of the eyes previously affected by optic neuritis and in a far lower percentage (approximately 60%) of visually asymptomatic eyes in patients with multiple sclerosis. Visual fields were abnormal in 40 eyes in the asymptomatic group (80%). This is a higher percentage than has usually been described in literature; e.g. Ellenberger and Ziegler (6) found an abnormal VF in 14% of their asymptomatic group. Static perimetry was extremely useful, especially in the asymptomatic group. By means of static perimetry we were able to obtain a more precise measure of the density of a scotoma (often unsuspected on the Friedmann visual field analysis).

In 16 eyes with a normal VECP an abnormal VF was detected; in only 2 eyes with a normal VF an abnormal VECP was found. There is no apparent explanation why the VECP is normal with an abnormal VF. It appears, however, that there is a high correlation of VECP and VF abnormalities when there are central as well as more peripherally localized VF defects.

As a final conclusion we would like to stress once more the fact that careful visual field assessment is very valuable in multiple sclerosis patients.

REFERENCES

1. Griffin, J. F. & S. H. Wray. Acquired color vision defects in retrobulbar neuritis. Amer. J. Ophthalmol. 86:193ff (1978).
2. Regan, D., R. Silver & J. Murray. Visual acuity and contrast sensitivity in multiple sclerosis: hidden visual loss. Brain 100:563ff (1977).
3. McAlpine, D., C. E. Lumsden & E. D. Acheson. Multiple Sclerosis. A reappraisal. Livingstone, Edinburgh (1965).
4. Duwaer, A. L. & H. Spekreyse. Latency of luminance and contrast evoked potentials in multiple sclerosis patients. Electroencephal. Clin. Neurophysiol. 45:244ff (1978).
5. Spekreyse, H., A. L. Duwaer & F. E. Posthumus Meyes. Contrast evoked potentials and psychophysics in multiple sclerosis patients. In: Human Evoked Potentials. Ed. by D. Lehmann and E. Callaway. Plenum Publishing Company (1979).
6. Ellenberger Jr., C. & S. B. Ziegler, Quantitative perimetry and visual evoked potentials in multiple sclerosis patients. In: Second International Visual Field Symposium. Tübingen, 1976. Ed.: E. L. Greve. Dr. W. Junk b.v. Publishers, The Hague, The Netherlands (1977).

Authors' address:
Department of Ophthalmology
Wilhelmina Gasthuis
University of Amsterdam
1e Helmersstraat 104
1054 EG Amsterdam
The Netherlands

QUANTITATIVE PERIMETRY IN OPTIC SUBATROPHY FROM PREVIOUS OPTICAL NEURITIS IN MULTIPLE SCLEROSIS

A. SERRA & C. MASCIA

(Cagliari, Italy)

ABSTRACT

The present report deals with patients suffering from multiple sclerosis (MS) with and without optic neuritis. We tested central visual function (visual acuity, colour discrimination, cortical evoked potential), peripheral vision (isopter and profile perimetry) as well as ocular motility (fusional amplitude).

The attack of neuritis is found to deteriorate both central and peripheral vision. Significant differences are found between the affected eye and the contralateral non-affected eye. The time elapsed after the detection of MS seems to be responsible for some contradictory effects: a slight improvement of central visual acuity and on the other hand a deterioration of the perimetric profile even in the contralateral eye without episodes of neuritis.

At last a dot-gram is suggested, to give an idea of the overall level of deterioration of visual function, in every patient: here the responses to various tests are weighted according to four step scales.

We tested a sample of 41 patients (ranging in age from 17 to 37 years), suffering from multiple sclerosis (MS). In the history of 21 of these patients, an attack of optic neuritis (ON) was recorded. This was not the case for the other 20 ones. We are mainly interested in the after-effects of the attacks of neuritis. For this, in addition to qualitative reports about the aspects of the optic disc, we gathered quantitative data about functional impairments concerning both central vision (visual acuity, colour discrimination, pattern evoked potential) and peripheral vision (both isopter and profile perimetry).

RESULTS

Visual acuity. The attack of neuritis is followed by a long-term reduction in visual acuity (VA).

Colour discrimination. The total score (TS) from the F-M 100-hue test is found to be abnormal in the majority of our patients [1-2-4-5-7]; the TS increases when the pattern of the response evolves from a tritan-tetartan defect to a R-G axis defect and to an anarchic tracing (Fig. 1). The distribution of the response patterns across the samples of patients with or without neuritis is shown in Table 1.

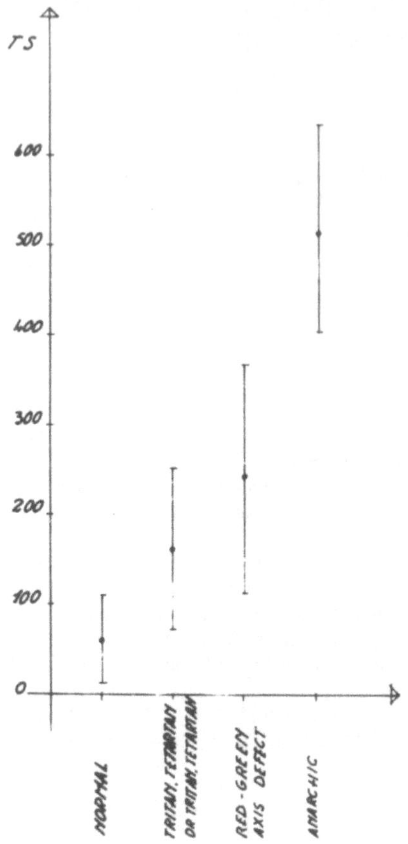

Fig. 1.

Relation between colour discrimination and visual acuity. The correlation [7] between VA and TS′ (that is the total score corrected for age effect according to Verriest's normal standard) is found to be significant. The equation of the linear fit was found to be:

$$TS' = -430\ VA + 600$$

(our slope being very close to that produced by Verriest for his MS patients).

Table 1. Number of MS patients showing some 100-Hue response patterns.*

	Y-B axis (tritan, tetartan, trit./tetart.)	R-G axis	Anarchic
Without neuritis	47	15	6
With neuritis	1	6	6

* Right and left eyes are tested separately. Some patients give normal 100-Hue responses. They are not considered here.

Interocular functional differences in cases of monolateral attacks of optic neuritis. Colour discrimination is worse (higher TS) in eyes after attack of optic neuritis than in contralateral eyes with no history. Similarly, visual acuity is worse in the attacked eye [3], in nine out of 13 patients at least.

Influence of time (d) after detection of MS. There seems to be a slight mean improvement in visual acuity as time after MS detection increases. This does not seem to be the case for colour discrimination (Table 2).

Table 2. Mean visual acuity (VA) and Total Score (TS'), corrected for age effect) for samples of subjects according to the time (d) elapsed since the detection of MS.

d (years)	VA	TS'
Less than 1	0.67 ± 0.34	341 ± 105
2-3	0.68 ± 0.37	253 ± 159
4-6	0.70 ± 0.22	256 ± 190
7-8	0.94 ± 0.13	353 ± 212

Evoked potentials. Both pattern (checkerboard) and blank evoked potentials are recorded monopolarly, in the transient state [8]. A negative wave (N1), peaking before 100 ms, and a positive wave (sometimes bi-peaked, P1 and P2), culminating between 100 and 200 ms are considered. Latencies to peak, for the tested patients, are compared to those of a normal sample.

Interocular differences in culmination times. Responses recorded from either eye of patients with monolateral attacks of optic neuritis are compared to those of patients suffering from multiple sclerosis without optic neuritis. For this, we estimated the differences in culmination times P1-N1 and P2-P1. Right eye estimates, for MS patients, are plotted versus left eye estimates. Dashed area in Fig. 2 denotes the range mean ± standard deviation across the MS sample. Asterisks and open circles refer to patients with optic neuritis. The time elapsed after the MS detection (within brackets) does not seem a relevant factor in this connection.

Isopter perimetry. Responses recorded by means of the Goldmann perimeter [6] (target II/2) lead to the results shown in Table 3, where labels n, MC etc. refer to a classification made by us after inspection of the responses: n for normal; MC for pericaecal scotoma; SC for central scotoma; DQ for quadrant defect, SCC for centro-caecal scotoma.

Table 3. Number of MS patients showing the labelled isopter responses.

	n	MC	SC	MC + SC	MC + DQ	SCC
Without neuritis	36	2	0	0	2	0
With neuritis	8	11	1	3	2	1

n = normal; MC = pericaecal scotoma; DQ = quadrant defect; SC = central scotoma; SCC = centro-caecal scotoma.

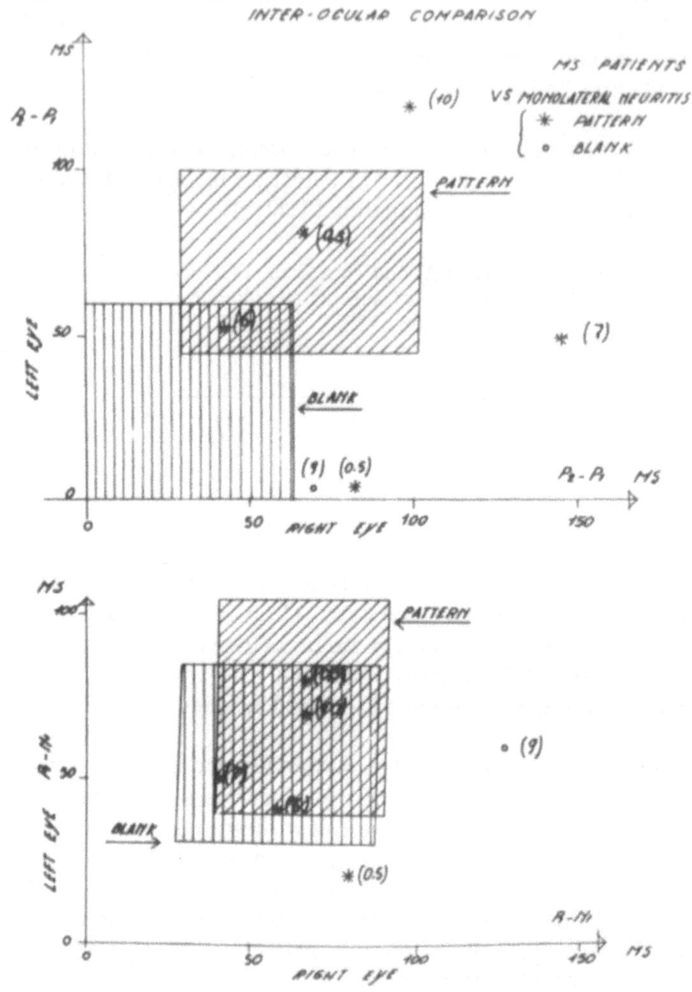

Fig. 2.

Profile perimetry. In patients with monolateral attack of optic neuritis some interesting results are found to assess the deviations from normality of the profiles were recorded along the horizontal meridian. If the MS detection is rather recent, the profile for the contralateral eye is practically normal while that of the attacked eye is not. If the date of MS detection is not recent, both profiles are abnormal. There is probably an effect of the MS, even if not revealed by a manifest attack (Fig. 3).

Overall evaluation of patient's responsiveness. To evaluate the overall effects of the disease on both central and peripheral vision of each patient, including ocular motility (fusional amplitude), we scored the severity of the defects according to four point scales.

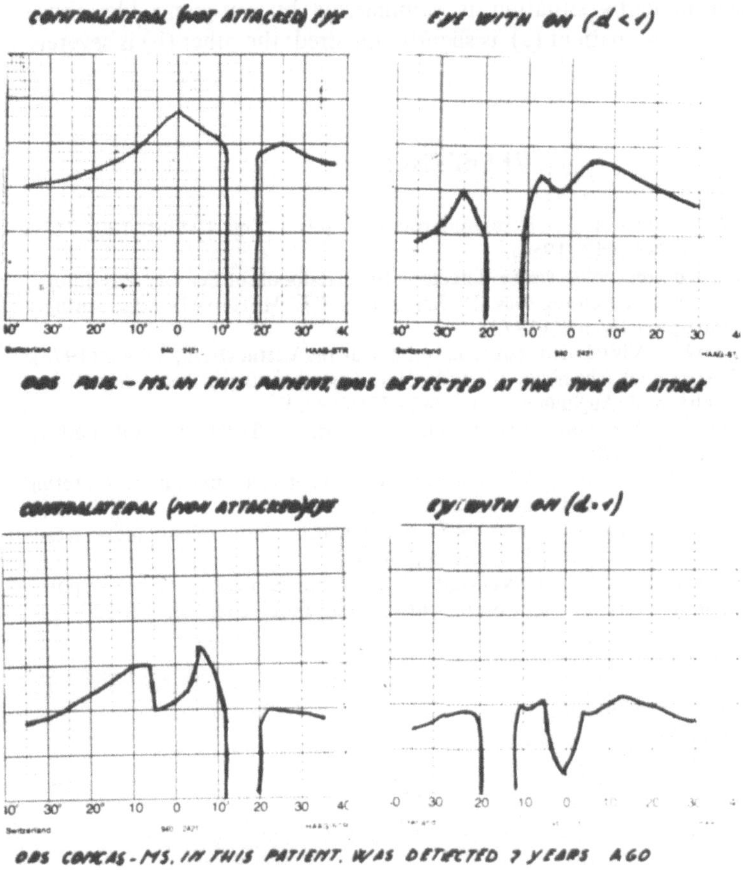
CONTRALATERAL (NOT ATTACKED) EYE
EYE WITH ON (d<1)
CONTRALATERAL (NON ATTACKED) EYE
EYE WITH ON (d<1)
OBS CONCAS - MS. IN THIS PATIENT. WAS DETECTED 7 YEARS AGO

Fig. 3.

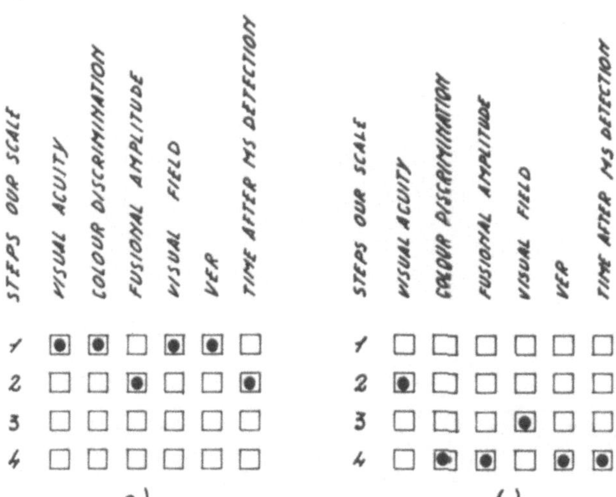
STEPS OUR SCALE
VISUAL ACUITY
COLOUR DISCRIMINATION
FUSIONAL AMPLITUDE
VISUAL FIELD
VEP
TIME AFTER MS DETECTION
1
2
3
4
a)
b)

Fig. 4.

Thus, each patient's situation is summarized by dot-grams like those shown in Fig. 4. One patient (a), is slightly impaired; the other (b) is severely impaired.

REFERENCES

1. François J. & G. Verriest. Les dyschromatopsies acquises. Ann. Oculist. 190: 713–746; 812–813; 893–943 (1957).
2. Gruetzner P. Acquired color vision defects – In: Handbook of Sensory Physiology, Vol. VII/4, Visual Psychophysics, D. Jameson and L. M. Hurvich, Eds., Springer Verlag, Berlin, pp. 643–659 (1972).
3. Khachaturova, N. K. Visual disturbance in optic neuritis. Vestn. Oftal., 57–60 (1973).
4. Nagel, E. Einige Beobachtungen über die Farbensinnstörungen bei retrobulbärer Neuritis – Klin. Mbl. Augenheilk. 431: 742–751 (1905).
5. Ohta, Y. Studies on the acquired anomalous color vision – Tagungsber. int. Farbtag Color, 69: 88–96 (1970).
6. Tate, W. & J. R. Lynn. Principles on Quantitative Perimetry. Testing and Interpreting the Visual Field. Grune and Stratton, New York (1977).
7. Verriest, G. Les déficiences acquises de la discrimination chromatique. Mém. Acad. Roy. Méd. Belg. II Sér., Tome IV, Fasc. 5 (1964).
8. Wilderberger, H. G. H. & G. M. H. Van Lith. Color vision and visually evoked response (VER) in the recovery period of optic neuritis. Mod. Probl. Ophthal., 17: 320–324 (1976).

Authors' address:
Cattedra di Ottica Fisiopatologica
dell'Università degli Studi di Cagliari
I-09100 Cagliari
Italy

DIFFERENCES IN THE VISUAL EVOKED POTENTIALS BETWEEN NORMALS AND OPEN-ANGLE GLAUCOMAS

BERNARD SCHWARTZ & SRIRAM SONTY

(Boston, Mass., U.S.A.)

ABSTRACT

Significant differences were found in the interocular latencies of the visual-evoked potentials between 11 normals and 20 open-angle glaucoma patients with visual field loss in one eye. A checkerboard pattern comprised of 40 minute checks was projected on the macular region through a dilated pupil over a 9° field by means of a direct viewing hand-held ophthalmoscope. The checks were alternated at 8 reversals per second. All patients had visual acuities of 20/40 or better in each eye. The visually-evoked potential was elicited under steady state conditions and averages were obtained of 64 sweeps. The differences in latencies between eyes were measured. The glaucomatous groups showed larger differences. in latencies than the normals.

INTRODUCTION

The visually-evoked potential (VEP) has become established as a diagnostic aid in optic nerve pathology (5, 15). The most reproducible change in the VEP is a latency delay, and abnormally long delays have been reported in various disorders of the optic nerve.

Since glaucomatous optic nerve disease can be regarded as a form of optic neuropathy, the measurement of the VEP in glaucoma may prove to be useful in the diagnosis and evaluation of visual field loss. Several previous studies on measurement of the VEP in glaucoma have been inadequately controlled for effects of pupil size and age (3, 6, 9–11). It was the purpose of our study to control for these factors and to evaluate the association of changes in the VEP with visual field loss by comparing the differences of latencies between eyes of the glaucomatous patient with visual field loss in only one eye to the differences between normal eyes.

MATERIALS AND METHODS

Eleven normals and 20 primary open-angle glaucomas with uniocular field loss were selected for study. Normal patients were defined as those with

Doc. Ophthal. Proc. Series, Vol. 26, ed. by E. L. Greve & G. Verriest

pressures below 21 mm Hg on two or more examinations with normal optic discs and visual fields as evaluated by static and kinetic methods with the Goldmann perimeter. Glaucomatous patients were defined as those with ocular pressures 21 mm Hg or greater determined on 2 or more examinations, open angles on slitlamp gonioscopy with glaucomatous optic disc changes and visual field changes. All glaucomatous patients were on therapy for glaucoma at the time of the examination. All patients had visual acuity of 20/40 or better in each eye (Table 1). Any patient with a history of neurological disease was excluded from the study. The maximum ocular pressure was determined by reviewing the patient's chart. Percent area of the optic disc for both cupping and pallor were measured by a series of transparent templates superimposed upon kodachrome photographs of the optic disc. Cupping was determined from stereophotographs and pallor from single photographs (12). Visual field loss was graded (Table 2).

An ophthalmoscopic stimulator was designed to project a checkerboard pattern reversal stimulus of 9° field size with 40 minute sized checks onto the retina. A central 2° steady light was used for fixation. The checks were presented at an alternation rate of 8 reversals per second. The luminance of the ophthalmoscopic stimulator was 7.1 candles per square meter. Silver electrodes were placed on the earlobes and the active electrode was placed 1 cm above the inion on the midline. The patient was asked to fixate at the central 2° light in the ophthalmoscopic stimulator. All pupils were dilated with cyclopentolate hydrochloride 1% and phenylephrine 2.5% drops. Sixty-four sweeps were used for each stimulus and these were averaged by a Nicolet averaging computer. The interocular latency difference for each subject was determined by calculating the average difference between eyes in latency of the eight corresponding positive peaks of the wave forms. Positive values indicate that the eye with the greater defect was associated with a longer latency than the fellow eye. Negative values indicate the converse. For glaucomas the difference was calculated as the eye with the loss of visual field minus the eye with no visual field loss. For normals the difference was calculated as the right eye minus the left eye.

Statistical analysis was done using 2-tailed non-parametric tests (14). For comparison of frequency distributions, the Wilcoxon matched-pair signed-rank test was used. A p less than 0.01 was chosen for significance.

RESULTS

The eleven normal patients had a median age of 65.3 years while the 20 glaucomatous patients' mean age was 67.3. For the normals, two patients were 40–49 years, two were 50–59, six were 70–79 and one was 80–89. For the glaucomas, one was 40–49, four were 50–59, eight were 60–69, six were 70–79 and one was 80–89. There was no significant difference between the frequency distributions of the ages of these groups. Tables 1 and 2 show the distribution of visual acuities and visual field loss for the normal and glaucomatous groups.

Table 1. Distribution of visual acuities for normal and glaucomatous patients and visual field loss

	Normals	Primary open angle glaucomas
20/40	0	3
20/30 or 20/25	7	12
⩾ 20/20	4	5
Total	11	20

Table 2. Distribution of visual field loss for glaucomatous patients

Type of visual field loss	Grade No.	No.
Paracentral scotoma	1	6
Nasal step	2	4
Nasal or temporal step with paracentral scotoma	–	2
Arcuate scotoma	3	5
Arcuate scotoma and step	4	1
One quadrant loss	5	2
Total		20

Figure 1 shows the distribution of interocular latency differences for both the normal and the glaucomatous groups. The glaucomas had significantly greater interocular latencies than the normals. However, there is some overlap between the two groups.

DISCUSSION

Ophthalmoscopic stimulators have been previously designed for control of fixation using light as a stimulus for the study of the VEP in amblyopia (7, 13). Our design incorporated a checkerboard pattern.

Our results indicate increased interocular latency differences in glaucomatous patients with field loss only in one eye compared to a similar group of age-matched normal patients. Previous studies of glaucomatous patients have also shown increased latencies (1, 3, 6, 9–11). However, there was inadequate control for age or for pupil size especially with glaucomatous patients on miotic therapy. Increased latencies with age have been demonstrated (4). With our technique, using the ophthalmoscopic stimulator, all pupils were dilated and accurate fixation obtained by projecting the checkerboard pattern on the macular area.

Our studies primarily measured differences between eyes in an effort to obtain as rigid control conditions as possible by using one eye in the patient as a control without visual field loss. Others have also studied glaucomatous

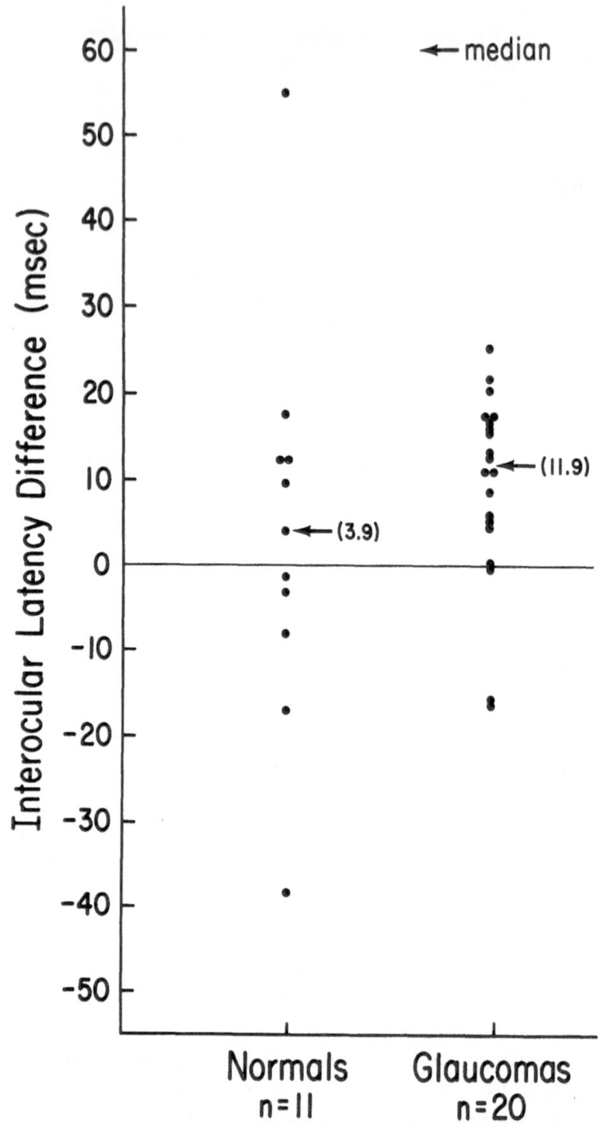

Fig. 1. Scatter plot of interocular latency differences for normal and glaucomatous eyes.

patients with visual field defects only in one eye and have observed differences in the VEP between the eyes (9, 11). It would obviously be of greater advantage to determine absolute latencies. However, before these can be termed 'normal' or 'abnormal' a large normal population would have to be measured.

Since our patients all had 20/40 vision or better, there is relatively little influence of degree of visual acuity which has been shown in other studies (15). This was also obviated by using the patient's correction whenever required in focusing the ophthalmoscopic stimulator checkerboard pattern on the retina.

Since the visually-evoked potential primarily represents macular function, it is surprising that such changes in interocular latency were obtained. The changes of the visual fields of the patients did not appear to encroach upon the macula. The check size which we used does extend beyond the macular area and thus some visual field loss could have been detected. Other disturbances of macular function have been noted in glaucoma patients, primarily color vision defects (8) and contrast sensitivity (2).

Further studies will have to be done to determine the sensitivity of the VEP in determining degrees of visual field loss. Perhaps by changing the stimulus pattern, the sensitivity could be improved so that smaller degrees of visual field loss could be detected. This method obviously has advantages as being an objective assessment of the optic nerve and may be useful in clinical situations where visual fields cannot be obtained. Furthermore, it would be most interesting to determine whether changes in the VEP occur in ocular hypertensive eyes with no visual field loss. Such studies are now in progress.

ACKNOWLEDGMENTS

We wish to thank John Kern for constructing the ophthalmoscopic stimulator and Drs. Samuel Sokol and Vernon L. Towle for counsel and for reviewing the manuscript.

Supported in part by an unrestricted grant from Research to Prevent Blindness, Inc., New York, New York.

The work for this paper was done while Dr. Sonty was a glaucoma fellow at Tufts New England Medical Center.

REFERENCES

1. Abe, H. & K. Iwata. Checkerboard pattern reversal VER in the assessment of glaucomatous field defects. Acta Soc. Ophthalmol. Jap. 80: 829–841 (1976).
2. Atkin, A., I. Bodis-Wollner, M. Wolkstein, A. Moss & S. M. Podos. Abnormalities of central contrast sensitivity in glaucoma. Am. J. Ophthalmol. 88: 205–211 (1979).
3. Cappin, J. M. & S. Nissim. Visual evoked responses in the assessment of field defects in glaucoma. Arch. Ophthalmol. 93: 9–18 (1975).
4. Celesia, G. C. & R. F. Daly. Effects of aging on visual evoked responses. Arch. Neurol. 34: 403–407 (1977).
5. Halliday, A. M. Visually evoked responses in optic nerve disease. Trans. Ophthalmol. Soc. UK 96: 372–376 (1976).
6. Huber, C. & T. Wagner. Electrophysiological evidence for glaucomatous lesions in optic nerve. Ophthal. Res. 10: 22–29 (1978).
7. Inoue, J., K. Takeo & I. Akiba. The visual evoked potentials to focal illumination of the retina by direct view ophthalmoscopy. Acta Soc. Ophthalmol. Jap. 67: 1145–1160 (1973).
8. Lakowski, R. & S. M. Drance. Acquired dyschromatopsias: The earliest functional losses in glaucoma. Documenta Ophthalmologica Proceedings Series 19: 159–165 (1979).
9. Levy, N. S. & L. Korhnak. The monocularly elicited visual evoked response in chronic glaucoma. Ann. Ophthalmol. 10: 551–555 (1978).
10. Mierdel, P. & E. Marré. Objective detection of reversible deficiencies in glaucoma. Ophthalmologica 177: 276–279 (1978).

11. Neetens, A., Y. Hendrata, J. Van Rompaey, M. C. Rubbens & C. Verschueren. VER and subclinical optic pathway damage. Bull. Soc. Belge Ophtal. 185: 83–98 (1979).
12. Schwartz, B. Correlation of pallor of optic disc with asymmetrical visual field loss in glaucoma, XXIIe Concilium Ophtalmologicum, Paris, 1974, Acta, vol. 2, pp. 632–638. Paris, Masson Publishers (1976).
13. Shipley, T. The visually-evoked occipitogram in Strabismic amolyopia under direct-view ophthalmoscopy. J. Pediatr. Ophthalmol. 6: 97–112 (1969).
14. Siegel, S. Non-parametric Statistics for the Behavioral Sciences. New York, McGraw-Hill Book Company (1956).
15. Sokol, S. Visually-evoked potentials: Theory, techniques and clinical applications. Surv. Ophthalmol. 21: 18–44 (1976).

Authors' addresses:
Bernhard Schwartz, M.D.
Sriram Sonty, M.D.
Dept. of Ophthalmology
New England Medical Center Hospital
and
Tuft University School of Medicine
171 Harrison Avenue
Boston, MA 02111
U.S.A.

PATTERNS OF VISUAL FIELD ALTERATIONS FOR LIMINAL AND SUPRALIMINAL STIMULI IN CHRONIC SIMPLE GLAUCOMA

FRITZ DANNHEIM

(Hamburg, F.R.G.)

ABSTRACT

The findings of 100 eyes with circumscript glaucomatous alterations evaluated by liminal and supraliminal stimuli are presented. Nerve fibre defects may be found in any part of the central or peripheral visual field including the centro-caecal area. Myopic eyes are more likely to develop defects in uncommon locations. The peripheral field may be exclusively affected, most often nasally. Defects in the nasal visual field reveal a second pattern of distribution corresponding to the vulnerability of the nerve fibres with the longest course from the ganglion cells to the optic disc. A non-linear scale for perimetric plots favouring the central field without excluding the periphery has definite advantages.

INTRODUCTION AND METHOD

The knowledge of the frequency distribution of glaucomatous visual field alterations may facilitate the choice of an adequate testing procedure. To this aim we have analysed 100 eyes of 90 patients with definite visual field defects due to chronic glaucoma belonging to stage I–III of the Aulhorn classification (1). All fields had been evaluated with a Tuebingen perimeter and a Rodenstock peristat in a careful static and kinetic manual test. Supraliminal stimuli were used to search for changes of sensation (4). One fifth of eyes had been examined with the OCTOPUS computer perimeter in addition.

RESULTS AND COMMENT

All 100 findings were divided into 6 groups according to the localisation of the major defect:

1. Changes in both the Bjerrum area and the nasal peripheral field occurred in 37 of the 100 eyes (Fig. 1). Since it is inconvenient to apply two different scales on two sheets for the central and peripheral field we designed a non-linear scale which adequately represents the central portion without excluding the periphery (Fig. 2).
2. Isolated scotomata in the Bjerrum area as the only glaucomatous defect have been found in 18 of 100 eyes, even though this location was described as the classical type of early damage (1, 2).

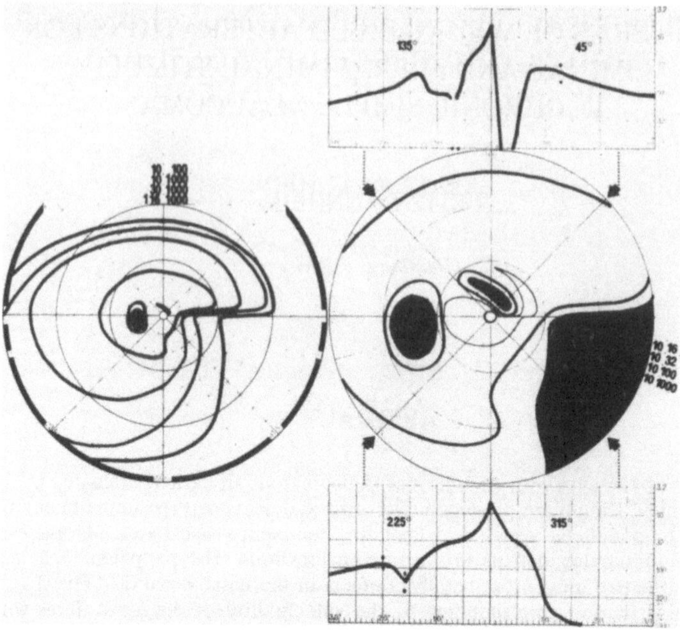

Fig. 1. Small paracentral Bjerrum defect and large nasal nerve fibre defect in central static and kinetic (right) and peripheral kinetic perimetry (left).

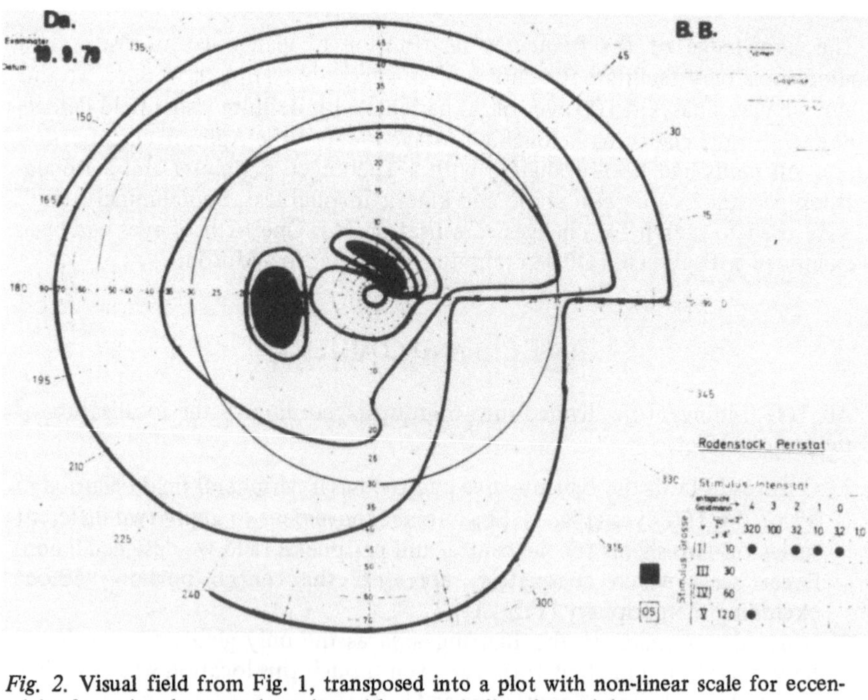

Fig. 2. Visual field from Fig. 1, transposed into a plot with non-linear scale for eccentricity favouring the central portion without excluding the periphery.

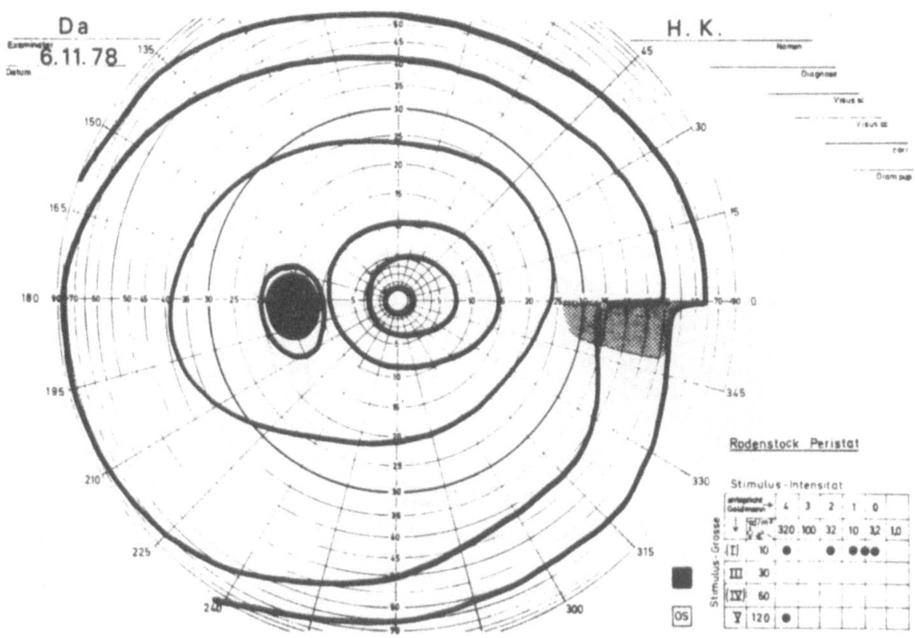

Fig. 3. Peripheral nasal step with unaffected central field. Zone with disturbance of sensation of supraliminal stimuli marked as grey. Scale as in Fig. 2.

3. Depression of sensitivity nasally with or without localized defects as the only alteration have been observed in 26 out of 100 eyes. A sector-shaped zone of change of sensation for supraliminal stimuli was regularly present (Fig. 3). This localisation which was regarded as rarely affected in an earlier report (2), was exclusively involved outside of the central field in 4 of these eyes (Fig. 3), which would have missed detection of the defect with campimetric devices.
4. Temporal peripheral defects (3, 4, 5, 6) have been present in 5 eyes as dominant feature and in 2 eyes as additional defects (Fig. 4), making up 7 of 100 eyes.
5. The area above or below the blind spot was with 4 out of 100 eyes least often affected, even though this localisation was estimated as most typical for early glaucomatous damage in older reports (7 among others). In all these fields the defect was separated from the blind spot for the smallest brightest target. This means that we never observed an isolated enlargement of the blind spot as an early glaucomatous sign (see also 2).
6. The centro-caecal field is generally regarded as most resistant to glaucomatous damage. We found isolated defects in this particular area in 10 of the 100 eyes (Fig. 4), in 2 of them being the only alteration (5).

Vertical steps (8) were never observed in this study. A video-tape analysis of all 100 findings (Fig. 5) reflects a similar frequency distribution for stage I (27 eyes), II (45 eyes) and III (28 eyes). This classification (1) is based on isolated paracentral defects as the only early glaucomatous alteration.

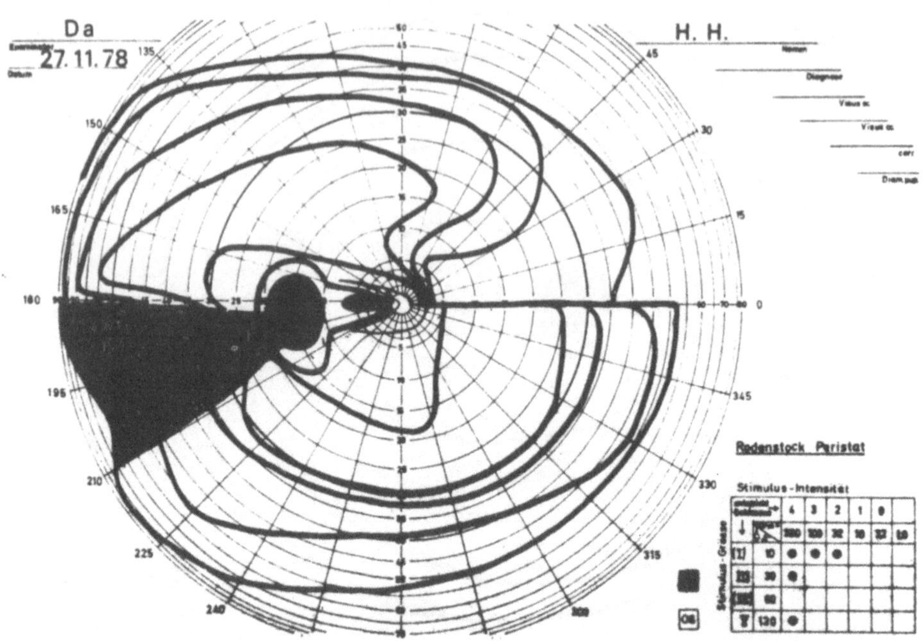

Fig. 4. Dense isolated centro-caecal and nasal defect and relative temporal defect. Zone of disturbance of sensation indicated only in the temporal field (grey). Scale as in Fig. 2.

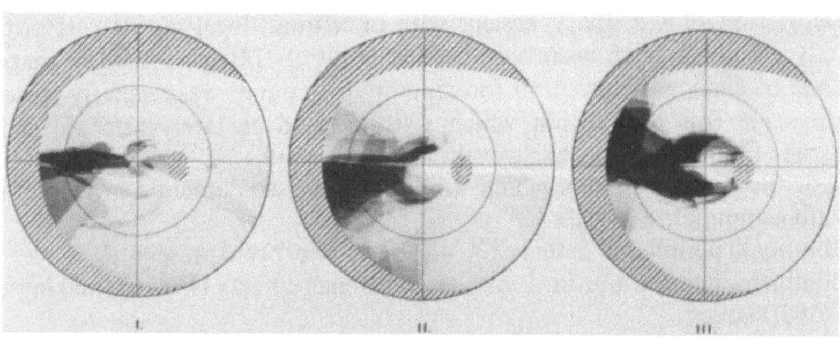

Fig. 5. Frequency distribution evaluated by video-tape analysis of 100 glaucomatous visual fields, divided into stage I (27 eyes), II (45 eyes) and III (28 eyes). Nasal field with highest frequency (marked darkest), followed by the Bjerrum area, the centro-caecal field, the temporal periphery and the area above or below the blind spot. Superior para-central defects more closely to fixation than inferior ones. Scale for eccentricity as in Fig. 2.

Depressions of sensitivity in the nasal field cannot properly be classified as long as they are separated from the blind spot. With our arbitrary division according to the affected area a high frequency of defects in the nasal visual field (5) is present in all 3 stages (Fig. 5). This may relate to a specific vulnerability of those nerve fibres within a bundle which travel the longest distance from the ganglion cells to the optic disc. This second pattern may be present in combination with the nerve fibre pattern (Fig. 6).

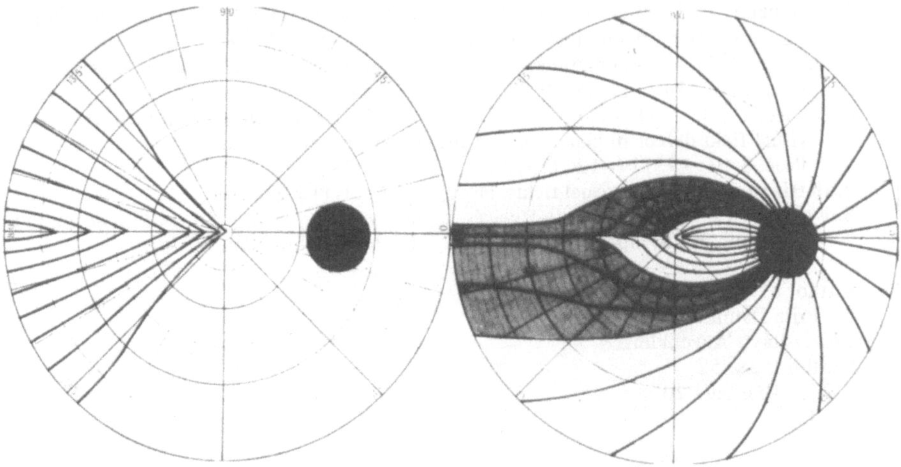

Fig. 6. Pattern of nerve fibre bundles as represented in the central visual field (right), most frequently affected bundles marked grey. Second pattern of distribution of glaucomatous defects in the nasal visual field (left).

Superiorly the defects tend to lie closer to fixation and inferiorly in the nasal periphery (Fig. 5, 6), as already described by Aulhorn (1). An evaluation of refraction of the 100 eyes disclosed a statistically significant difference in favour of higher myopia for the eyes with temporal and centro-caecal defects as compared to the ones with isolated Bjerrum defects (3, 5).

The presented frequency distribution confirms the one reported by Drance and co-workers (6) and deviates only in the addition of centro-caecal defects (5). Thus no part of the visual field should be excluded from the search for glaucomatous damage, and special emphasis should be placed on the nasal visual field.

ACKNOWLEDGEMENTS

The author is indebted to the Claere Jung Foundation for the donation of an OCTOPUS computer perimeter. He also wants to express his appreciation to members of the Institute for Mathematics and Analysis of Data in Medicine, University of Hamburg: Prof. Dr. K. H. Hoehne and his assistants provided with the video-tape computer analysis of visual fields, and Dr. R. Fehr gave valuable support in statistical analysis of data.

REFERENCES

1. Aulhorn, E. & H. Karmeyer. Frequency distribution in early glaucomatous visual field defects. Docum. Ophthal. Proc. Series 14: 75–83 (1977).
2. Aulhorn, E. & H. Harms. Early visual field defects in glaucoma. In: Glaucoma, Symp. Tutzing Castle 1966, pp 151–186. Karger, Basel (1967).
3. Brais, P. & S. M. Drance. The temporal field in chronic simple glaucoma. Arch. Ophthal. (Chic.) 88: 518–522 (1972).

4. Dannheim, F. Liminal and supraliminal stimuli in the perimetry of chronic simple glaucoma. Docum. Ophthal. Proc. Series 19: 151–157 (1979).
5. Dannheim, F. Verteilungsmuster glaukomatöser Gesichtsfeldstörungen. Der Augenspiegel 25: 514–525 (1979).
6. Drance, S. M., M. Fairclough, B. Thomas, G. R. Douglas & R. Susanna. The early visual field defect in glaucoma and the significance of nasal steps. Docum. Ophthal. Proc. Series 19: 119–126 (1979).
7. Harrington, D. O. The visual fields. Mosby, St. Louis (1971).
8. Lynn, R. Correlation of pathogenesis, anatomy, and patterns of visual field loss in glaucoma. In: Symp. on glaucoma, chap. IX. Mosby, St. Louis (1975).

Author's address:
Dr. Fritz Dannheim
Universitaets-Augenklinik
Martinistrasse 52
D-2000 Hamburg 20
F.R.G.

RECEPTIVE FIELD-LIKE PROPERTIES TESTED WITH CRITICAL FLICKER FUSION FREQUENCY
Perimetric analysis

EMILIO C. CAMPOS & SAMUEL G. JACOBSON

(Modena, Italy/Boston, Mass., U.S.A.)

ABSTRACT

A new psychophysical function reflecting receptive field-like properties has been described. It is based on measurement of the critical flicker fusion frequency (CFF) for a small target centered within a circular background, the size of which is varied as the test parameter. The foveal CFF function has a characteristic V-shape similar to that of the conventional sustained-like function.

A perimetric analysis of the CFF function at 2°, 5° and 10° in the nasal and temporal visual fields shows that with increasing eccentricity the general shape of the function is maintained. The minimum, however, shifts toward larger background sizes and the areas of interaction tend to increase. At 10° in the periphery, the function flattens and deteriorates. The perimetric behaviour of the CFF function is compared with that of the sustained-like function. Clinical application of this function is suggested mainly for diseases of the fovea.

INTRODUCTION

The receptive fields of individual neurons in the visual system have been well studied with physiological techniques in animals. Properties thought to derive from these basic visual units recently have been studied in man with psychophysical techniques (2). Both a sustained-like and a transient-like function have been demonstrated. These psychophysical tests have been investigated primarily perimetrically and in subjects with discrete retinal lesions (2).

A new psychophysical function based on the determination of critical flicker fusion frequency (CFF) was described recently (1). The CFF was measured for a tiny test target centered on a circular background (of fixed luminance), the size of which was varied as the test parameter. The CFF function, like the sustained function, has an interaction zone within which summation-like and inhibition-like components are present.

Campos and Bedell (1) studied the CFF function at the fovea. In this paper, we report a perimetric analysis of this function.

METHODS

Apparatus. Details of apparatus similar to that used in the present experiments have been published previously (Campos and Bedell, 1978). In brief,

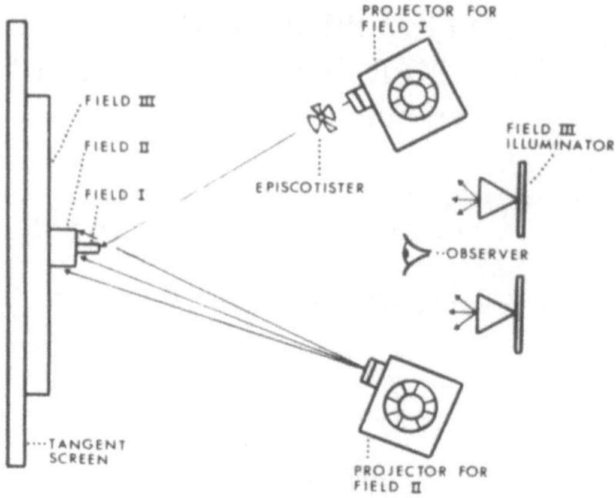

Fig. 1. Schematic diagram of the apparatus. Arrows represent light pathways.

three fields were projected onto a tangent screen located 125 cm in front of the subject (Fig. 1). Field III was the general background and provided low photopic adaptation at 0.68 log cd. m^{-2}. Field II was a circular target imaged by a Kodak carousel projector. The range of sizes for Field II was that used for the conventional sustained-like function and was equivalent to the range of Goldmann perimetric targets. Luminance of Field II was 0.95 log cd. m^{-2}, the optimal level for the CFF function (1). Field I was a tiny circular flickering target provided by a Kodak carousel projector and an episcotister (light-dark cycle, 1 : 1), which interrupted the light beam. The sizes of Field I used at the different loci in the visual field were as follows: 0° and 2° – 0.57 (min of arc)^2; 5° – 1.68 (min of arc)^2; and 10° – 1.89 (min of arc)^2. The luminance of Field I could be adjusted in 0.1 log unit steps with neutral density filters.

Procedure. CFF functions were determined monocularly for the fovea and for 2°, 5° and 10° along the horizontal meridian of both nasal and temporal visual fields. Prior to the CFF determinations, the increment threshold of Field I on Field III was measured with Field I flickering at 4 Hz. Luminance of Field I was adjusted to 1.0 log unit above this increment threshold. CFF for Field I was determined then as a function of the size of Field II using a modified method of limits. Each threshold represents the mean of at least one ascending and one descending judgment.

RESULTS AND DISCUSSION

Four normal subjects with best corrected monocular visual acuities of 6/6 were tested perimetrically for the CFF function. Fig. 2 shows representative data from the nasal and temporal visual fields of one subject. CFF is plotted against the log area of Field II. The foveal function has the typical U- or V-shape. High CFF values were obtained with the smallest and largest sizes of Field II, while the minimum CFF occurred at 1.81 log (min of arc)^2. An

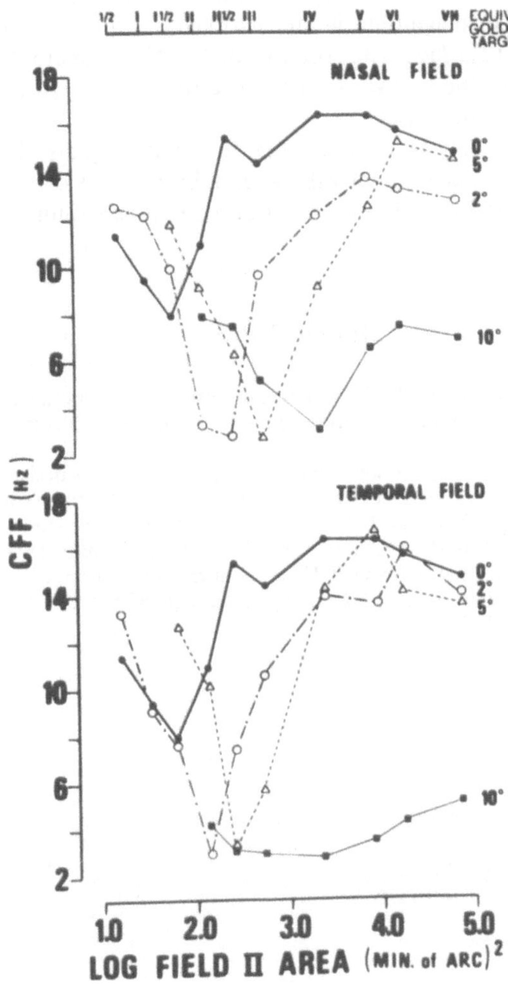

Fig. 2. CFF functions at the fovea and at 2°, 5° and 10° along the horizontal meridian in the nasal field (upper graph) and temporal field (lower graph) of one subject.

asymptote of the function at larger sizes of Field II is present. These characteristics of the foveal CFF function are similar to those already described by Campos and Bedell (1).

The CFF function in the periphery retains the characteristic shape. However, with increasing eccentricity from the fovea, the minimum of the function shifts towards larger sizes of Field II. A tendency for increased areas of interaction also occurs at eccentric loci, and by 10° in the periphery the function becomes less well defined and nearly flat. This pattern of results was present equally in the nasal and temporal visual fields and was consistent in the different subjects.

A similarity exists between the CFF function and the sustained-like function in that both functions show the tendency for an increase in center- and surround-like areas with eccentricity. On the other hand, the sustained-like function increases in magnitude in the periphery, while the CFF function actually decreased (2). This deterioration in the CFF function presumably can be attributed to the known decrease in critical flicker fusion frequency with increasing eccentricity (3).

This perimetric analysis of the CFF function suggests that the most interesting clinical application of this psychophysical test of receptive field-like properties would be in the investigation of lesions within the central 5° of the visual field.

REFERENCES

1. Campos, E. C. & H. E. Bedell. Critical flicker fusion frequency as an indicator of human receptive field-like properties. Invest. Ophthalmol. & Visual Science 17: 533–538 (1978).
2. Enoch, J. M. & E. C. Campos. New quantitative perimetric tests designed to evaluate receptive field-like properties in diseases of the retina and optic nerve. In: Electrophysiology and Psychophysics: Their Use in Ophthalmic Diagnosis, ed. S. Sokol, International Ophthalmology Clinics, Little Brown, Inc., Boston (1980).
3. Van de Grind, W. A., O.-J. Grüsser & H. U. Lunkenheimer. Temporal transfer properties of the afferent visual system. In: Handbook of Sensory Physiology. Vol. VII/3A, Springer-Verlag, Berlin (1973).

Authors' addresses:

Emilio C. Campos, M.D.
Dept. of Ophthalmology
University of Modena
Via del Pozzo 71
41100 Modena
Italy

Samuel G. Jacobson, M.D., Ph.D.
Massachusetts Eye and Ear Infirmary
Harvard University
Boston MA
U.S.A.

FLICKER FUSION IN PERICOECAL AREA

GIOVANNI CALABRIA, ENRICO GANDOLFO,
GIUSEPPE CIURLO & PIETRO ROSSI

(Genoa, Italy)

ABSTRACT

The pericoecal area is known to be the site of some early defects of the visual field. Flicker fusion frequencies, on turn, have been reported to be often altered when more classical perimetric examination results are still unchanged. This work is intended to report 'normal' values for flicker fusion frequencies in this area based on the examination of four normal subjects.

INTRODUCTION

The assessment of flicker fusion frequencies (F.F.F.) appears a sensitive means of investigation of the pericoecal area and looks a promising means for understanding the earliest impairments in visual function that take place in this critical area of the visual field.

In this work we describe a standardized technique for pericoecal flicker perimetry, together with the results obtained in normal subjects.

MATERIAL AND METHOD

Four healthy subjects aged from 27 to 31 years were examined.

We used the flickering device for the Goldmann perimeter previously described by two of us (1). The examination concerned:

- The threshold luminance for the target area of 1.4 mm^2 was determined with a statical method in each of the points shown in Fig. 1.
- The target luminance was increased 0.4 log unit, according to the criteria previously described (2).
- The flicker fusion frequency for each target size in each point was then determined. A sampling presentation was used: for every point 10 measures were made.

The results were evaluated to assess:

- The mean value and the standard deviation within each set of measures.
- F.F.F. variations related to the target size and its position. The significance of the differences were evaluated by means of the Student's t test.

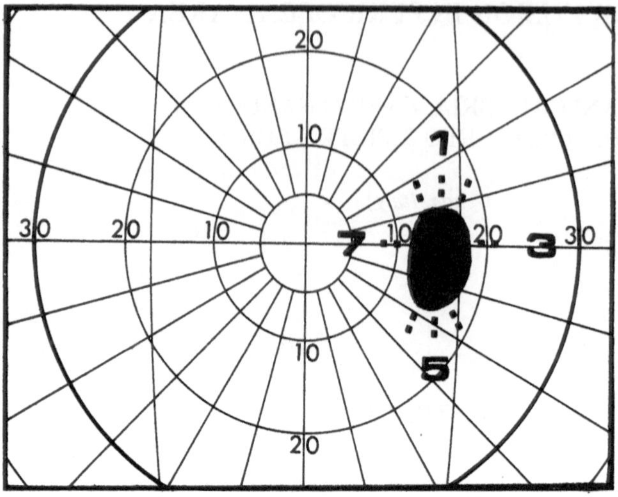

Fig. 1. Pattern of the tested points

RESULTS (Table 1)

- The scatter in the F.F.F. is fairly low.
- The F.F.F. does not change significantly according to the tested point or to the target diameter.

CONSIDERATIONS

The following considerations may be drawn on the technique used and its results.

Technique. The main drawback of our technique is the low number of tested points. This is mostly due to the long time needed for this kind of examination. However, if flicker perimetry of the pericoecal area must become a rather handy examination, at least for investigative purposes, the number of tested points can hardly be further increased. The double ring pattern of the examined points looks suitable to detect both generalised and localised alterations in C.F.F.

Results. The following points can be stressed:

- F.F.F. determination in the pericoecal area is a very accurate and reliable test: the scatter of the results is actually low.
- Even if light thresholds are quite uneven the time resolution properties of all the retinal points tested are quite steady. This result is strictly bound to the photometric features of the stimulus. It must be stressed that the F.F.F. in each point does not change with the target size. The steadiness of the F.F.F. for 'threshold' stimuli throughout the pericoecal area bears two practical consequences:

Table 1. Results.

Number	1		2		3		4		5		6		7		8	
Points	I	O	I	O	I	O	I	O	I	O	I	O	I	O	I	O
Anna P.	19,2 ±3	21 ±2,6	20,3 ±4	21,1 ±4,6	21,2 ±3,7	23,2 ±4,1	20,8 ±4,1	18,1 ±3,1	18,7 ±4,1	21,2 ±3,1	20,9 ±2,7	21,3 ±3,1	20,2 ±3,0	21,7 ±2,7	21,2 ±3,1	22,1 ±4,1
Carmen B.	18,7 ±3,1	19,9 ±2,1	21,6 ±3,1	22,3 ±3,7	19,8 ±2,7	20,9 ±1,9	19,1 ±2,3	21,3 ±3,1	21,4 ±2,1	22,3 ±3,1	21,9 ±2,9	22,4 ±3,1	22,3 ±3,1	21,3 ±4,1	23,1 ±3,1	24,1 ±2,9
Federico B.	18,1 ±3,1	18,3 ±4,2	21,3 ±3,1	22,3 ±2,9	21,3 ±3,1	18,1 ±3,2	19,6 ±3,1	20,2 ±4,1	21,3 ±3,1	22,1 ±4,3	23,4 ±3,1	21,2 ±3,4	22,2 ±3,1	21,3 ±3,2	18,6 ±4,1	19,9 ±2,7
G. Carlo S.	19,3 ±4,2	22,3 ±3,1	22,3 ±2,8	22,3 ±3,1	24,2 ±3,1	24,3 ±3,8	22,2 ±3,1	23,2 ±3,1	24,2 ±3,4	21,9 ±3,6	19,9 ±2,8	18,9 ±3,1	20,6 ±4,1	21,2 ±4,2	20,3 ±2,3	19,9 ±3,3

Legends: The mean value and the standard deviations of the F.F.F. obtained in each point with targets of 1,4 mm^2. I = inner circle; O = outer circle.

a) every localized deflection should be regarded as a pathological finding.
b) temporal resolution alone can be specifically investigated. Alterations in photometrical equivalences should not lead to differences in F.F.F. values obtained with targets of different sizes, unless temporal resolution is affected together with spatial summation.

CONCLUSIONS

Our work has shown that:

- Flicker perimetry of the pericoecal area may become a practical and useful tool for clinical investigations.
- Temporal resolution and spatial summation can be separately investigated. Therefore, flicker perimetry may throw further light on the actual vision impairment in the early phases of those diseases in which pericoecal area visual field is involved.

REFERENCES

1. Ciurlo, G., P. Rossi & G. Suetta. Nuovo apparecchio per la flicker-perimetria. Min. Oftal. 20: 61–68 (1978).
2. Zingirian, M., G. Ciurlo, P. Rossi & C. Burtolo. Flicker fusion and spatial summation. (in press).

Author's address:
Giovanni Calabria
University Eye Clinic
Viale Benedetto XV
16132 Genoa
Italy

ACUITY PERIMETRY

CHARLES D. PHELPS, PAUL W. REMIJAN & PIERRE BLONDEAU

(Iowa City, Iowa, U.S.A.)

ABSTRACT

Measurement of peripheral visual acuity may provide useful clinical information not obtainable from classical light sense perimetry. We have designed and built a new laser interferometer which allows us to test visual acuity at various eccentricities from zero to 20° and along any meridian. The test field is round, one degree in diameter, and contains alternating red and black stripes. The orientation and separation of the stripes can be varied, as can the intensity of the background illumination. The subject is asked if he can detect the striped pattern and, if so, its orientation.

The light source is a helium neon laser. A holographic phase grating separates the light into two coherent, equal strength, spherical waves diverging from a single point. The waves are focused near the nodal point of the subject's eye and form interference fringes on the retina. The fringes are not 'focused'; they occur wherever the waves overlap. Thus visibility of the fringes is virtually independent of the eye's refraction and is not impaired by minor media opacities.

INTRODUCTION

Visual acuity may be defined as the ability of the visual system to resolve fine detail. This ability is greatest for foveal vision and declines towards the periphery of the visual field (4). The measurement of foveal or central acuity, of course, is an integral part of every eye examination. It should not be forgotten, however, that the extrafoveal retina also has measurable acuity. The measurement of extrafoveal or peripheral acuity is a curiously neglected area of clinical visual function testing. Although many investigators, using a variety of techniques, have measured peripheral acuity in normal research subjects, almost nothing is known about alterations of peripheral acuity in diseases of the eye or visual pathways.

In this paper we describe a prototype instrument which allows us to test extrafoveal visual acuity. This instrument, which we call an acuity perimeter, measures resolution acuity at any location in the central 40° of the visual field. It uses for its acuity target a sinusoidal grating. The grating, a pattern of red and black stripes, is created on the retina by the interference of two laser beams.

METHODS

The acuity perimeter is a compact instrument with outside dimensions of 60 × 45 × 18 cm. It is mounted on a stand which is adjustable for height. The subject or patient sits in front of the instrument and looks into an eyepiece (Fig. 1). All controls are mounted on top of the instrument and are easily accessible to the examiner who stands next to the instrument.

The subject sees in Maxwellian view a uniformly illuminated round background field. The background illumination is produced by a white light source which is focused in the subject's entrance pupil. Thus, the amount of background flux entering the eye is independent of pupil size. The size of the background, which is limited by the eyepiece aperture, is 40°. The luminance of the background can be varied from 0.015 to 15.0 asb, allowing acuity testing to be done under either scotopic or photopic conditions.

In the center of the background field is a round fixation light, 1/2 of a degree in diameter. The color and intensity of the fixation light, can be varied. For routine testing, we use a dim white fixation light, somewhat brighter than the background illumination. Light from the fixation source leaves the instrument eyepiece as a 2 mm collimated beam. In order to see the fixation target, the subject must adjust the lateral position of his eye so that his pupil accepts the fixation source energy. Longitudinal adjustment of the subject's eye is also required so that the pupil accepts the background flux without vignetting. When the fixation source and unvignetted background appear simultaneously, the eye pupil is properly positioned for presentation of acuity targets out to ±20° eccentricity. The criteria for proper eye position is unambiguous, and most subjects naturally seek the correct eye position.

The acuity test target is one degree in diameter. It consists of a $(\text{sine})^2$ wave grating of alternating red and black stripes. The separation of maxima can be continuously varied from 1.5′ (resolution angle of 0.75′. grating frequency of 40 cycles/°, Snellen equivalent of 20/15) to 40′ (resolution angle of 20′, grating frquency of 1.5 cycles/°, Snellen equivalent of 20/400). The stripes can be oriented in any direction; stop-positions indicate the vertical, horizontal, and two oblique orientations. The acuity target can be presented along any meridian at 1° intervals from fixation to 20° eccentricity.

If desired, the acuity target can be presented continuously, but we prefer to present it intermittently. The target presentation is accurately timed with a variable speed electromagnetic shutter which allows the presentation time to be changed from 1/0 to 32 sec.

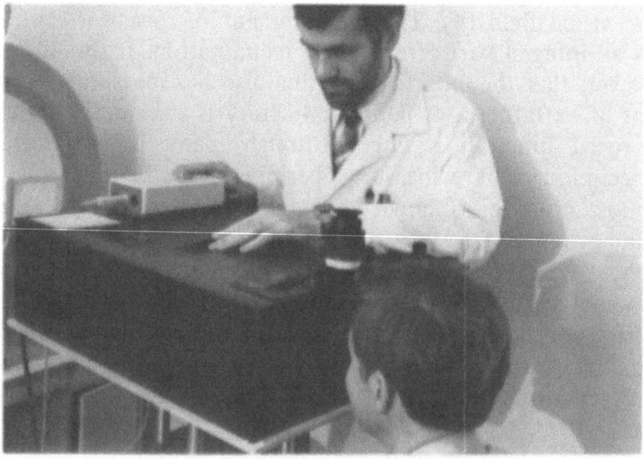

Fig. 1. Acuity perimeter: subject looking into viewing eyepiece.

The acuity perimeter is a modification of an earlier instrument which used laser interference fringes to measure central acuity (3). The new instrument, too, can be used to test central acuity. When testing centrally, the field of interference fringes can be varied in size from 1/2 degree to 40°. However, for peripheral measurements, the acuity target size is fixed at one degree.

The light source for the interference fringes is a 0.9 mW cylindrical helium-neon gas laser which operates in the standard gaussian transverse mode. Its maximum output in irradiance levels on the retina is about 350 nW. Thus it easily meets Bureau of Radiological Health safety standards for a class 1 laser device.

A holographic phase grating separates the laser light into two coherent, equal strength, spherical waves diverging from a single monochromatic point source. The two diffracted waves are focused near the nodal point of the subject's eye and form interference fringes on the retina. The optical geometry and its relationship to fringe separation are discussed in an article describing the original instrument for measuring central acuity (3).

The present instrument differs in design from the first by incorporating four additional features.

1. Fringe spacing is controlled by moving the holographic grating with respect to a fixed coherent point source. Such an arrangement provides a constant target irradiance at all acuity settings.
2. Fringe orientation is achieved by rotating the holographic grating. The natural field limitations of a standard dove prism image rotator are incompatible with the wide field requirements of the acuity perimeter.
3. A calibrated focusing eyepiece adjustment is provided for subjects requiring refractive correction. The focusing adjustment permits optimum visual resolution of the relatively small 1° target boundaries without alteration of the eyepiece focal length.
4. Beams from the holographic grating are collimated before reaching the test target aperture.

The necessity of an eyepiece focusing adjustment can be explained by considering the diameter of laser beams propagating through the vitreous and illuminating the retina. The fringe pattern is formed at any location within the eye where the two laser beams overlap. Relatively large targets of 5° or greater produce two large diameter beams within the eye. These large beams overlap sufficiently at the retina even when subjects have severe refractive errors. With the small 1° targets used in the acuity perimeter, the two laser beams within the eye are quite small in diameter and will not completely overlap at the retina of an eye exhibiting large refractive errors. Therefore, with tiny 1° targets, an adjustment is required to maximize the small area of overlap at the retina. The beam overlap area at the retina is a maximum when the target boundary is clearly resolved by the subject. The fixation source is in the plane of the target apertures and can be used as a target for the focusing adjustment prior to the presentation of laser fringe targets.

Movement of the subject's eye towards or away from the instrument affects neither the fringe spacing nor the target position in the field of vision. The eyepiece collects collimated laser beams emerging from the target aperture and forms two coherent points of light at its rear focal plane. Light emanating from these twin point sources propagates through space, forming fringes in any area of overlap common to both beams. When the sources formed by the eyepiece are located near the nodal point of the eye, the two beams propagate through the vitreous and form fringes on the retina. If the subject's eye is moved away from the eyepiece so that the twin sources are formed at the cornea, the beams are projected over a longer distance before reaching the retina. At first the formation of coarser fringes on the retina might be suspected, but the movement of point sources to the cornea and away from the nodal points also increases the angle between interfering beams. Increasing the fringe projection distance produces coarser fringes while increasing the beam interaction angle produces finer fringes. These two effects nullify each other and result in an invariant fringe spacing on the subject's retina. A similar analysis applies when the point sources are formed deeper within the eye. Thus, fringe spacing perceived by the subject is unaffected by variations of eye position along the optical axis.

Invariant target position within the field is achieved by collimating the laser beams prior to interception by the target aperture and using a constant focal length eyepiece.

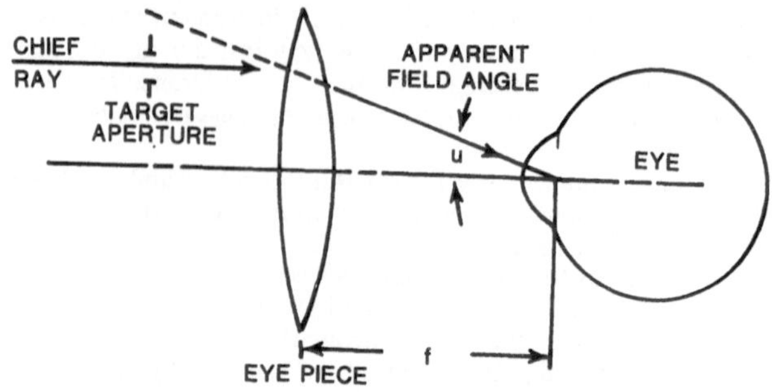

Fig. 2. Invariance of target position in field of vision.

With collimated beams, the chief ray passing through the target aperture strikes the eyepiece lens at the same height regardless of the aperture to eyepiece distance which is varied during focussing adjustment. The apparent field angle of the acuity target is invariant as shown in Fig. 2. Eye movement toward and away from the eyepiece is simply limited to positions which will allow complete transmission of both laser beams by the eye's pupil.

Acuity perimetry can be performed with any natural pupil size. The point source separation within the eye pupil is given by the formula $S = (\lambda/\sin \theta\nu)$ where S is the separation in millimeters; λ is 0.0006328 mm, the laser wavelength; and $\theta\nu$ is the angular subtense between stripes. For a Snellen equivalent target of 20/15, the point separation in the pupil is 1.4503 mm; for a Snellen equivalent target of 20/20, the point separation is 1.0877; and for a Snellen equivalent target of 20/400, the point separation is 0.0544 mm.

COMMENT

Acuity perimetry differs from conventional perimetry in that acuity rather than light sense is the visual function tested. Resolution acuity is a more complex visual function than simple light sense. It requires, at a minimum, integration of information from at least three percipient units. One limiting factor in acuity is probably the population density of ganglion cells (1, 6). It is possible that certain diseases, such as glaucoma, which cause a diffuse loss of ganglion cells and their axons, may impair acuity before interfering with light sense. It is this possibility which was the impetus for the construction of this instrument.

Laser interference fringes are an excellent acuity target for measurement of peripheral acuity. They are not focused and thus are not influenced by off-axis refractive aberrations such as coma and astigmatism of oblique incidence. Minor degrees of cataract do not impair fringe formation. Other investigators have used targets such as Snellen letters and Landolt rings for the measurement of peripheral acuity. Perception of these targets, of course, depends on proper focusing. The refraction of the eye may vary from one part of the retina to another. Snellen letters test not only resolution but also recognition. An interference fringe target, thus, is more likely to test retinal resolving power alone and not be influenced by optical or psychological factors.

Some background illumination is necessary if the eye is to remain light adapted. Peripheral acuity, like central acuity, decreases with dark adaptation (2). Background illumination has the disadvantage that it reduces the contrast of the interference fringes which, if the background were not illuminated, would be 100%. We are currently conducting studies to determine the optimal background illumination for clinical testing.

It was necessary in this instrument to choose one field size for the test target. A small target was desirable because it would restrict the area of the retina to be tested. On the other hand, the smaller the target, the fewer the number of stripes per target. This is particularly crucial with coarse gratings. Our compromise for this instrument was to use a one degree test field. With the widest separation of stripes (20/400 Snellen equivalent), only one and a half cycles are contained in the one degree field.

In acuity perimetry, as in classical light sense perimetry, one can plot acuity isopters (Fig. 3) and acuity profiles (Fig. 4). Testing is done with static presentation. The subject is asked if he can detect the striped pattern and, if so, the orientation of the stripes. For the two acuity fields illustrated here, the subject was required at each locus tested to identify the orientation correctly at least three out of five randomly selected presentations. He was

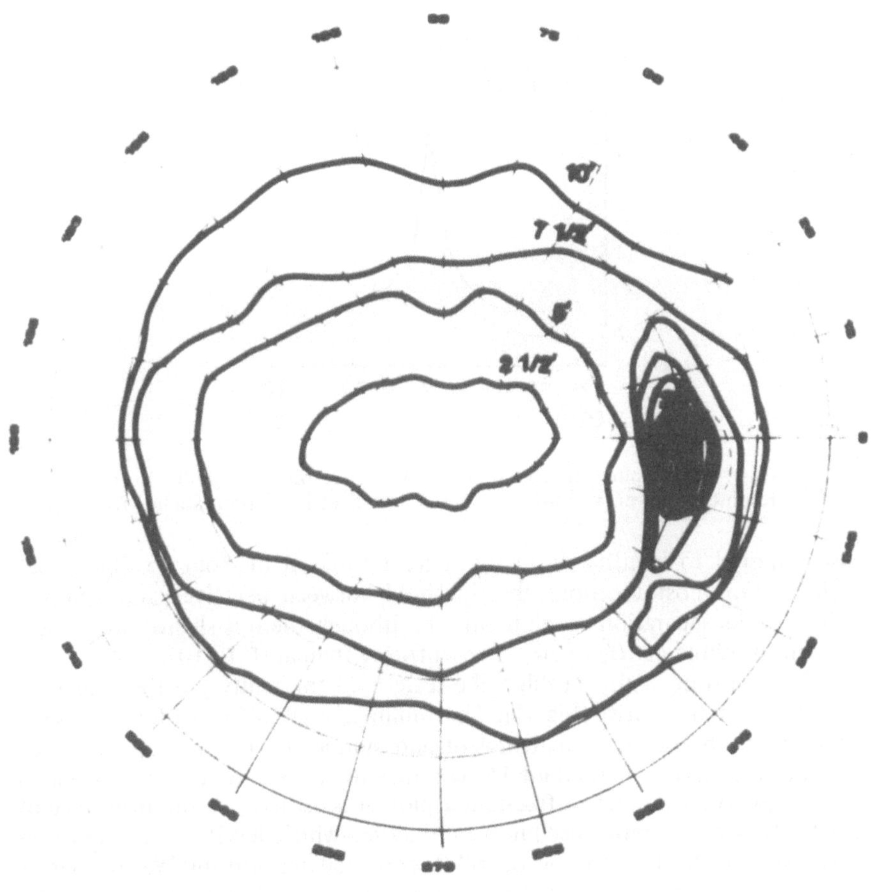

Fig. 3. Acuity isopter plot.

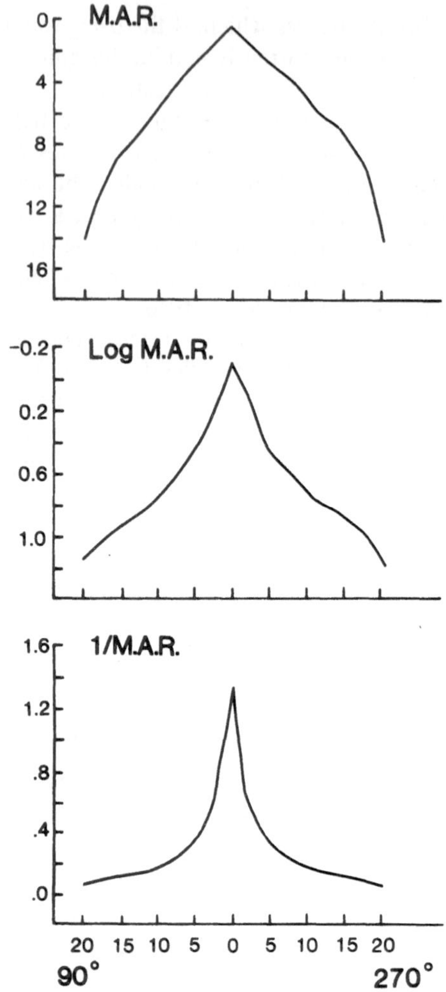

Fig. 4. Acuity profile plots: upper: minimal angle of resolution; middle: log of minimal angle of resolution; lower: reciprocal of minimal angle of resolution (Snellen fraction).

also required to identify correctly at least three of the four possible orientations. For most locations the threshold between perceived and non-perceived stripe separations is quite abrupt although there is slightly more variance in threshold at 10° to 20° of eccentricity than at 0° to 10°.

When plotting acuity profiles, the scale used for acuity greatly influences the shape of the curve (Fig. 4). The minimal angle of resolution (MAR), a plot of thresholds, is straightforward and simple. It shows a gradual linear decline from fixation to about 15° eccentricity with a more steep decline in the periphery. The Snellen fraction, a plot of sensitivity, is the reciprocal of MAR. It shows a rapid decline near fixation which levels off to approach zero asymptotically. The log of MAR, as noted recently by Westheimer, is the best representation of just noticeable differences (5) and its curve has a shape in between the other two curves. Use of the Snellen fraction places so much emphasis on acuity changes near fixation, that it is difficult to exhibit alterations from normal acuity in the less sensitive areas of the field away from fixation. We have chosen to use MAR rather than log MAR for our routine testing because it can be plotted directly without an additional computation.

Further studies are currently being conducted to determine in normal subjects the influence on peripheral acuity of stimulus orientation, stimulus duration, stimulus intensity, background intensity, and practice.

ACKNOWLEDGEMENT

We are indebted to Thomas W. Smith, M.D., and Hansjoerg E. Kolder, M.D., Ph.D., for their helpful suggestions and encouragement.

REFERENCES

1. Frisén L. & M. Frisén. A simple relationship between the probability distribution of visual acuity and the density of retinal output channels. Acta Ophthalmol. 54: 437–444 (1976).
2. Mandelbaum, J. & L. Sloan. Peripheral visual acuity, with special reference to scotopic illumination. Am. J. Ophthalmol. 30: 581–588 (1947).
3. Smith, T. W., P. W. Remijan, W. Remijan, H. E. Kolder & J. Snyder. A new test of visual acuity using a holographic phase grating and laser. Arch. Ophthalmol. 97: 752–754 (1979).
4. Wertheim, T. Über die indirekte Sehschärfe. Ztsch. Psychol. Physiol. Sinnesorg. 7: 172–189 (1894).
5. Westheimer, G.: Scaling of visual acuity measurements. Arch. Ophthalmol. 97: 327–330 (1979).
6. Weymouth, F. W. Visual sensory units and the minimal angle of resolution. Am. J. Ophthalmol. 46(II): 102–113 (1958).

Authors' address:
Department of Ophthalmology
University Hospitals
Iowa City, Iowa 52242
U.S.A.

VISUAL FIELD STUDIES WITH FUNDUS PHOTO-PERIMETER IN POSTCHIASMATIC LESIONS

Y. OHTA, M. TOMONAGA, T. MIYAMOTO & K. HARASAWA

(*Tokyo, Japan*)

ABSTRACT

We have developed a new method of recording the isopter on the fundus photograph under direct observation or TV-monitoring under infrared illumination. We examined 17 cases with visual field defects in post-chiasmatic lesions manifesting as bitemporal or homonymous hemianopsia and papilledema. The results were compared with those by Goldmann perimeter, U-O test chart and Amsler charts. In cases with bitemporal hemianopsia, macular sparing detected by U-O test chart and Amsler charts appeared as vertical splitting lines located in the hemianoptic side of the fovia with the present technique.

INTRODUCTION

At the 3rd International Visual Field Symposium, we introduced a new technique of fundus photo-perimetry which enabled us to record the visual field on a fundus photograph after direct observation by TV-monitoring (5).

With this device, we examined the visual field defects of post-chiasmatic lesions, such as papilledema, bitemporal hemianopsia, homonymous hemianopsia, etc., and also drew comparisons between pre and post craniotomy. We compared the visual field changes obtained from the above examination with those from quantitative kinetic perimetry by the Goldmann perimeter (G.P.), U-O test (Umazume-Ohta's central scotometric plate test) and Amsler chart test and discussed the results (1, 4).

MATERIALS AND METHOD

The fundus photoperimeter (F.P.P.) we developed was employed in the present experiment. While background luminance was fixed at 0.24 $cd.m^{-2}$, luminance of the stimulus was varied from 0.85 $cd.m^{-2}$ to 76.36 $cd.m^{-2}$. Although the latter can be changed continuously, we singled out several levels. All of the targets were set 19′ wide. There were 17 subjects in all; 8 cases of brain tumor, 1 case of disseminated sclerosis, 2 cases of head blow, 4 cases of intracranial vascular disturbance and 2 cases of opticochiasmal arachnoiditis. Twelve of them underwent craniotomy. The 5 cases without craniotomy

Table 1. Examination results

Case	Sex	Age	Diagnosis	Visual acuity	Period from operation to examination	Papilla findings	G. P.	F. P. P.
1	M	28	Left antero temporal lobe glioma	R.V. = 1.0 (n.c.) L.V. = 1.2 (n.c.)	9 months	R.: L.: Temporal papillae yellowish white	Right homonymous hemianopsia	
2	M	8	Right antero temporal lobe tumor	R.V. = 1.2 (n.c.) L.V. = 0.8 (1.2)	Preop 14 days	R.: L.: Papillaedema	Enlargement of blind spot	
3	F	33	Sellar craniopharyngioma	R.V. = 0 L.V. = 0.03 (0.04)	7 years	R.: L.: Pale papillae	R.: Could not be measured L.: Temporal hemianopsia	
4	M	57	Sellar craniopharyngioma	R.V. = 0.5 (0.9) L.V. = 0.1 (0.4)	8 months	R.: Normal L.: Pale papilla	Bitemporal hemianopsia	
5	F	27	Sellar meningioma	R.V. = 0.7 (10) L.V. = 0.04 (1.0)	5.5 months	R.: L.: Papillae yellowish white	Bitemporal hemianopsia	
6	F	40	Pituitary adenoma	R.V. = 30cm/mm L.V. = 0.07 (0.5)	10 months	R.: L.: Pale papillae	Bitemporal hemianopsia	
7	M	53	Pituitary adenoma	R.V. = 0.4 (0.5) L.V. = 1.0 (n.c.)	Preop 11 days	R.: L.: Normal	R.: Enlargement of blind spot L.: Temporal hemianopsia	
8	F	44	Right sphenoidal meningioma	R.V. = 0.8 (1.0) L.V. = 1.2 (n.c.)	1 month	R.: L.: Papillae irregular border	Enlargement of blind spot	
9	F	40	Disseminated sclerosis	R.V. = 1.0 (n.c.) L.V. = 1.5 (n.c.)		R.: Papilla white L.: Papilla yellowish white	Right homonymous hemianopsia	
10	M	28	Left head blow	R.V. = 1.5 (n.c.) L.V. = 1.5 (n.c.)		R.: L.: Normal	Right superior homonymous quadrantanopsia	
11	M	30	Left head blow	R.V. = 2.0 (n.c.) L.V. = 1.2 (n.c.)		R.: L.: Normal	Left homonymous hemianopsia	
12	M	26	Idiopathic intracranial bleeding	R.V. = 0.5 (12) L.V. = 0.3 (1.2)	2 months	R.: L.: Normal	Left homonymous hemianopsia	
13	M	26	Right occipital aneurysma	R.V. = 0.8 (1.2) L.V. = 0.4 (1.2)	4.5 years	R.: L.: Papillae irregular border	Left inferior quadrantanoptic scotoma	
14	M	23	Intracranial vascular disturbance	R.V. = 1.5 (n.c.) L.V. = 1.5 (n.c.)		R.: L.: Normal	Right homonymous hemianopsia	
15	M	72	Intracranial vascular disturbance	R.V. = 0.6 (0.8) L.V. = 0.6 (1.0)		R.: L.: Papillae yellowish white	Bitemporal hemianopsia	
16	M	52	Opticochiasmal arachnoiditis	R.V. = 0.3 (1.2) L.V. = 0.1 (0.3)	Preop 4 days	R.: L.: Papillaedama	Enlargement of blind spot	
17	M	25	Opticochiasmal arachnoiditis	R.V. = 0.02 (n.c.) L.V. = 0.08 (n.c.)	Preop 2 months	R.: L.: Pale papillae	Centrocecal scotoma	

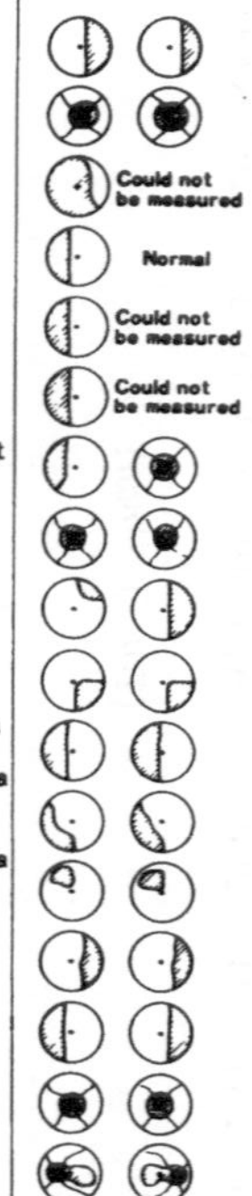

consisted of 1 case of disseminated sclerosis, 2 cases of head blow, and 2 cases of intracranial vascular disturbance.

RESULTS

Table 1 shows the experimental data of all 17 cases. All the cases except 9, 10, 11, 14, 15 underwent surgery. In the table, G.P. stands for results with the Goldmann perimeter and F.P.P. for results with the fundus photo-perimeter.

Figures 1 through 6 show part of the results obtained by the G.P., U-O test and Amsler chart test. Fig. 1 shows Case 2, an 8-year-old boy in which a right antero-temporal tumor was diagnosed. Fundus diagnosis was papilledema. The lower figures show the findings a month after the operation. A comparison between the pre-operative and post-operative observations shows a reduction of 10.46 cd. m^{-2}-isopter and a decrease of scotoma with an improvement of papilledema.

Fig. 2 shows Case 4, a 57-year-old man in whom a diagnosis of sellar craniopharyngioma had been made. The visual field change demonstrates bitemporal hemianopsia. In this figure, 8 months after craniotomy, we found macular sparing in the left fundus by U-O test and Amsler chart test. As for the fundus field detected by F.P.P., splitting was found in the hemianoptic

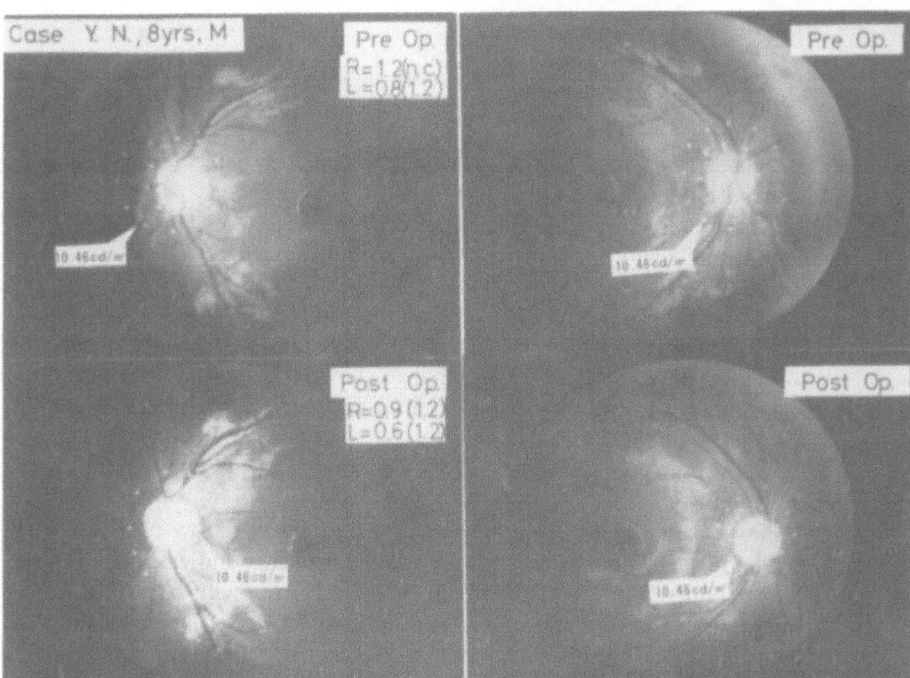

Fig. 1. Case 2, male, 8: Right antero temporal tumor. Top: Before craniotomy. Bottom: After craniotomy.

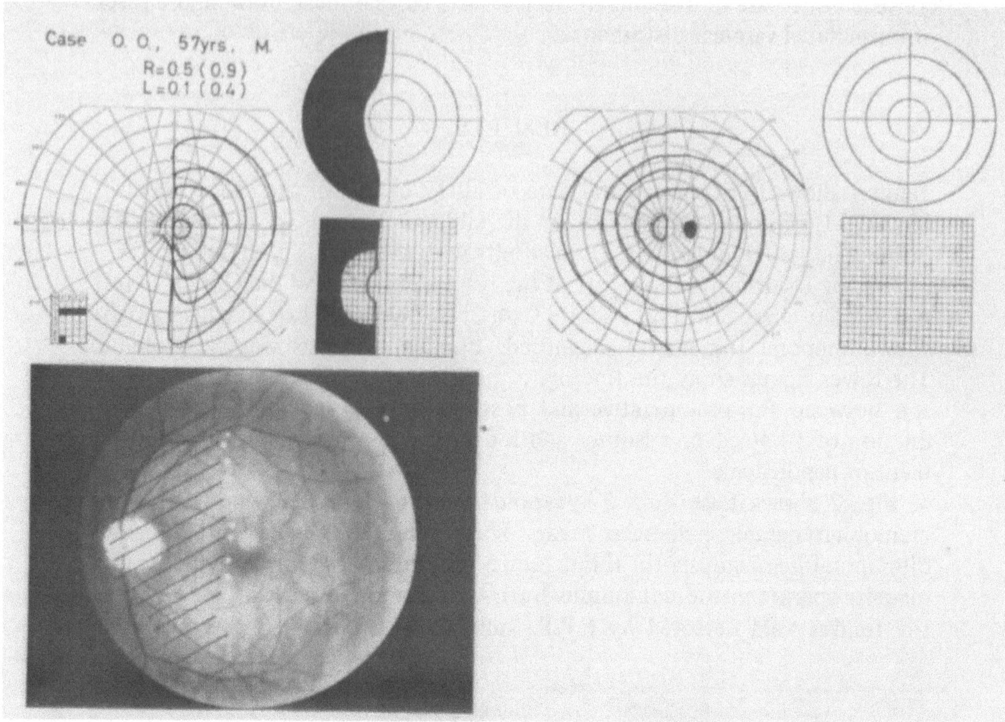

Fig. 2. Case 4, male, 57: No abnormality. 8 months after craniotomy for sellar craniopharyngioma.

side of the fovea as vertical lines. The visual field in the right eye improved after the operation and showed no abnormality. Here we must add that the slant lines in the color film were filled in afterward for easy discrimination of the hemianoptic side and this was performed in all other cases.

In Case 10 (Fig. 3), a 28-year-old man suspected of epilepsy after a head injury. CT scan and CAG findings were normal, but EEG indicated an abnormal pattern of waves similar to that of epilepsy. The patient was not submitted to craniotomy. The visual field change shows right superior homonymous quadrantanopsia, and that of F.P.P. almost corresponds with the results of G.P., U-O test and Amsler chart test.

The inside isopter was measured as 76.36 cd. m^{-2}, and the outside isopter 0.85 cd. m^{-2} in both eyes.

Fig. 4 shows Case 11, a 30-year-old man who received a blow on the left temporal lobe in a traffic accident. The visual field change indicates the left homonymous hemianopsia, and the visual field by F.P.P. yields two splitting lines: namely, with the luminance of the stimulus at 76.36 cd. m^{-2} a splitting line is found on the left in both eyes and at 0.85 cd. m^{-2} on the right with an enlargement of the hemianopsia with regard to visual field changes in U-O test and Amsler chart test, macular sparing is found in both eyes.

A diagnosis of idiopathic hemorrhage of the right occipital lobe was made in a 26-year-old male case (Case 12, Fig. 5). A high density area was found in

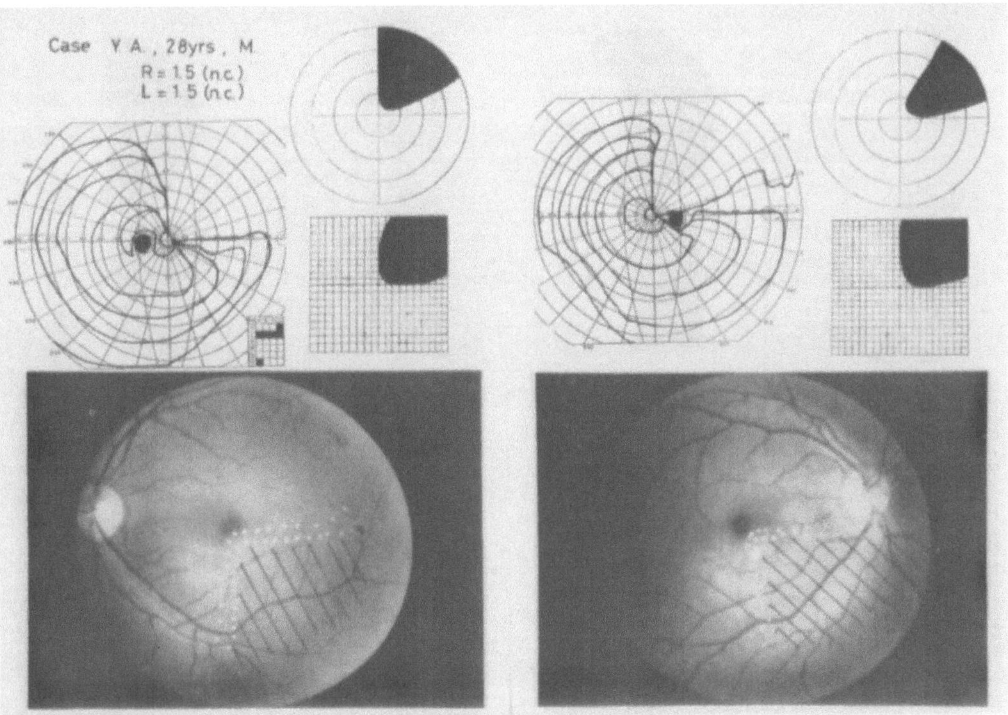

Fig. 3. Case 10, male, 28: Head blow.

the right occipital lobe by CT scan, and it was identified by craniotomy as blood coagulation. This patient consulted our outpatient department complaining of pulsating pain of the right temporal lobe and left hemiplegia. The visual field change indicates the left homonymous hemianopsis; and the result of the visual field examination by F.P.P. with the luminance of the stimulus at 76.36 cd. m^{-2}, practically coincides with those of the visual field measured by G.P. and the visual field change detected by U-O test and Amsler chart test.

DISCUSSION

In the present clinical experiment we employed a background luminance of 0.24 cd. m^{-2} and set the luminance of the stimulus at a maximum of 76.36 cd.m^{-2} and at a minimum of 0.85 cd.m^{-2}. These luminance values were reckoned most suitable with reference to several preparatory experiments we had carried out. As a result, they proved highly effective in the detection of hemianopsia and papilledema. Our method of fundus photo-perimetry completely eliminates the incomplete fixation pointed out in other methods of fundus perimetry such as G.P., U-O test and Amsler chart test, and will make it possible to perform fundus detection in those subjects who have difficulty

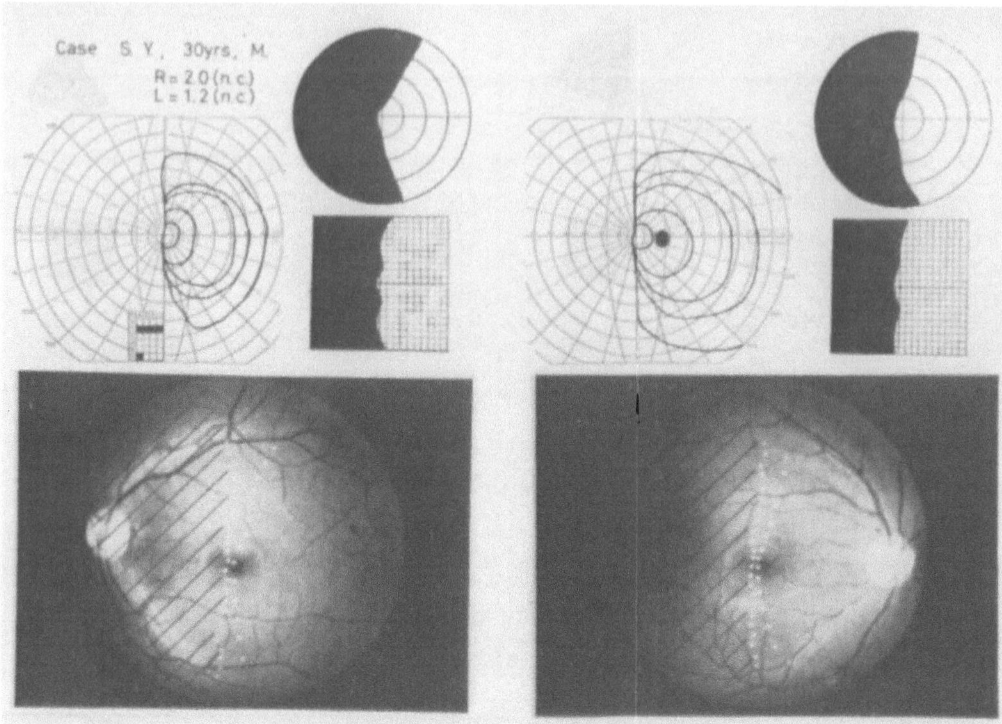

Fig. 4. Case 11, male, 30: Head blow.

in forming stable fixation – that is, our method is profitable for observing patients with unstable fixation and macular sparing (6).

To date, macular sparing has been thought of from the standpoint of niveau diagnosis pertaining to visual pathway injury. In hemianopsia, it is believed that when the optic radiation in the upper part of the lateral geniculated body or the area strata above the optic radiation is injured, the boundary line which vertically divides the visual field enters the hemianoptic portion in a semicircle at the visual point. It is this assumption that has supplied grounds for our diagnosis.

Duke-Elder has introduced theories of many researchers in regard to the cause of macular sparing (2). The histological experiment on a monkey's severed optic tract by Stone reports a case of macular sparing, with visual pathway injury at the lower part of the lateral geniculate body (7). Although there are many cases in which macular sparing is found, the fact that it is not immediately related to niveau diagnosis of visual pathway injury should be considered. Actually, the visual field by our F.P.P. demonstrated a vertical splitting line which swayed the fovea and which was exactly the same case when we observed macular sparing by U-O test and Amsler test.

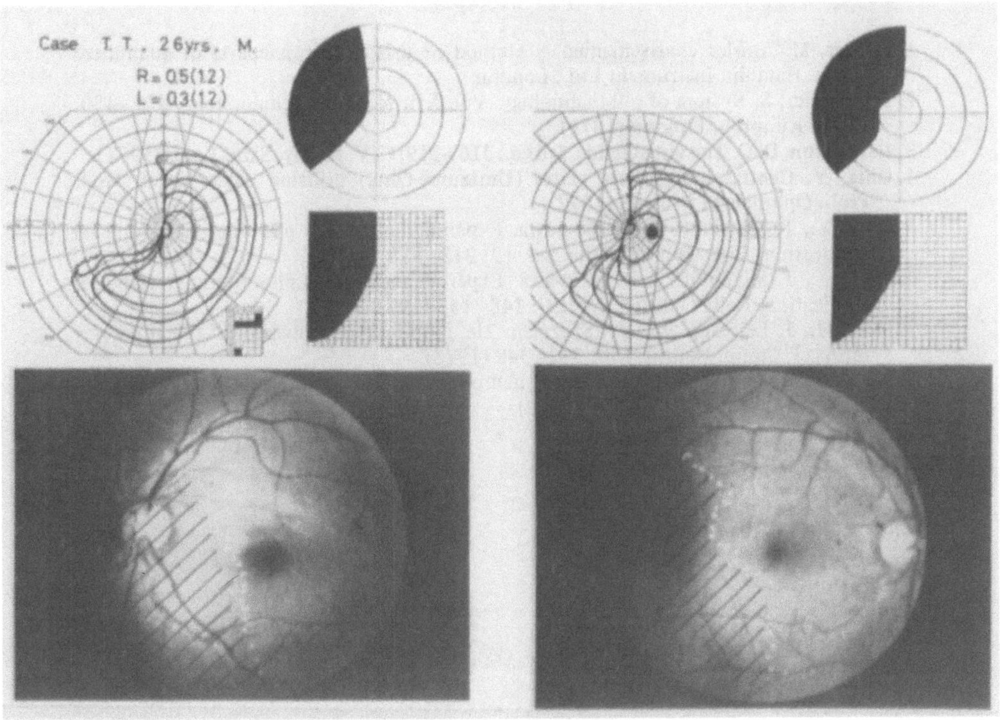

Fig. 5. Case 12, male, 26: Idiopathic hemorrhage of the right occipital lobe.

CONCLUSION

We performed visual field examinations in 17 cases of visual pathway injury postchiasmatic lesion with a new method of recording the isopter on the fundus photograph after direct observation by TV-monitoring. As a result of fundus photo-perimetry, macular sparing appeared in the form of a vertical splitting line in hemianopsia and it was identified as a vertical line slanting into the hemianopsia with reduced luminance of the stimulus.

With this technique, it is possible to obtain perfectly stable fixation which is most important in visual field examination.

REFERENCES

1. Amsler, M. Amsler charts manual – Method of using the test charts of qualitative vision. Hamblin Instrument Ltd., London.
2. Duke-Elder, S. System of ophthalmology. Vol. XII: Neuro-Ophthalmology, 427–430, Henry Kimpton, London (1971).
3. Harrington, D. O. The visual fields. 3rd ed., 316–319, C. V. Mosby, Saint Louis (1971).
4. Ohta, Y. Central scotometric plates (Umazume-Ohta) utilizing color vision. Mod. Prob. Ophthal. 11: 40–48 (1972).
5. Ohta, Y., T. Miyamoto & K. Harasawa. Experimental fundus photoperimeter and its application. Doc. Ophthal. Proc. Ser. 19: 315–358 (1978).
6. Ohta, Y., T. Miyamoto & K. Harasawa. Experimental fundus photoperimeter and its application. Folia Ophthal. Jap. 30: 148–153 (1979).
7. Stone, J., J. Leicester & S. M. Sherman. The naso-temporal division of the Monkey's retina. J. Comp. Neurol. 150: 333–348 (1973).
8. Walsh, F. B. & W. F. Hoyt. Clinical neuro-ophthalmology. 3rd ed., Vol. 1: 78–81, Williams & Wilkins, Baltimore (1969).

Authors' address:
Department of Ophthalmology
Tokyo Medical College
7-6-1, Nishishinjuku
Shinjuku-ku
Tokyo 160
Japan

FLICKER FUSION AND SPATIAL SUMMATION

M. ZINGIRIAN, G. CIURLO, P. ROSSI & C. BURTOLO

(Genoa, Italy)

ABSTRACT

Flicker fusion frequencies in the central and paracentral retina were studied for liminar and supraliminar stimulations with targets of different size. Statistical analysis of the results obtained in a relatively large series of patients allows a good standardization of 'normal' values for healthy people. Furthermore, the evaluation of the results lends insight into the relationships between temporal resolution and spatial summation.

INTRODUCTION

Flicker fusion alterations have been shown to often precede the corresponding scotomata of classic perimetry. The results of such experiments are, however, difficult to evaluate and compare with each other, mainly because of the different experimental conditions in which the test was carried out by the different examiners.

Our work was aimed to the following purposes:

- Standardize the photometric conditions of flicker perimetry.
- Report of the results obtained in the central visual field in healthy people.
- Discuss some of the physiological implications of our results.

MATERIAL AND METHOD

Four healthy subjects, with normal visual acuity and field were examined. Their age ranged from 27 to 31. A Goldmann perimeter was equipped with an electrically driven semicircular sector to obtain flickering of the target. This device was described, together with its main features, in a previous paper (1).

The flicker fusion frequency (F.F.F.) was determined at the fixation point and along the horizontal meridian at the following eccentricities: 3° – 5° – 10° – 15° – 20°. The examination was carried out at a photopic adaptation level and followed these steps:

- Assessment of the threshold luminance for non-flickering targets with a surface diameter of 1/16, 1/4, 1, 4, 15, 64 mm^2, at each of the tested positions.
- Increase of the target luminance by 0,4 L.U. above threshold levels.
- Determination of the F.F.F. for each target stimulus size surface in every

point. A sampling method of presentation was used and a set of 10 measures was obtained in each point.
- The F.F.F. was re-measured in each position for each stimulus with a luminance value corresponding to the threshold at 25° eccentricity.

The following parameter was calculated from the data obtained:

- mean value and standard deviation for every set of measures.

RESULTS (see Table 1)

- Flicker fusion frequencies can be determined with great accuracy in the central visual field with a fairly low scattering of the values.
- The F.F.F. for a 'threshold' target of a given size is fairly constant throughout the whole central retina.
- Photometrically equivalent stimulation are fused at the same frequency.
- When the same flickering target is used to test different retinal points the flicker fusion frequency values slightly rise from the periphery to the fovea.

CONSIDERATIONS

Some considerations on the technique used, the results and their physiological implications will be discussed.

Technique. The 0.4 L.U. increase of the threshold luminance results from a 0.3 L.U. increase needed to avoid the disappearance of the target at the F.F.F. frequency, according to the Talbot and Plateau law, and a further 0.1 L.U. increase in order to avoid the uncertain perception of a liminal stimulus. Therefore, all flickering targets actually realised supraliminal stimulations. This drawback is unavoidable, but we think that the sampling presentation of the stimuli should minimize its actual influence over the results.

Results. Flicker perimetry with 'threshold' stimuli appears a handy, reproducible and accurate test, at least within the central visual field.

The F.F.F. is fairly steady throughout the tested area, and it does not change when targets of different diameter are used. The assessment of this 'temporal plateau' is strictly bound to the features of the stimuli: photometrically equivalent stimulations are fused at the same frequency. Therefore the temporal resolution of the visual field is mainly related to the strength of the flickering stimulation and appears to be independent from spatial summation.

Isolated increases in the target size or in its luminance after the stimulus strengthen and change the F.F.F., according to the Granit and Harper or Ferry and Porter laws, respectively. This condition is realised when different retinal areas are tested with the same stimulus: the central areas will actually receive a more supraliminal stimulation than the peripheral ones and the temporal resolution will correspondingly appear higher.

Table 1. Results.

Target size (mm^2)										
1/16	18,9±1,8 18,9±1,8	21,7±1,7 24,7±3,1	20,6±2,1	19,9±1,6 24,4±3,1	22,1±2,1 25,3±4,1	20,8±2,3 23,8±19,5	19,8±2,4	21,7±1,9 23,7±19,9	20,8±1,8	19,8±1,5 19,8±1,5
1/4	17,1±1,8 17,1±1,8	20,7±2,9 23,8±1,8	21,7±1,8	18,9±2,0 24,6±2,1	21,8±1,4 25,6±3,7	22,4±1,7 25,7±2,1	21,5±1,4	21,6±2,1 22,6±3,5	23,5±2,1	19,6±1,7 19,6±1,7
1	19,9±1,7 19,9±1,7	21,2±1,8 24,6±3,6	19,8±1,7	20,9±1,8 24,4±2,6	21,9±2,1 26,7±4,1	22,3±3,6 23,8±2,2	22,7±3,7	23,6±1,9 24,1±2,5	22,7±1,9	21,8±3,7 21,8±3,7
4	17,8±2,6 17,8±2,6	20,6±2,3 23,4±3,5	19,4±1,1	20,7±2,8 25,8±3,7	23,6±3,1 29,1±5,1	22,7±1,9 24,6±3,7	20,7±1,8	22,9±2,1 23,9±2,4	22,8±1,9	19,9±1,9 19,9±1,9
16	19,8±1,7 19,8±1,7	20,9±1,8 23,7±2,7	19,8±1,8	18,9±2,1 25,7±3,7	20,9±1,5 25,8±3,1	21,9±2,1 24,6±3,7	19,8±2,1	21,8±3,0 23,7±2,9	22,9±1,9	18,9±1,9 19,9±1,9
64	20,9±3,5 20,9±3,5	21,8±2,7 24,1±2,7	20,8±2,1	20,8±1,9 23,9±2,8	22,8±1,8 25,7±2,5	22,9±3,1 24,8±3,7	18,9±1,9	21,9±1,7 20,8±5,9	22,8±2,6	20,8±1,6 20,8±1,6
Eccentricity (degrees)	20	10	5	3	0	3	5	10	15	20

Legend. Upper line: F.F.F. for threshold targets. Lower line: F.F.F. for the 20° eccentricity threshold target at 10°, 3°, 0 eccentricities.

CONCLUSIONS

- If the standardized photometric conditions of a Goldmann perimeter are used, flicker perimetry can become a fairly exact testing of the temporal resolution properties of the visual system.
- The temporal resolution is mainly related to the level of the stimulus and is not influenced by spatial summation. Photometrically equivalent 'threshold' stimulations are fused at the same frequency throughout the central visual field.

REFERENCE

1. Ciurlo, G., P. Rossi & G. Suetta. Nuovo apparecchio per la flicker-perimetria. Min. Oftal. 20: 61–68 (1978).

Author's address:
University Eye Clinic
Viale Benedetto XV
16132 Genoa
Italy

THE AULHORN-EXTINCTION PHENOMENON
Suppression scotomas in normal and strabismic subjects

V. HERZAU

(Tübingen, F.R.G.)

ABSTRACT

The extinction phenomenon after Aulhorn was used to measure the spread of suppression in binocular rivalry with a modified method. The new method permits the tested person to observe how the suppression scotoma emerges and after 2–3 seconds vanishes. In squinters with large deviation the extinction phenomenon is not elicitable in all cases and only to a very limited extent in the region between the monocular centres in the binocular visual field. But, cases with microstrabismus showed quite normal rivalry outside of their fixation point scotoma. The cause for the different findings was attributed to the difference in function of retinal points with the same image in squinters.

If both eyes are stimulated with different images, binocular rivalry occurs. A special form of rivalry represents the extinction phenomenon after Aulhorn (1). Here both eyes are successively stimulated with monocular images. If both stimuli fall on corresponding retinal points, the impression of the first stimulated eye will be extinguished at the moment of the stimulation of the second eye. Not only does the extinction occur if the stimuli are falling on corresponding retinal points, but also if the second stimulus is adjacent to this area.

The maximal distance of both stimuli, at which extinction will be observed is a measure for the spread of suppression which derives from a retinal point of one to the other eye in binocular rivalry. This maximal distance is a function of the eccentricity of the examined retinal points. The maximum distance is about 0.5° for stimuli close to the fixation point and 2–8° for stimuli presented 8° away from the fixation point.

The described method requires many single measurements for the determination of one extinction area and is therefore not useful for examinations of most patients. Therefore, we used a simplified modification of successive monocular stimulation for examination of suppression. The purpose of these investigations was to examine the phenomenon of binocular rivalry in normal persons and squinters with anomalous retinal correspondence.

METHOD

The tested person looks through a phase-difference-haploscope to a fixation point (10′, 100 asb) on a white wall (luminance 10 asb) at 1.5 m distance. To the tested eye a large grid pattern is presented as the first stimulus (diameter 60°; dark strips: 10 asb, 0.4° in width, angular distance between the stripes: 2°; contrast 1:10). The fellow eye is stimulated in intervals with the second, extinction stimulus (diameter 1°, 1 000 asb). The tested person has to observe if extinction around the second stimulus occurs and has to determine the position and the size of the extinction field. In squinters the deviated eye was examined; the second stimulus was presented to the leading eye.

RESULTS

a) Normal subjects

All normal tested persons could observe, after a short training period, a defect in the grid pattern around the second stimulus (Fig. 1a). The determination of the size of the extinguished area requires very good observation ability and steady fixation. Most often this was possible only after several repetitions. Especially difficult was the judgement at an eccentricity of the second stimulus of over 8°. Beyond 20° the extinction phenomenon is no longer elicited with certainty (Awaya, 1978, and personal observations).

The defect in the grid pattern develops after a scarcely perceptible latency and fades away after 2–3 sec. A non-moving extinction stimulus causes a round scotoma, while a moving stimulus seems to pull a suppression trail (Fig. 1b). This trail phenomenon is very impressive but not useful for quantitative examinations, because here the judgement of the spread of suppression is especially difficult and it is only possible to measure the vertical limits of the suppression.

Exceptionally, after the presentation of the extinction stimulus no suppression was observed, or after the development of a typical extinction area, an additional large suppression scotoma with bizarre borders, occurred. These exceptions were not taken into consideration.

Fig. 2 shows the horizontal and the vertical spread of the extinction area of 2 normal persons for 2 different distances of the extinction stimulus from the fixation point. As Aulhorn (1967) has already shown for the maximal vertical distances, the spread of suppression increases with the eccentricity of the second stimulus. This slope is also demonstrable by means of calculation of the sizes of the extinction areas despite a large scatter in the answers. The size was calculated as the product of the half of the horizontal diameter and half of the vertical diameter of the extinction area multiplied by π (Fig. 3).

Orientation examinations showed clearly that the spread of suppression additionally depended on the size and luminance of the extinction stimulus. Systematic examinations in this regard are still to be done.

In the usual test the extinction stimulus was presented monocularly to the non-examined eye. However, the extinction phenomenon was also elicitable with a binocular extinction stimulus, but its perception was reported to be less clear by most observers.

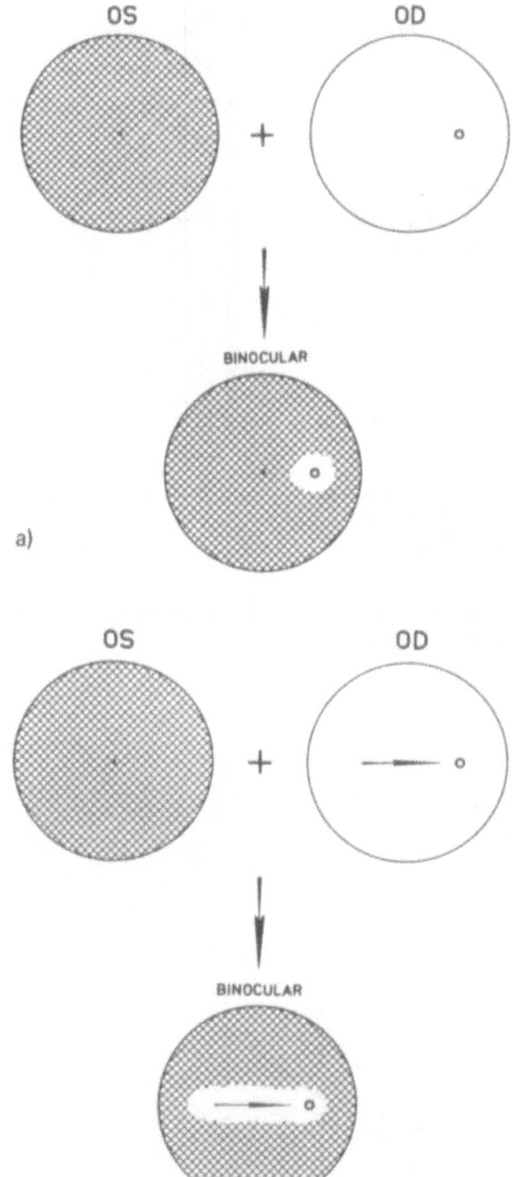

Fig. 1. Extinction phenomenon on the monocular grid.
a) with a stationary extinction stimulus;
b) with a moving extinction stimulus.

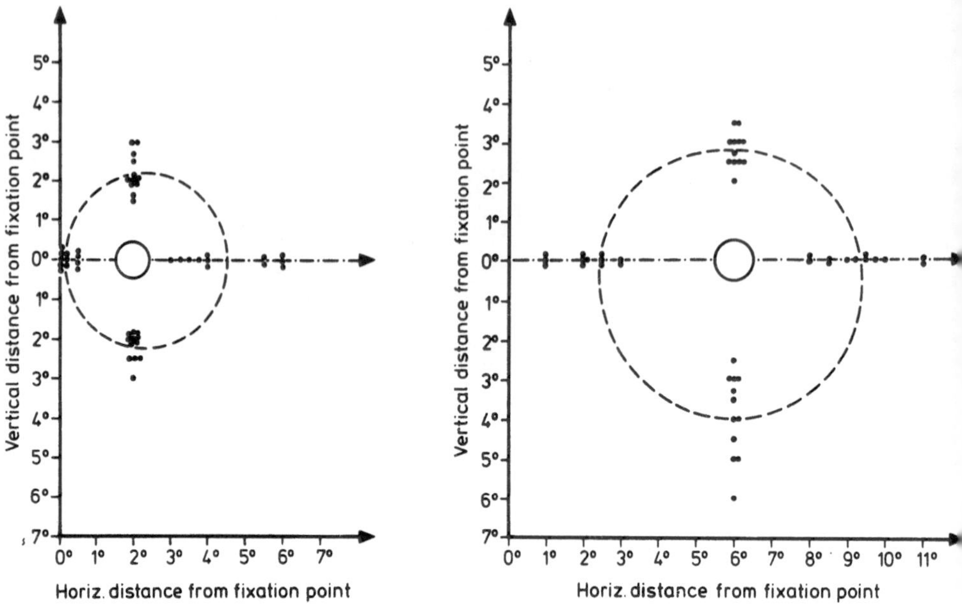

Fig. 2. Mean size of extinction area for 2° (left) and 6° (right) eccentricity of the extinction stimulus. 2 subjects, 6 sessions.

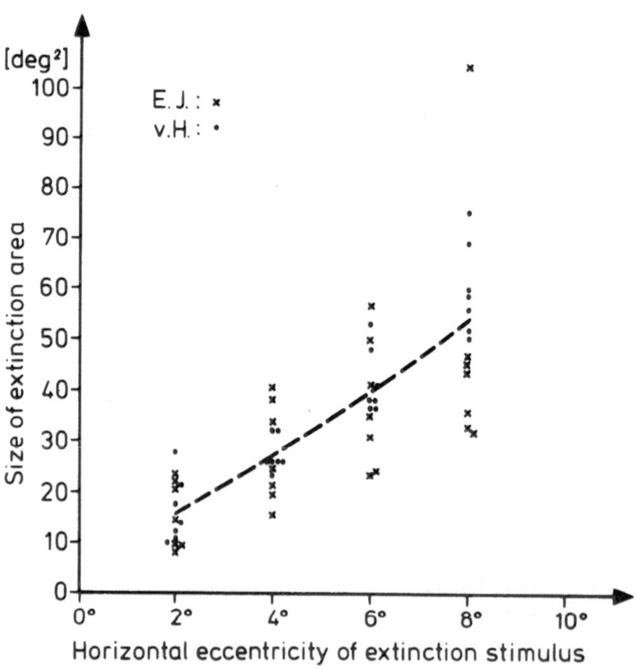

Fig. 3. Size of extinction area for various eccentricities of the extinction stimulus in 2 normal subjects.

b) Squinting patients

Twenty patients with manifest strabismus and harmonious anomalous correspondence were examined with the described method. Only 10 patients perceived distinct extinction areas and were able to describe them. Six patients observed no extinction at all.

Fig. 4a shows the typical findings of a patient with esotropia. The angle of deviation is 14°. The delineated plane corresponds to the size of the tested

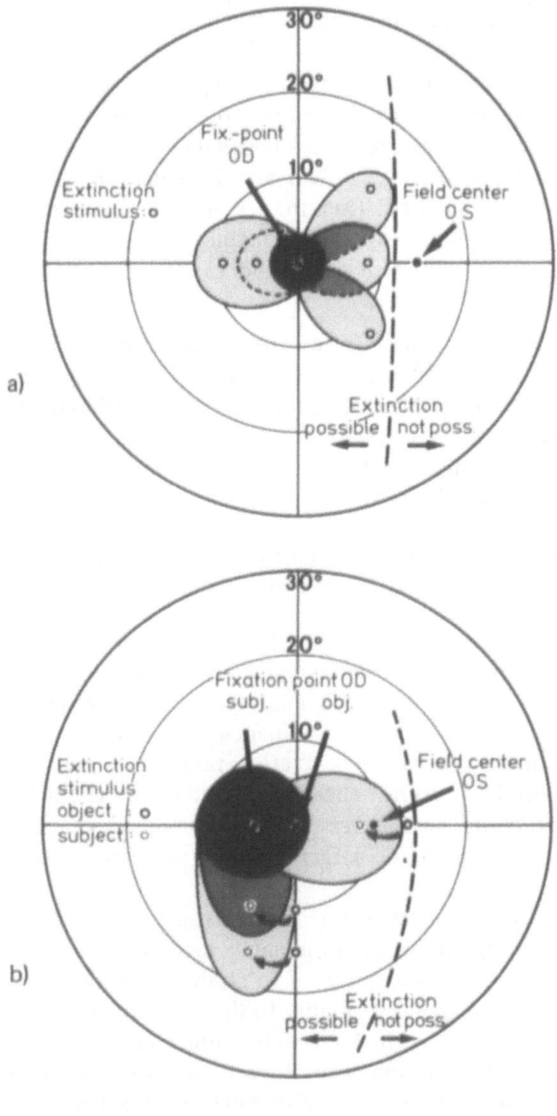

Fig. 4. Extinction phenomenon in strabismus convergens; visual acuity: OD/OS: 1.0.
a) patient with HARC;
b) patient with DARC.

field and the monocularly presented grid pattern. The right eye looks at the central fixation point; the visual field centre of the deviated eye is located 14° to the right of the fixation point. The monocular grid pattern is visible only to the deviated left eye. Around the fixation point there is a steady defect in the pattern corresponding to the fixation point scotoma, which is typical for anomalous correspondence. Additionally, the location of several extinction stimuli for the right eye and the corresponding extinction areas for the left eye are shown. In comparison with the normal extinction phenomenon there are 3 striking differences:

1. The extinction areas are not circumscribed but are always connected to the fixation point scotoma.
2. The suppressed areas do not vanish spontaneously at all locations. The reappearance of the suppressed area was observed only in the neighbourhood of the visual field centre of the deviated eye.
3. There exists a binocular visual field area in which no suppression of the deviated eye can be elicited. Then the second stimulus is visible in the grid pattern without a suppression halo. Inability to suppress relates to the central visual field of the deviated eye or at least to the peripherally adjacent area.

Fig. 4b shows a further example of esotropia. The angle of squint is 10°; the retinal correspondence is disharmonious. Therefore, the images of the fixating right eye are shifted to left in the grid pattern. Accordingly the extinction areas are also displaced.

Up to now, all examined patients with a moderate or a large convergent deviation, ARC, and the ability to observe an extinction phenomenon showed similiar behaviour. Also, at other points than those shown, similiar extinction phenomena were elicited. They are omitted for clarity. Though if the second stimulus were located too far peripherally no definite suppression could be observed.

In patients with exotropia, an extinction phenomenon was elicited in only some cases, but they all showed similar behaviour. The steady fixation scotoma was much larger and often hemianopic in character (Fig. 5a).

In the border zone between the dominance areas of each eye an extinction stimulus causes an increase of this fixation point scotoma. Stimuli located further in the periphery do not elicit suppression. The visual field centre of the deviated eye could be suppressed only in some cases. The size of the extinguished area seems to be larger than in normals or in patients with esotropia.

A single exception was observed in one exotropic patient. He demonstrated an extinction phenomenon in the dominance area of the deviated eye as well as the phenomenon typically observed in strabismic patients (Fig. 5b). The shape of the suppressed area was similiar to that of normals.

The described findings with large extinction areas which are connected to the fixation point scotoma were found only in cases with deviations greater than 5°. Patients with convergent micro-strabismus showed a normal extinction phenomenon outside of their fixation point scotoma. Only in cases with deep amblyopia was the size of the suppressed area of the deviated eye increased as shown by Aulhorn (1).

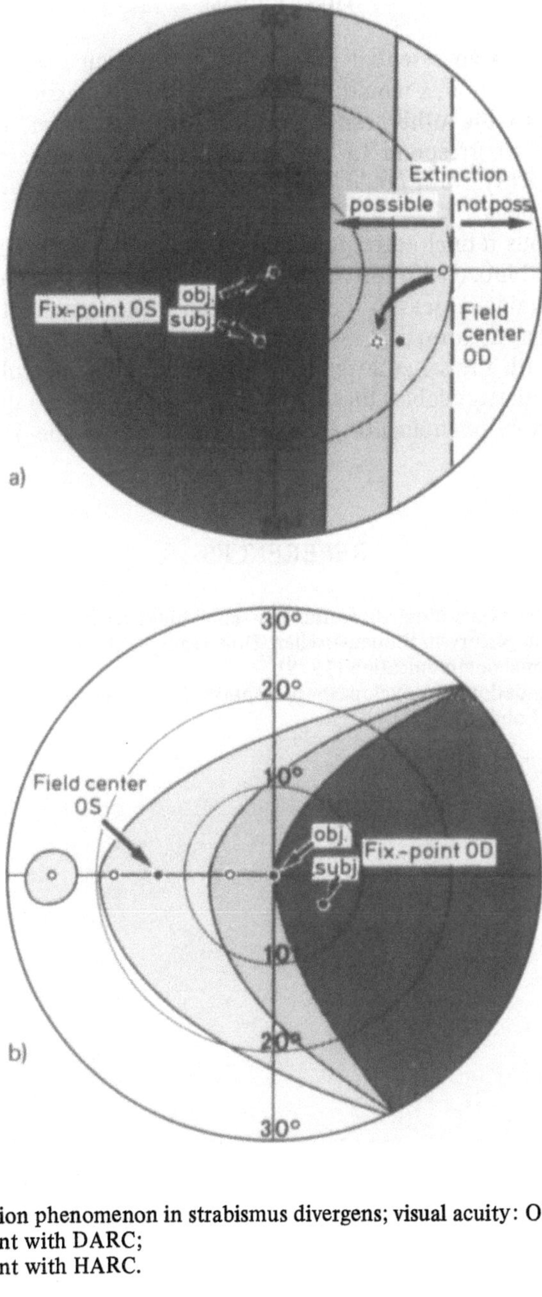

Fig. 5. Extinction phenomenon in strabismus divergens; visual acuity: OD/OS: 1.0.
a) patient with DARC;
b) patient with HARC.

DISCUSSION

Binocular rivalry is an essential part of normal binocular vision. Using the extinction phenomenon, a remarkable spread of the suppression which derives from one eye to the other can be demonstrated. However, the necessary cross-connections correspond to the maximal fusion of disparate images as found by Julesz (3). So it could be possible that the same neurons are used for both phenomena.

The anomalous retinal correspondence of squinters with a large deviation permits such a binocular interrelation only to a very limited extent. Only between the dominant areas of the two eyes can a certain extinction phenomenon be elicited as in normals. I assume that the large difference in function of retinal points with the same image prevents functioning binocular linkage. It is therefore understandable that only in cases of microstrabismus can a normal extinction phenomenon be elicited outside of the fixation point scotoma.

REFERENCES

1. Aulhorn, E. Die gegenseitige Beeinflussung abbildungsgleicher Netzhautstellen bei normalem und gestörtem Binocularsehen. Doc. Ophthal. 23: 26–61 (1967).
2. Awaya, S. Personal communication (1978).
3. Julesz, B. Foundations of cyclopean perception. The University of Chicago Press, Chicago and London (1971).

Author's address:
V. Herzau
Universitäts Augenklinik
Schleichstrasse 12
D-7400 Tübingen
F.R.G.

SPATIAL SUMMATION IN THE FOVEAL AND PARAFOVEAL REGION

OSAMU MIMURA, KAZUTAKA KANI & TOSHIO INUI

(Nishinomiya, Japan)

ABSTRACT

Spatial summation effects have been studied in several retinal loci between 0° and 10° from fovea in normal and abnormal subjects using fundus controlled perimetry. Results of spatial summation were as follows: in normal subjects, spatial summation curves have two asymptotes – one shows complete spatial summation and the other shows no summation; in the fovea of amblyopic eye, spatial summation curves represent abnormal gradient with small target; in the eye of optic neuritis patient, spatial summation curves utterly lack the region of complete spatial summation immediately after the visual acuity returned to normal. These results suggest that our new instrument applied to evaluation of visual field in clinical practice is also available for analysis of human abnormal vision function in relation to pathogenesis.

INTRODUCTION

Spatial summation is one of the most basic and essential mechanisms of the visual function, and has been studied in psychophysics and electrophysiology using several procedures. These procedures, however, are so complicated that they are not suitable for clinical use. Therefore, we have developed a new method using fundus controlled perimeter for clinical application.

In this article, a new instrument is shown and spatial summation effects in the fovea and parafoveal region are presented in normal and abnormal subjects.

MATERIALS AND METHODS

Apparatus

Trials were conducted on a new modified fundus controlled perimeter which was originally designed by Kani & Ogita (3). The block diagram is shown in Fig. 1. The fundus image is focused on the plane B where the infrared Wratten filter was placed. A pinhole was made on the filter with Nd-YAG laser processing device. The light emitted by the light source A passed through this pinhole and illuminates the retina as a stimulus. Stimulus, background and fixation light beams were set up in a Maxwellian view arrangement. The light

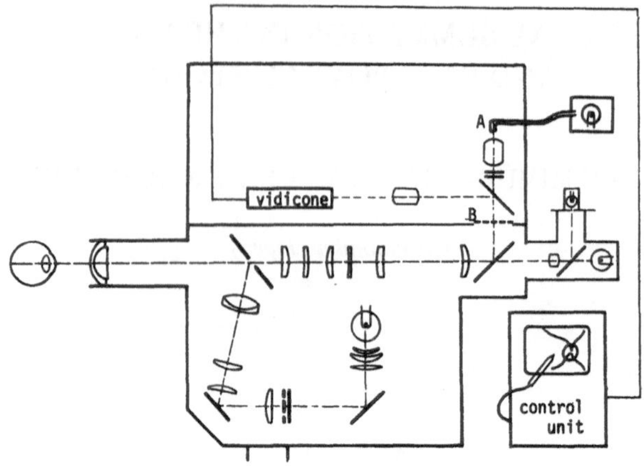

Fig. 1. Block diagram of the new instrument.

passed through the central part of the subject's pupil with 1.5 mm in diameter. Subject's fundus picture and target position on the retina could be monitored by means of infrared television system. Subject's head was fixated with a chin and forehead rest, preventing any horizontal and vertical head movements.

The fixation point at the center of background was a red spot of 7 minutes or 20 minutes in diameter. The background was illuminated by a single tungsten lamp, and a light balancing filter was used to raise the colour temperature of the projected light to 6000 K. The background subtended a circular visual field of 30° in diameter and the luminance was 10 apostilbs (5.6 trolands). Target spot was also illuminated by a single tungsten lamp and the colour temperature was the same as the background. Target intensity could be changed with neutral density filters (Kodak Wratten No. 96) by steps of 0.1 log unit. Exposure duration of the target was controlled by an electromechanical shutter and it was 200 ms in this experiment. The principal experimental variables were target size and retinal locus. Target sizes used here were 1.2, 2.7, 3.1, 6.4, 10, 13, 21, 28, 33, 60 and 79′ in diameter. Spatial summation determinations were made at the position of retinal eccentricities, 0, 1, 2, 4, 5 and 10° on the horizontal meridian of the temporal part of the subject's retina. Fixation light was turned off in the case of spatial summation determination at fovea.

Procedure

Subject's pupil was dilated with a mydriatic, 0.5% Tropicamide. The subject was allowed approximately twenty minutes for the background adaptation. At the start of the experiment, the subject was instructed to press the key in their right hand if the target was seen, and to do nothing otherwise. The subject was told to be sure the fixation point was in good focus before initiating each session. The trials were self-paced. The subject began each trial by pressing the key in their left hand, which triggered the target. Throughout each session, the examiner monitored if the target spot was fallen on the vessel.

Subjects participated in eleven experimental sessions, each of which corresponded to one of the target sizes selected randomly. A session consisted of five blocks of ten or twenty trials. Prior to each session, five trials were performed so that target intensity was set up to the vicinity of the threshold. Ten or twenty data were collected by the up-down method and 50% threshold, at which 50% 'Yes' responses were obtained, was determined from the probability-seeing curve.

Subjects

One normal subject and three abnormal subjects participated in this experiment. The visual acuity of the normal subject, H.K. (27-year-old man) was more than 1.0 for both eyes without correction. Two abnormal subjects, suffering from intractable amblyopia, were M.H. (26-year-old woman) and J.K. (29-year-old woman). The visual acuity of these patients was 0.05 in amblyopic eye and 1.2 in non-amblyopic eye without correction. The other abnormal subject, suffering from the bilateral retrobulbar optic neuritis, was N.K. (30-year-old woman). The visual acuity of the patient improved from 0.02 to 1.2 on both eyes after treatment with corticosteroid for two weeks.

RESULTS

The results of these experiments are illustrated in Figures 2 to 7. Figure 2 shows the spatial summation curves in normal subject H.K., in which log

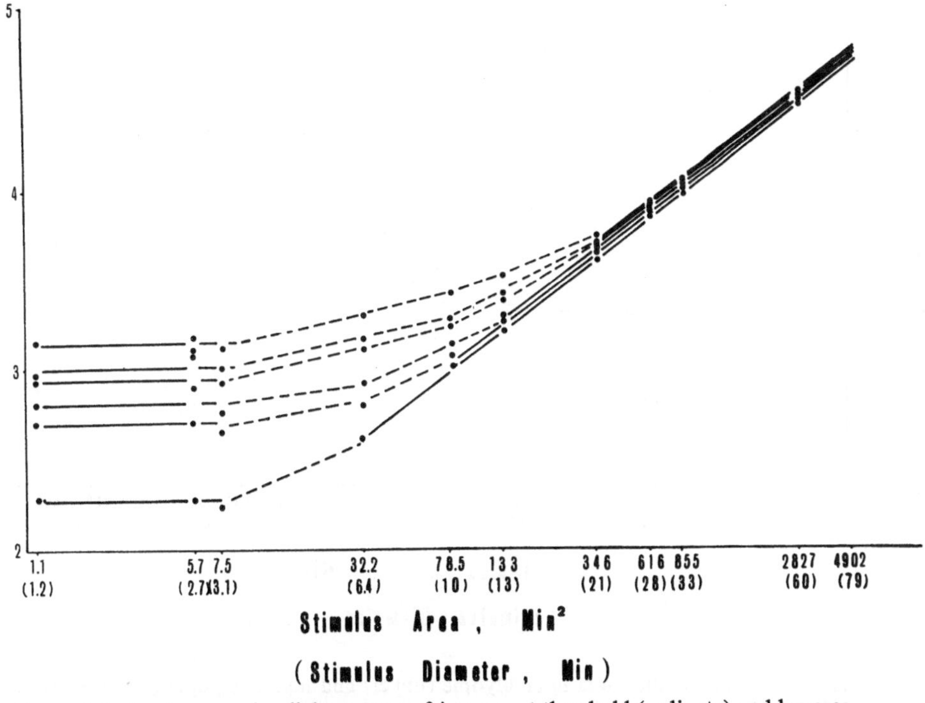

Fig. 2. Relation between log light energy of increment threshold (ordinate) and log area of stimulus (abscissa) at six different eccentricities in normal subject H.K.

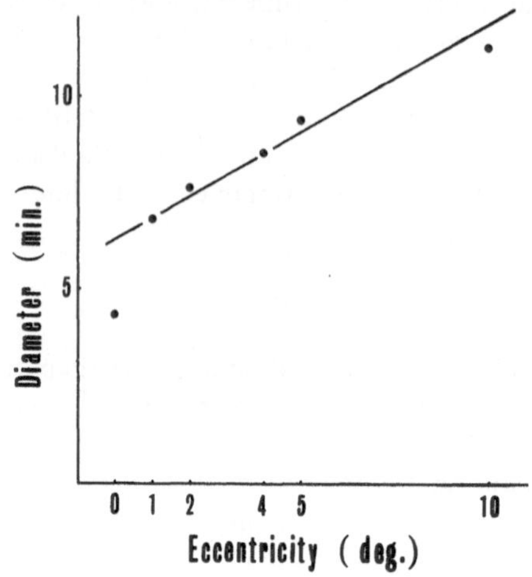

Fig. 3. Relation between critical size diameter (ordinate) and retinal eccentricity from fovea (abscissa) in subject H.K.

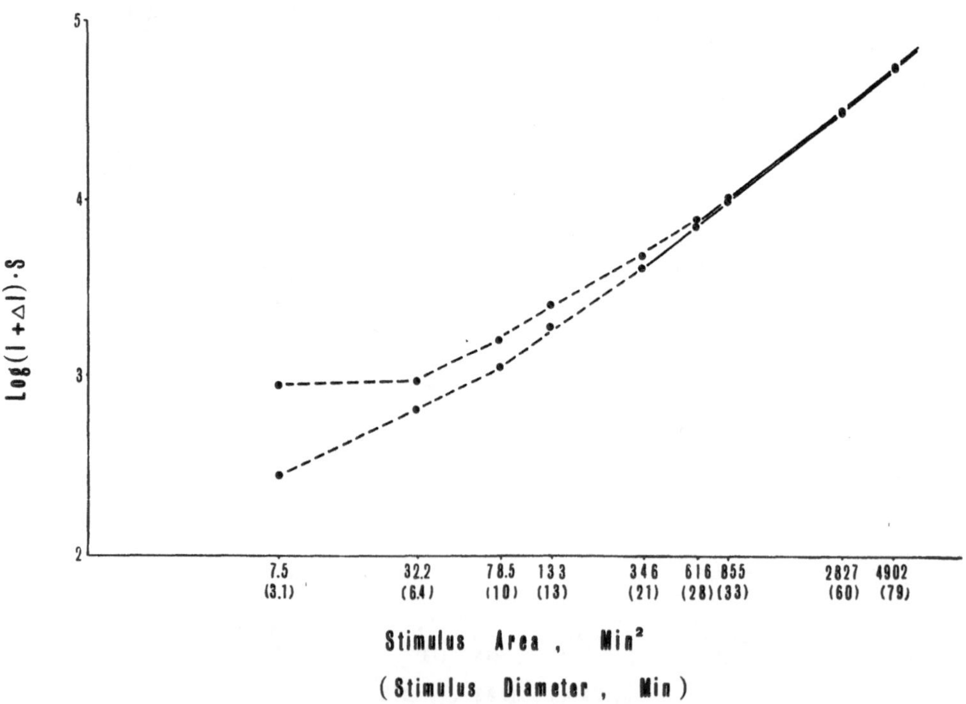

Fig. 4. The data at the fovea in amblyopic (upper) and non amblyopic (lower) eyes in subject H.M.

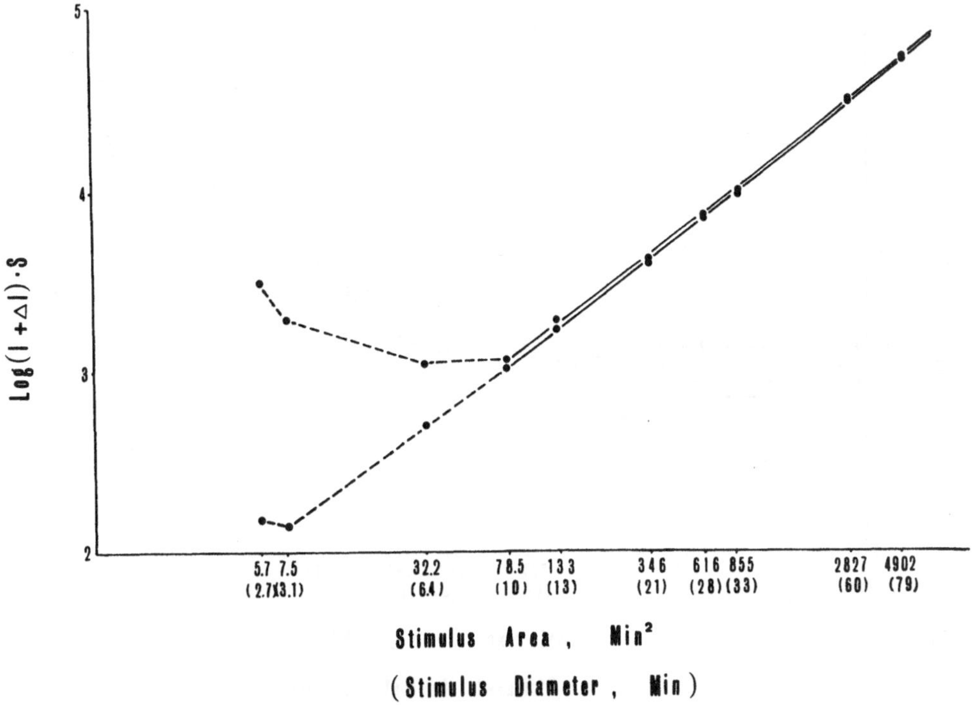

Fig. 5. The data at the fovea in amblyopic (upper) and non amblyopic (lower) eyes in subject J.K.

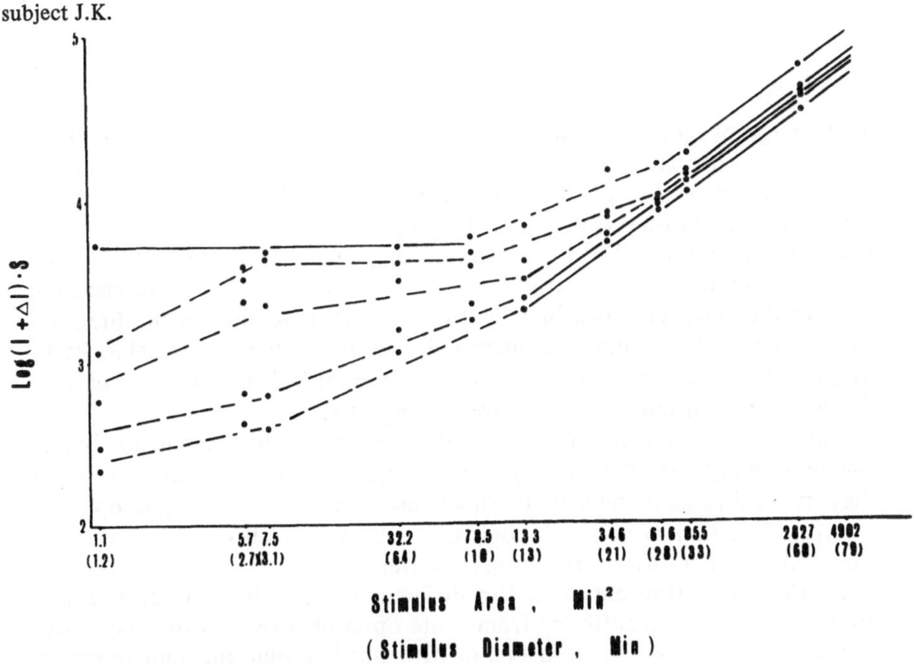

Fig. 6. The data at five different eccentricities, 1, 2, 4, 5 and 10 degrees, in subject N.K., suffering from acute optic neuritis, at three days after recovery of vision.

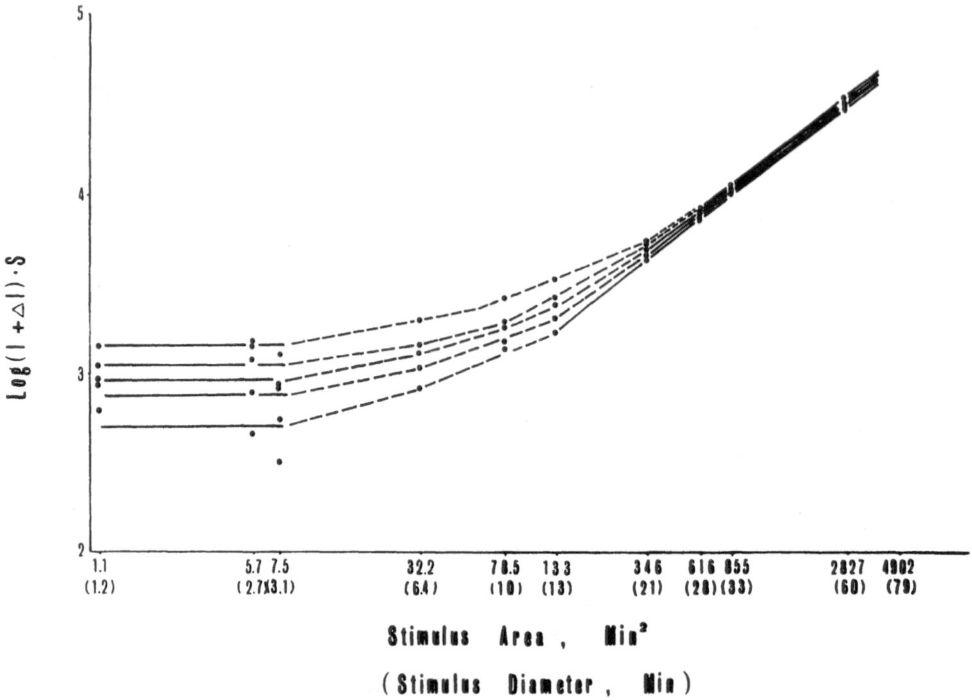

Fig. 7. The data in subject N.K. at two weeks later.

light energy of increment threshold plotted against log area of stimulus at six different eccentricities. The data of increment threshold show a certain regularity, in which with very small stimuli they are parallel to the abscissa, and with large stimuli they approach a slope of 45°. Thus, the sensitivity curves have two asymptotes. The former shows complete spatial summation and the latter, no summation. We termed the stimulus diameter at the intersecting point of the two asymptotic lines as critical size diameter. Increment threshold energy of complete summation increased monotonically with retinal locus up to 10 degrees from the fovea. Fig. 3 shows the critical size diameter plotted against the eccentricity from the fovea in subject H.K.

Figs. 4 and 5 show the spatial summation curves at the fovea in amblyopic and non amblyopic eyes in subject H.M. and subject J.K., respectively. In these two subjects, increment threshold energy at the fovea in amblyopic eye is larger than that in non amblyopic eye with very small stimuli. With large stimuli the former differs little from the latter.

Spatial summation curves at five different eccentricities (1, 2, 4, 5 and 10°) in subject N.K., suffering from acute optic neuritis, at three days after recovery of vision is shown in Fig. 6. With small stimuli, incomplete spatial summation occurred instead of complete summation. Two weeks later, spatial summation curves became completely normal (Fig. 7).

DISCUSSION

Spatial summation, one of the most basic and essential functions for vision, has been studied in normal and abnormal subjects (1, 2, 6). The importance of analysing spatial summation effects needs no longer to be emphasized. It was supported that the psychological properties of spatial summation were closely related to the receptive field organization of the retinal ganglion cells. Most of these experimental systems, however, are so delicate and complicated that they are not acceptable for clinical applications. Furthermore, not all of them are suitable for analysing in patients poor central fixation.

The advantages of fundus controlled perimetry (4) used in the present experiment are as follows:

By the television image we can easily grasp (1) whether the light beam passes through the center of the pupil, (2) where the stimulus falls, (3) whether the retinal locus is free from the vessels or retinal diseases, and (4) whether the eye does not move during the stimulation.

In normal subject H.K., the sensitivity curves have two asymptotes as shown in Fig. 2. Two asymptotes mean complete spatial summation and non summation, respectively. Our results are in nearly complete agreement with others (2, 6). From these results, the conclusion can be drawn that the fundus controlled perimeter is reliable for analysing spatial summation effects.

There have been few studies concerning foveal sensitivity in eccentrically fixating eyes. Using the fundus controlled perimetry, we can easily examine foveal function in patients with poor fixation. In amblyopic subjects, the sensitivity curves at the fovea in non amblyopic eyes are similar to those at the fovea in normal subject. In amblyopic eyes, the sensitivity curves at the fovea are similar to those at the parafoveal or peripheral retina in normal subject.

The fact that the receptive field size in amblyopic eye is larger than that in non amblyopic eye in experimental animal has gained wide acceptance. While a proposal of this fact to extend to human is very attractive, it still lacks direct experimental support. Our findings in this experiment could show this possibility, although it needs still more thorough researches.

In subject N.K., the data of increment threshold show lack of complete summation at three days after recovery of vision (Fig. 6), and normal summation effects at two weeks after recovery of vision. Why have the data of increment threshold no regularity with small stimuli? The suggestion for this problem is controversial (5). We attempted to explain the lack of complete summation in this patient on the basis of dysfunction of energy transmission rather than abnormality of visual field, such as sieve like defect.

The simplicity of this technique, availability and lack of discomfort, and ability to perform in subjects with fixation instability, make it clinically useful as a guide to the analysis of the visual function.

ACKNOWLEDGEMENTS

We wish to thank Prof. J. Imachi and Prof. Masashi Shimo-oku for their kind and helpful instructions.

REFERENCES

1. Flynn, J. T. Spatial summation in amblyopia. Arch. Ophthalmol. 78: 470–474 (1967).
2. Glezer, V. D. The receptive fields of the retina. Vision Res. 5: 496–525 (1965).
3. Kani, K. & Y. Ogita. Fundus controlled perimetry. Folia Ophthalmol. Jpn. 30: 141–147 (1979a).
4. Kani, K. & Y. Ogita. Fundus controlled perimetry. The relation between the position of a lesion in the fundus and in the visual field. Docum. Ophthal. Proc. Series 19: 341–350 (1979b).
5. Mimura, O., K. Kani & T. Inui. Spatial summation – its clinical application. Folia Ophthalmol. Jpn. 30: 1543–1547 (1979).
6. Wilson, M. F. Invariant features of spatial summation with changing locus in the visual field. J. Physiol. 207: 611–622 (1970).

Authors' address:
Department of Ophthalmology
Hyogo College of Medicine
Mukogawa-cho, 1-1, Nishinomiya
Hyogo, 663
Japan

COMPARISON OF SPATIAL CONTRAST SENSITIVITY WITH VISUAL FIELD IN OPTIC NEUROPATHY AND GLAUCOMA

YUSAKU TAGAMI, TAKAHIRO ONUMA, KUNIYOSHI MIZOKAMI & YOSHIMASA ISAYAMA

(Kobe, Japan)

ABSTRACT

The contrast sensitivity functions (CSFs) were disturbed in recovered optic neuropathy and early glaucoma cases with the visual acuity of more than 1.0 in the conventional acuity tests, and gradually decreased as the atrophic states of the maculopapillar bundles developed ophthalmoscopically. The statistical analysis revealed that the static visual fields were also disturbed when the CSFs were decreased in these cases. Both of the CSFs and the static field were useful for the detection of abnormal central vision.

INTRODUCTION

During the last decade psychophysical analysis had demonstrated that measurement of spatial contrast sensitivity is one of the most reliable methods for general description of an entire visual system (3). By studying the contrast sensitivity functions (CSFs), it is possible to detect a deficiency of visual functions not determined in the conventional acuity tests. Recently, disturbances of the CSFs were described in optic neuropathy (1, 3, 7, 12) and glaucoma cases (2), however, there was not specific mention of their correlations with the visual fields which have been widely used in clinical opthalmology.

In optic neuropathies, a close relationship was found between the static visual fields and the atrophic states of the maculopapillar bundles under red-free light (10, 11) and also it was documented that the CSFs decreased as the atrophy of the maculopapillar bundles developed (6).

It is then of interest to compare the detection ability of the CSF test with that of static perimetry in recovered optic neuropathy and early glaucoma cases with the visual acuity of more than 1.0 in the conventional acuity tests.

SUBJECTS AND METHODS

21 patients (27 eyes) with recovered optic neuropathies were studied after a minimum of 2 months the patients regained the visual acuity of over 1.0 by the conventional acuity tests. 6 patients (6 eyes) with ocular hypertension

Doc. Ophthal. Proc. Series, Vol. 26, ed. by E. L. Greve & G. Verriest

and 12 patients (12 eyes) with primary open-angle glaucoma with the visual acuity of over 1.0 were also used for this study. In glaucoma cases, kinetic visual fields showed only paracentral scotomas with or without slight nasal steps.

In all cases, the CSFs were examined and compared with the atropic states of the maculopapillar bundles under red-free light. In 12 cases with optic neuropathy and 6 cases with glaucoma, the CSFs were compared with the macular sensitivity examined by Tübinger's static perimetry and with the foveal sensitivity determined by Quantitative Maculometry with direct fundus examination (5), which maintained the polite central fixation during the measurements. The age range of the patients was 19–50 years with a median of 36.5 years.

1. Contrast sensitivity functions (CSFs)

A laser interferometer (retinal visual acuity and MTF tester, EA-250M, Takata Co., Tokyo) was used for this study. This interferometer is described in detail in Sugimachi *et al.* (9). Light from a He-Ne laser was divided into two beams and focused into two small focal images in the observer's pupil. The resulting interference pattern appeared to the observer as a vertical and red sine-wave grating that filled a circular test field subtending an angle of 5 degrees in a dark surrounding. The spatial frequency and the contrast could be varied by maintaining a constant mean retinal illuminance of 300 trolands. The constant sensitivity was examined at each spatial frequency of 1.5, 2, 3, 4, 5, 6, 10, 14, 20 and 30 cycles/degree. The sensitivity was determined by raising the contrast from a subthreshold level at a selected spatial frequency until a pattern was just visible to the observer. The measurements were carried out more than 6 times, then the mean and the standard deviation were calculated. The contrast sensitivity was determined monocularly with the natural pupil, and when the observer had a refractive error of more than ±2D, suitable contact lenses were used during the measurements.

The results from 30 normal subjects with the age range of 16–50 years (mean 34.0 years) were used as the normal controls.

The contrast sensitivity at each spatial frequency of the patients was divided by that of the control function, then added together and averaged. The results were used for the attenuation ratio of the CSFs.

2. Red-free fundus photography

The atrophic stages of the maculopapillar bundles under red-free light in recovered optic neuropathy were described in detail in a recent paper (11). The atrophic stages of the maculopapillar bundles were classified into stage 1 (normal state or only slight diffuse atrophy), stage 2 (moderate diffuse atrophy) and stage 3 (severe diffuse atrophy).

3. Macular sensitivity by Tübinger's static perimetry

The field was examined using a 7′ white stimulus with the background illumination of 10 asb. The sensitivities of 7 points, all inside 3 degrees from 0 degree, were determined at every 1 degree on the horizontal meridian. The sensitivities were averaged, and the result in each patient divided by the mean of that in 12 normal controls (age range 22–48 years, mean 35.2 years) was used for the attenuation ratio of the macular sensitivity.

4. Foveolar sensitivity by quantitative maculometry

The sensitivity at 0 degree was examined using a 6.37′ white stimulus with the background illumination of 250 asb. The sensitivity in each patient divided by the mean of that in 12 normal controls (age range 22–48 years, mean 35.2 years) was used for the attenuation ratio of the foveolar sensitivity.

RESULTS

1. CSFs and atrophic stages of maculopapillar bundles

The means of the CSFs in each atrophic stage of recovered optic neuropathy and the normal controls are illustrated in Fig. 1 for spatial frequencies. Similarly, the means of the CSF in ocular hypertension and early glaucoma cases are illustrated in Fig. 2. The CSFs in the normal controls had a bell-shaped, high and low frequency attenuation with a peak sensitivity at 3 cycles/degree.

The results of the CSFs were analysed by the student's t-test at each

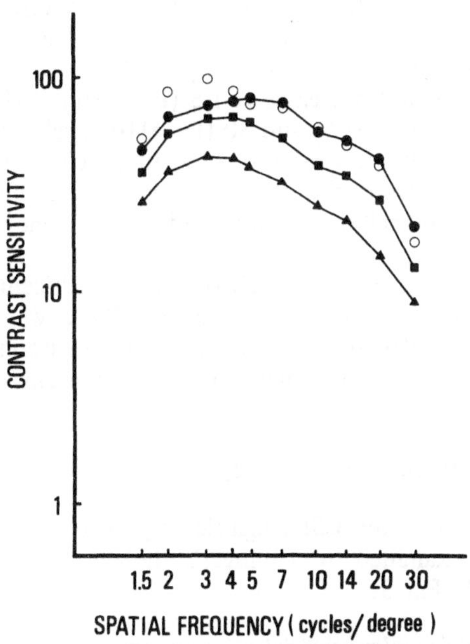

Fig. 1. Spatial contrast sensitivity functions (CSFs) in recovered optic neuropathy with various atrophic stages of maculopapillar bundles and the normal controls. ○, normal controls; ●–●, atrophic stage 1; ■–■, atrophic stage 2; ▲–▲, atrophic stage 3.

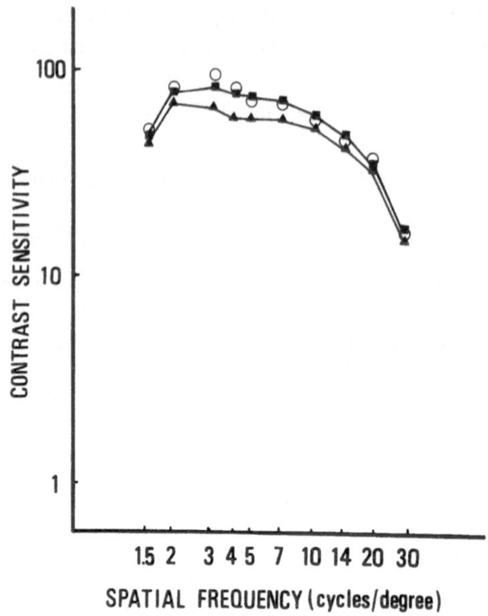

Fig. 2. CSFs in ocular hypertension, early glaucoma and the normal controls. ○, normal controls; ●—●, ocular hypertension; ▲—▲, early glaucoma.

examined spatial frequency in regard to the difference between the control and the patient's groups. In atrophic stage 1 of recovered optic neuropathy, the sensitivity was significantly decreased only at 3 cycles/degree ($P < 0.01$), as compared with the normal controls. In atrophic stage 2, the sensitivities were slightly decreased at all spatial frequencies, however, the statistical analysis revealed significant decreases at 1.5 ($P < 0.01$), 2 ($P < 0.01$), 3 ($P < 0.01$), 4 ($P < 0.05$), 7 ($P < 0.05$) and 30 ($P < 0.01$) cycles/degree. The sensitivities were significantly decreased at all spatial frequencies ($P < 0.01$) in atrophic stage 3. Even when the atrophic stages of maculopapillar bundles developed to stage 3, the bell-shaped, high and low frequency attenuation was not changed.

In early glaucoma cases, the sensitivity was significantly decreased at 3 ($P < 0.01$) and 4 cycles/degree ($P < 0.05$). There were no significant differences between ocular hypertension cases and the normal controls. The maculopapillar bundles in early glaucoma cases were almost normal states (stage 1) under red-free light.

2. CSFs and macular sensitivity by Tübinger's static perimetry

The attenuation ratio of the CSFs significantly correlates with that of the macular sensitivity examined by Tübinger's static perimetry ($r = 0.48$, $P < 0.01$) as illustrated in Fig. 3.

3. CSFs and foveolar sensitivity by quantitative maculometry

The attenuation ratio of the CSFs has no significant correlation with that of the foveolar sensitivity determined by Quantitative Maculometry ($r = -0.11$),

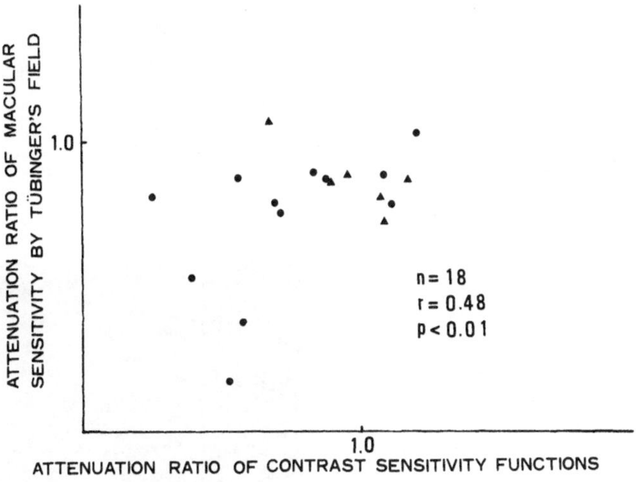

Fig. 3. Correlations between CSFs and macular sensitivity by Tübinger's static central field, •, recovered optic neuropathy; ▲, early glaucoma.

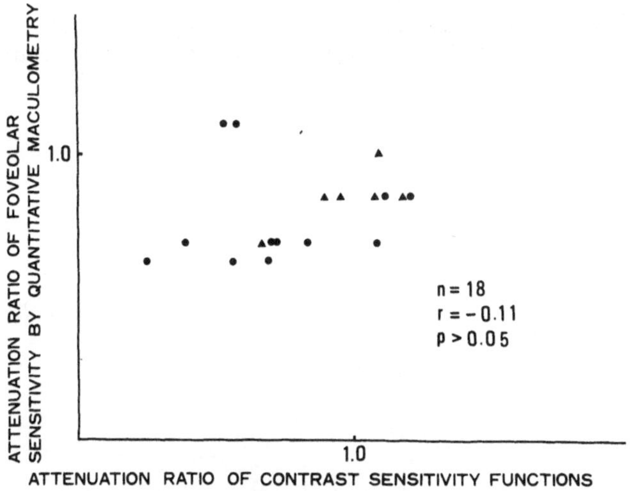

Fig. 4. Correlations between CSFs and foveal sensitivity by Quantitative Maculometry, •, recovered optic neuropathy; ▲, early glaucoma.

as illustrated in Figure 4. The foveolar sensitivities have relatively good values even when the CSFs are disturbed.

CASE REPORTS

For example, the CSF and Tübinger's static central field in a case of recovered optic neuropathy and early glaucoma are given in Figs. 5 and 6.

In a recovered optic neuropathy case, the CSF is decreased at all spatial frequencies and the Tübinger's static field shows a paracentral depression. In

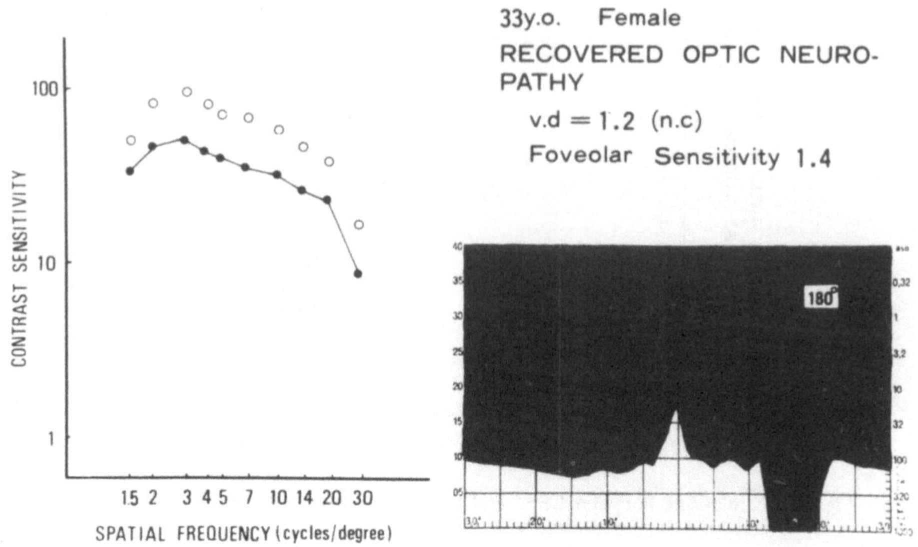

Fig. 5 CSF and Tübinger's static field in a case of recovered optic neuropathy. The foveal sensitivity by Quantitative Maculometry was 1.4 (the mean of the normal control 1.4).

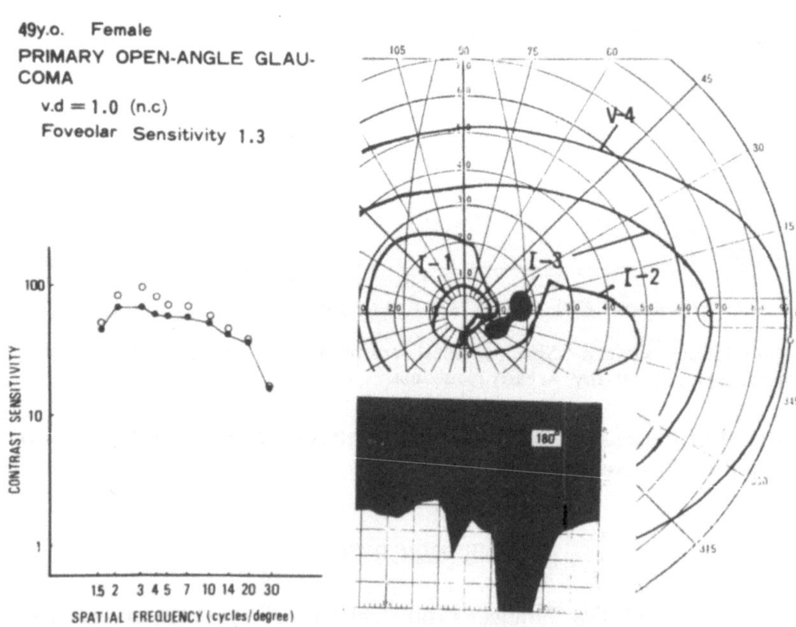

Fig. 6 CSF, Goldmann's kinetic field and Tübinger's static field in a case of early glaucoma. The foveal sensitivity by Quantitative Maculometry was 1.3 (the mean of the normal control 1.4).

an early glaucoma case, the CSF is slightly decreased at 3–4 cycles/degree and the Tübinger's static field shows a wedge-shaped paracentral depression. In each case, the foveolar sensitivity by Quantitative Maculometry is relatively good as compared with the normal controls.

DISCUSSION

The statistical analysis in the present study confirms our recent conclusion that the CSFs are disturbed in cases of recovered optic neuropathy and early glaucoma with good visual acuity, and gradually decrease as the atrophic states of the maculopapillar bundles develop ophthalmoscopically (6). In addition, the analysis also reveals the slight losses of the CSFs in the early stage of glaucoma, in which the central vision has been believed to be undisturbed until the late stages.

As to correlations between the CSFs and the visual field examinations, the sensitivity of the whole macular region examined by Tübinger's static field also decreased when the losses of the CSFs existed. However, the foveolar sensitivity examined by Quantitative Maculometry did not decrease even when the CSFs were disturbed. Most likely, the foveolar sensitivity corresponds to the good visual acuity in the conventional acuity tests (10). These facts indicate that the losses of the CSFs at the spatial frequency of 1.5 to 30 cycles/degree mainly correspond to the parafoveolar decreases in the static field tests in these cases.

In conclusion, both of CSF tests and accurate static visual field examinations are clinically useful for the detection of abnormal central vision in cases of optic neuropathy and glaucoma.

REFERENCES

1. Arden, G. B. & A. G. Gucukoglu. Grating test of contrast sensitivity in patients with retrobulbar neuritis. Arch. Ophthalmol. 96: 1626–1629 (1978).
2. Arden, G. B. & J. Jacobson. A simple grating test for results indicate value for screening in glaucoma. Invest. Ophthalmol. 17: 23–32 (1978).
3. Campbell, F. W. The transmission of spatial information through the visual system. The neurosciences third study program. 95–103, the MIT press, Cambridge, Massachusetts (1974).
4. Frisén, L. & T. Sjostrand. Contrast sensitivity in optic neuritis. Doc. Ophthalmol. Proc. Series 17: 165–174 (1978).
5. Isayama, Y. & Y. Tagami. Quantitative Maculometry using a new instrument in cases of optic neuropathies. Docum. Ophthalmol. Proc. Series 17: 237–242 (1977).
6. Isayama, Y., K. Mizokami & Y. Tagami. Spatial contrast sensitivity in optic nerve disorders. Jpn. J. Clin. Ophthalmol. 34: 293–300 (1980).
7. Regan, D., R. Silver & T. S. Murray. Visual acuity and contrast sensitivity in multiple sclerosis: hidden visual loss. Brain 100: 563–579 (1977).
8. Sekular, R. Spatial visuion. Ann. Rev. Psychol. 25: 195–232 (1974).
9. Sugimachi, Y., M. Futenma, M. Itoi, A. Nakajima, T. Kawara & H. Ohzu. Apparatus to measure interference fringe visual acuity and modulation transfer function. Jpn. J. Clin. Ophthalmol. 30: 1319–1323 (1976).
10. Tagami, Y. Correlations between atrophy of maculopapillar bundles and visual functions in cases of optic neuropathies. Doc. Ophthalmol. Proc. Series 19: 17–26 (1979a).

11. Tagami, Y. Atrophy of maculopapillar bundles in recovered optic neuropathies. Jpn. J. Ophthalmol. 23: 301–309 (1979b).
12. Zimmerman, R. L., F. W. Campbell & I. M. S. Wilkinson. Subtle disturbances of vision after optic neuritis elicited by studying contrast sensitivity. J. Neurol. Neurosurg. Psychiat. 42: 407–412 (1979).

Authors' address:
Department of Ophthalmology,
School of Medicine,
Kobe University
Kusunoki-cho, 7-chome,
Ikuta-ku, Kobe, 650
Japan

RICHARDSON-CROSS-LECTURE

EARLY DISTURBANCES OF COLOUR VISION IN CHRONIC OPEN ANGLE GLAUCOMA

STEPHEN M. DRANCE

(*Vancouver, Canada*)

INTRODUCTION

I am honoured by the invitation to join that distinctive group of ophthalmologists who have been invited to present the Francis Richardson Cross Lecture. I accept this invitation on behalf of a team of colleagues and technicians who have worked with me over the years. Francis Richardson Cross was a remarkable person whose life spanned 83 years until his death in 1931 from influenza. He practised ophthalmology until he was 80 years old and at the age of 78 was still operating with skill and steadiness. Born in Somerset, he received his medical education in London where he was influenced by Lister. He held ophthalmic posts at the Royal Ophthalmic Hospital and at King's College Hospital and was an evening Lecturer in physiology and a part-time demonstrator in anatomy in London. In Bristol he joined the Department of Anatomy and was then appointed into general surgery at the Royal Infirmary before becoming an ophthalmic surgeon in the Eye Department of the Royal Infirmary which he founded, and at the Eye Hospital which was in poor shape until reorganized by him. Cross became the first Dean of Medicine in 1880 and subsequently held the post of Lecturer and Reader in Ophthalmology. His academic accomplishments included the annual oration of the Medical Society of London, the Bradshaw Lecture of the Royal College of Surgeons, the Long Fox Lecture in Bristol and the Doyne Memorial Lecture at the Oxford Congress. His bibliography includes general surgical as well as many ophthalmological subjects, among them many of interest to the International Perimetric Society.

He was a striking looking man, over six feet in height, and white hair through most of his life. He became Sheriff of Bristol, President of the Grateful Society, and President of the Bristol Dolphin Society, as well as a Councillor Clifton College. Almost 50 years have now gone by since his death but it is clear that we are honoring a remarkable ophthalmologist.

Chronic open glaucoma is a disease in which the optic nerve suffers characteristic damage ultimately manifested by both cupping and excavation associated with characteristic nerve fibre bundle defects of the visual field. This neuropathy is usually accompanied by various degrees of elevations of intraocular pressure which may be either associated with the disease or causative. The neuropathy can also occur without any demonstrable elevations of

Doc. Ophthal. Proc. Series, Vol. 26, ed. by E. L. Greve & G. Verriest

intraocular pressure presumably because of the many other factors with which intraocular pressure can interact. Fifteen percent of glaucoma patients with visual field defects show no clearly recognizable changes at the optic nerve head, but in the remaining 85% there is good correlation between the optic nerve head appearance and a visual field defect (3). In many the cup of the optic nerve head enlarges symmetrically prior to the development of characteristic nerve fibre bundle defects (1). This makes it clear that disc changes usually precede visual field defects, but that field defects may occur prior to the appearance of characteristic and recognizable features at the optic nerve head. In recent years studies of visual functions other than increment thresholds have been carried out to see if abnormal functions occur before a visual field defect takes place. Such changes might have a better correlation with the early subtle appearances of the optic nerve head. Contrast sensitivity (2) and receptive field-like functions (4) has been found to be abnormal in glaucoma suspects prior to visual field disturbances. Neither of these two have yet been prospectively validated for their predictive value. Increased scatter of increment threshold response, tested kinetically and statically, were found to be abnormal in localized areas of the visual field which subsequently developed nerve fibre bundle disturbances (6).

COLOUR VISION AND ITS RELATIONSHIP TO CHRONIC OPEN ANGLE GLAUCOMA

Disturbances of colour vision have been described in the glaucomas since 1881. A number of workers found that the yellow/blue end of the spectrum was disturbed in glaucoma, while others suggested that red/green disturbances accompany the disease (Table 1). Much of this work was done prior to the differentiation between angle closure glaucoma and chronic open angle glaucoma and it is therefore difficult to sort out the differences between these conflicting reports. Studies (5) with the Farnsworth Munsell 100-Hue Test and the Pickford Nicholson Anomaloscope of 248 eyes in 248 patients with elevated intraocular pressure and 194 eyes with varying severity of glaucomatous visual field defects showed a correlation between the severity of visual field defects and the disturbance of colour discrimination. Eyes with elevated intraocular pressure showed poorer colour discrimination than eyes with normal pressure in people of the same age. In those eyes on pilocarpine there

Table 1. Colour vision disturbances in glaucoma.

Red/green disturbance		Yellow/blue disturbance	
1924	Koellner	1881	Bull
1926	Engelking	1959	Francois & Verriest
1927	Speciale *et al.*	1961	Ourgaud & Etienne
1960	DuBois Poulsen & Magis	1967	Ayers
1966	Zimmerman	1968	Meduri *et al.*
		1971	Krill & Fishman
		1972	Grutzner & Scheicher
		1979	Lakowski & Drance

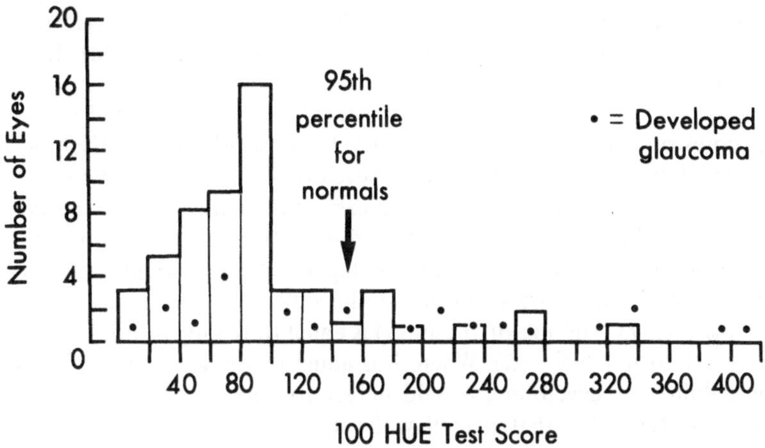

Fig. 1. Frequency distribution of eyes with elevated intraocular pressure followed for 5 years or more without developing a visual defect. The 100-Hue scores of the eyes that developed chronic open angle glaucoma during the follow-up period is also shown.

was poorer colour discrimination compared with untreated eyes. Nineteen percent of eyes with elevated intraocular pressure without pilocarpine had a colour score worse than the 95th percentile for normals, while in those on pilocarpine 50% had a score worse than the 95th percentile. In the advanced open angle glaucoma group 74% were above the 95th percentile for normals. With the Pickford Nicholson Anomaloscope the losses seemed to be most marked in the yellow/blue and blue/green part of the spectrum and were severe enough to amount to a Tritan or Tetartan defect.

We studied and followed 47 patients with elevated intraocular pressures who had their colour score examined more than 5 years earlier and who did not develop visual field defects during that period of time. In addition to that, 22 patients (24 eyes) developed field defects during the course of the 5 year follow-up. One eye of each of the 22 patients who developed open angle glaucoma were used to analyse the incidence of glaucoma in the groups with normal and poor colour discrimination (Fig. 1). Using the Chi Square test (Table 2) the incidence of glaucomatous visual field defects was significantly higher as the 100-Hue score increased. Of those whose 100-Hue scores was 100 or less, 19% developed visual field defects whereas of those whose

Table 2. 100-Hue scores of patients who developed glaucomatous field defects and ocular hypertensives followed for 5 years.

	100 Hue scores			
	0–100	101–200	>201	Total
No field defects	34	10	3	47
Field defects	8	4	10	22
Total	42	14	13	69

$\chi^2 = 15.43$ $P < 0.001$.

scores were over 200, 77% developed a field defect during the 5 year follow-up. These differences were statistically significant at the 0.001 level of probability.

We used Cox's method of logistical linear regression of the 100-Hue colour vision scores on the log of the odds of developing a field defect. Each person in the population has a probability of developing a nerve fibre bundle field defect. This probability appears to increase exponentially with the colour vision score (Table 2). The log of the probability of developing a defect is therefore approximately linear and the log of the probability of not developing a field defect is also linear. If the odds ratio of the i_{th} subject is $p_i/(1-p_i)$ then λi (the log of the odds) is equal to the log of $p_i/(1-p_i)$ and this is equal to $\alpha + \beta(x_i - \bar{x})$. Where λ is equal to the log of the odds, p_i is the probability of developing a field defect for the i_{th} patient and x_i the colour vision score for that person while $\bar{x}$ is the mean colour vision score for the group.

Utilizing the information from the 100-Hue tests the log odds (λ) is equal to $-1.9 + 0.005(x - 133.53)$. The probability that the slope was significantly different from zero is highly significant with a probability equal to 0.0062.

DISCUSSION

A number of visual functions have recently been shown to be abnormal in glaucoma suspects prior to the development of nerve fibre bundle defects of the classical type. In some of these, such abnormalities in contrast sensitivity and receptive field-like functions have not yet been shown to be followed by visual field defects but this is probable. Increased localized scatter of increment thresholds and colour vision disturbances reported in this paper have a validated predictive value of subsequent visual field defects compared with those in whom these visual functions were normal. As these visual function disturbances seem to occur earlier than the classical nerve fibre bundle defects it will be interesting to correlate them with the earliest tissue disturbances of the optic nerve head. Hopefully the change in structure would be accompanied by appropriate changes in function, even though the classical perimetric increment thresholds may not be sensitive enough to indicate such early functional disturbance. By utilizing the 100-Hue score of a suspect in the estimate of the log of the odds of developing a field defect one can work out the risks for the individual of developing subsequent visual field defects. This may have important prognostic value for an individual at risk. Although the risks of developing damage are much greater the more disturbed the colour score, some patients develop field defects with initial scores within the 95th percentile for the normal population. Even among those who already have the disease there are some whose colour scores show no abnormality, which would indicate that there are many patients in whom visual field disturbance is preceded by a disturbance in colour vision and others in whom no such disturbance precedes the field defect. The demonstration that there may be at least two mechanisms of developing a visual field defect in chronic open angle glaucoma should start research to explore if there are more mechanisms of damage which might explain some of the conceptual difficulties which we have had in understanding the disease.

REFERENCES

1. Anderson, D. R. & J. E. Pederson. The mode of progressive disc cupping in ocular hypertension and glaucoma. Arch. Ophthalmol. 98: 490 (1980).
2. Atkin, A., I. Bodies' Wollner, M. Wolkstein, A. Moss & S. Podos. In: Amer. J. Ophthalmol. 88: 205 (1979).
3. Drance, S. M., G. R. Douglas & M. Schulzer. A correlation of fields and discs in open angle glaucoma. Canad. J. Ophthalmol. 9: 391 (1974).
4. Enoch, J. M. & E. C. Campos. Analysis of patients with open angle glaucoma using perimetric techniques reflecting receptive field-like properties. Third International Visual Field Symposium, Tokyo. Doc. Opthal. Proc. Series. Ed. E. L. Greve. Junk Publishers, The Hague, p. 137 (1978).
5. Lakowski, R. & S. M. Drance. Acquired dyschromatopsias. The earliest functional losses in glaucoma. Third International Visual Field Symposium, Tokyo. Doc. Ophthal. Proc. Series. Ed. E. L. Greve. Junk Publishers, The Hague, pp. 173–159 (1978).
6. Werner, E. B. & S. M. Drance. Early visual field disturbances in glaucoma. Arch. Ophthalmol. 95: 1173 (1977).

Author's address:
Dr. S. M. Drance
2550 Willow Street
Vancouver V5Z 3N9
Canada

IS CLINICAL COLOUR PERIMETRY USEFUL?

ANDERS HEDIN & GUY VERRIEST

(Stockholm, Sweden/Ghent, Belgium)

ABSTRACT

Renewed interest has in recent years been paid to colour perimetry. The question has, however, been put forward whether perimetry with coloured targets is of any clinical value. The authors have therefore been asked by the IPS to present a report on 'the current status of colour perimetric testing and standards indicating specific diseases where colour provides information over and above that available when using white light perimetry'. This paper is a review of the current knowledge of the peripheral colour vision physiology and of studies where colour targets have given unique information. Because of space limitation, details of the physiology and of early studies are excluded; the reader is referred to recent papers by the authors (41, 85, 86).

What is colour perimetry? To some, it means measurements only in the periphery, i.e., outside the fovea. To others, it means measurements with the aid of a perimeter and includes the fixation point. Thresholds recorded are either chromatic or achromatic, a distinction of immense importance in studies outside the central part of the visual field. Other end-points are the hue variation or magnitude (or loss) of saturation of a coloured stimulus. All different tests will be covered in the paper, also foveal measurements, although we consider the extrafoveal visual field of primary importance when we talk about colour perimetry.

Some qualitative attributes of peripheral colour vision have been known since the beginning of the 19th century: colours lose saturation as they are moved outwards from the fixation point and most colours are subject to hue shifts. Quantitative aspects, on the other hand, have always been the subject of much debate, mainly because of the obvious dependence of the results on the experimental conditions. Examples of variables that need precise control are the state of adaptation and stimulus parameters like size, duration, luminance and chromaticity. Testing colour perception in the periphery is more complicated than foveal testing because of lower visual acuity and increased optical aberrations, rapid local adaptation (Troxler effect) and the uncertainty of peripheral visual judgements (62).

Ordinary colour vision tests unfortunately cannot be used in the periphery of the visual field (90). Outside 20–30°, pseudo-isochromatic plates are not read at all, and arrangement profiles become anarchic. Thus, for clinical studies of peripheral colour vision perimetric methods are necessary.

Doc. Ophthal. Proc. Series, Vol. 26, ed. by E. L. Greve & G. Verriest

PERIPHERAL COLOUR VISION PHYSIOLOGY

Colour discrimination at the retinal level

A prerequisite for understanding the psychology and psycho-physics of colour vision is some knowledge of the reactions at the cellular level. Naturally, human data are scarce, and some information must be deduced from studies of primates whose colour vision is similar to that of man.

According to the duplicity theory of vision, colour sense is mediated by cones and achromatic night vision by rods. In the peripheral field, however, rods do contribute to colour vision (73–76, 79, 80). Colour vision is mediated through a trichromatic receptor stage to an opponent response stage further centrally. At the receptor stage, there are three kinds of cones with maximum absorption of short wavelengths (B cones), medium wavelengths (G cones), or long wavelengths (R cones).

Some limit to the peripheral colour vision must be set by the total and relative number of cell elements in the different parts of the retina. The density of cones and ganglion cells steadily decreases from the fixation point outwards; most steeply within 10° (28). B cones are relatively less frequent; they are fewest in number in the fovea and densest at about 1°. From 5° to the outer periphery the proportion of the cone types are: B cones 13%, G cones 54%, and R cones 33% (55).

Retinal ganglion cells are divided according to their spectral response characteristics into colour-opponent and non-opponent classes. The latter class reacts with the same type of response to all wavelengths; reactions are phasic and the conduction velocity is high. Colour-opponent cells react with tonic maintained responses and their conduction velocity is lower. They are excited by some wavelengths and inhibited by others. Two or sometimes three cone types feed into each ganglion cell. In the parafoveal retina, rods also activate some opponent cells, and these can under dark adaptation change into non-opponent cells. Colour-opponent cells comprise the highest proportion near the fovea, non-opponent in the more peripheral part of the retina (1, 18, 19, 20, 32). It was recently shown that with sufficiently high flicker frequency colour-opponent cells can change to non-opponent cells with a different spectral response (33).

Little, if any, chromatic processing is thought to occur between the ganglion cells and cells of the geniculate nucleus. In the striate cortex, colour opponent cells have been found in 25–54% of the total number studied. Parafoveal cells are less frequently colour opponent than foveal cells (31, 32, 44).

Summarizing these data, we see that the density of cones and ganglion cells and the proportion of colour-opponent cells decrease with increasing distance from the fixation point. Impaired colour vision in the periphery is a logical consequence of these distributions.

Psycho-physics of peripheral colour vision

At the detection threshold, colour stimuli are seen coloured or colourless. In the latter case, colour perception is attained first at a higher intensity level.

The first threshold is then called the achromatic threshold and the second one is called the chromatic threshold. Between these is the photochromatic interval, which varies with stimulus characteristics, eccentricity and state of adaptation (72, 104).

In order that the stimulus shall be detected, the luminance threshold must be passed, i.e., a sufficient reaction of brightness-sensitive elements must be created. There is today firm evidence that brightness is mediated through both achromatic non-opponent and chromatic colour-opponent channels (38, 96). The contribution of the chromatic channels is the so-called chromatic brightness, which is relatively greater in the spectrum extremes (29). In order that the stimulus hue shall be identified, the chromatic brightness must reach a certain proportion of the total brightness response.* The spectral sensitivity is recorded by means of absolute thresholds, increment thresholds, brightness matching, or other methods (40, 48). The spectral sensitivity curve is not uniform, but varies with the relative response of the two brightness-mediating channels. In most situations, the threshold depends on the most sensitive of the two systems.

Flicker photometry and minimum border measurements provide monophasic curves pointing at about 555 nm and similar to the CIE V(λ) curve. These curves are supposed to depend on achromatic non-opponent channel activity. Another curve type, broader and with several humps and dips, is recorded when the absolute or increment thresholds are measured or using heterochromatic brightness matching. The humps are located at about 440 nm, 530 nm, and 600 nm. In these conditions, the colour opponent channels are also active, and the humps are claimed to show cone responses or interaction between cone mechanisms (69). Certain test situations favour the broader humped curve, as shown by King-Smith & Carden (45), Zrenner (112) and Ichikawa et al. (42). These are stimuli of long duration and large subtense and a high luminance background (Fig. 1). Possible reasons for this behaviour are greater spatial and temporal integration in the colour-opponent than in the non-opponent channels.

These data show that chromatic reactions can be studied using coloured stimuli and achromatic subject responses.

Under scotopic conditions, the spectral sensitivity does not vary with retinal eccentricity (apart from the pre-receptor absorption by, e.g., the macular pigment) and corresponds to the properties of rhodospin (47, 103).

The photopic spectral sensitivity varies, however, with retinal location. Lights of equal foveal brightness, i.e., lights equated for brightness according to the foveal luminosity function, may be drastically mis-matched when viewed peripherally (2).

The peripheral spectral sensitivity curves are, like the foveal, influenced by the test conditions. Thus, heterochromatic brightness matching, and absolute and increment threshold curves show several maxima (Fig. 2; 10, 11, 47, 70, 77, 82, 101, 102). Also, when increment thresholds are measured

* Recent papers on this matter were presented at the European Conference on Visual Perception, Noordwijkerhout, 1979 by a.o. Bauer & Cavonius and Burns, Smith, Pokorny & Elsner. A review on the detection and identification of coloured stimuli is that of Voke (94).

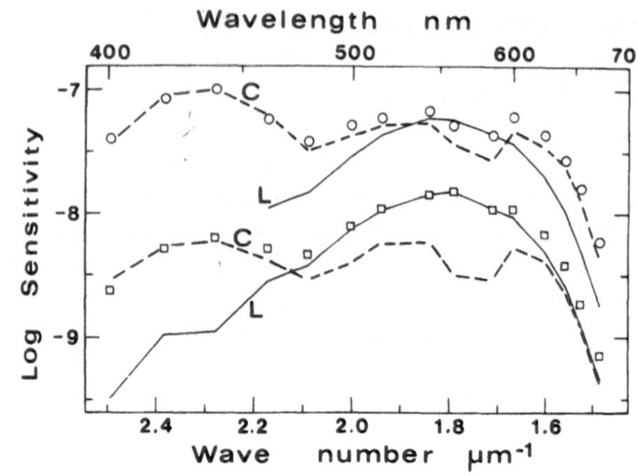

Fig. 1. Increment threshold spectral sensitivity curves; 1° test flashes on a 1000 td white background (symbols). Circles: 200 ms flashes; squares: 10 ms flashes. The curves show the deduced sensitivities of the luminance system (L, continuous curves), and the opponent-colour systems (C, dashed curves). (From King-Smith & Carden, 1976).

with the aid of a clinical perimeter calibrated in energies, irregularities of the curves appear (Fig. 3; 89).

The overall spectral sensitivity in the periphery differs from that of the fovea: short wavelength sensitivity is higher outside the fixation point (Figs. 2, 4; 2, 47, 70, 77, 97). This finding has been partly explained by the peripheral absence of the macular pigment. However, the main reason seems to be rod intrusion, even under conditions which foveally are considered purely photopic (74, 82, 100). Another possible reason is variations in the relative activity of the different cone classes (see below).

When results from several studies are put together, it is evident that short wavelength sensitivity increases from the fovea to about 10° and then possibly decreases (35, 107).

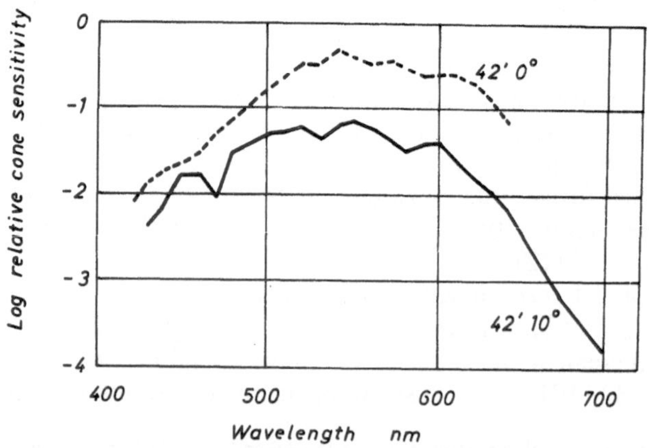

Fig. 2. Mean relative cone sensitivity curves. Dashed line: absolute thresholds of 42′ foveal stimuli. Continuous line: thresholds at the plateau of the dark adaptation curve at 10° eccentricity of 42′ stimuli. (From Sperling & Hsia, 1957).

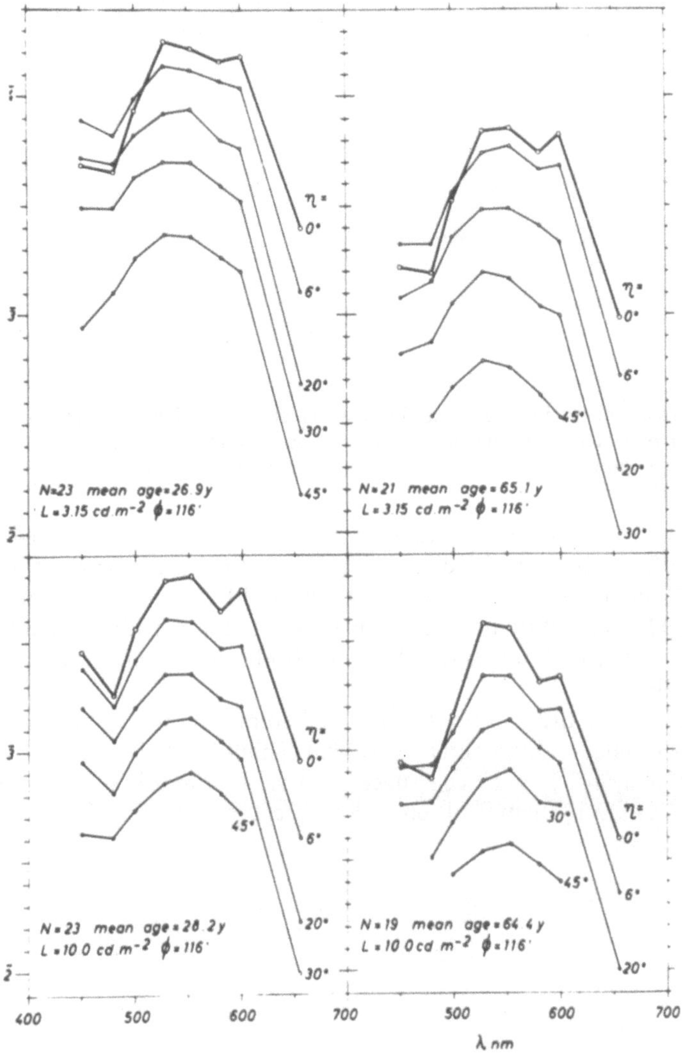

Fig. 3. Mean static achromatic thresholds to stimuli of different wavelength at different eccentricities as measured in the Tübinger perimeter. Low (upper curves) and high (lower curves) background luminance in younger (left two diagrams) and older (right two diagrams) subjects. (From Verriest & Kandemir, 1974).

In order to disclose the activity of a single cone class, chromatic backgrounds have been used to suppress the other two classes. Today, Wald's modification of Stiles' original method is mostly used; this technique comprises suppression of two cone classes with broad-banded coloured backgrounds (98). In the periphery, the method was used by Wald (99) and Wooten & Wald (108). The latter found that the sensitivity of all three cone mechanisms monotonically decreased from 7° outwards; the B cone mechanism was reduced to a greater extent, especially outside 40° (Fig. 5). The

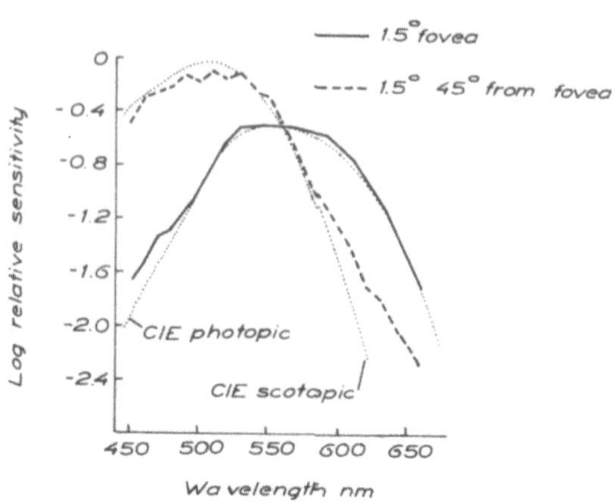

Fig. 4. Foveal and peripheral spectral sensitivity curves obtained with heterochromatic flicker at a photopic level. The curves have been equated at 560 nm. For comparison, the CIE photopic and scotopic curves have been added to the graph. (From Abramov & Gordon, 1977)

red and green components grew broader and more poorly separated peripherally. Results similar to Wooten & Wald's were recently shown by Obstfeld (67) for four meridians to an eccentricity of 30°. This author also found a considerable variability between individuals and for different colours and meridians. Chromatic backgrounds have also been used clinically, as will be discussed later.

The results of the two-colour threshold studies show that the dichromacy or monochromacy of the outer visual field cannot be explained by absence of cone mechanisms. It has been suggested that the impaired colour discrimination is caused by neural fusion and the great reduction of blue cones (102, 108).

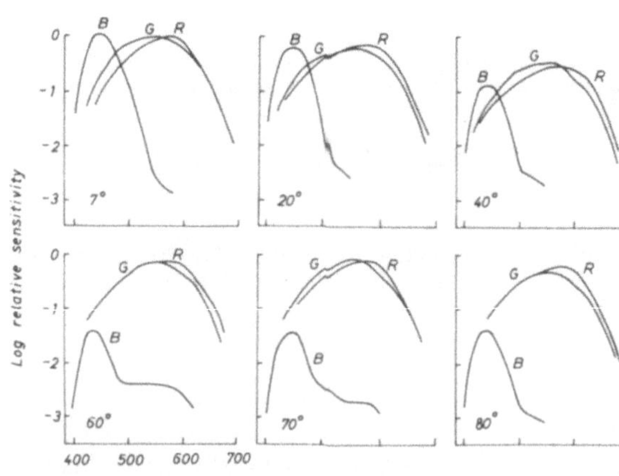

Fig. 5. Spectral sensitivities of the three colour mechanisms in the peripheral visual field of one normal trichromat. The maxima at the 7° locus have been arbitrarily brought to the same height; all other curves are relative to these maxima. (From Wooten & Wald, 1973)

As mentioned in the introduction, colour appearance varies with eccentricity. Not only are colours desaturated towards the periphery, but most colours also change their hue. Under certain test conditions, some colours are recognized at greater angles than others. In early studies, one searched the so-called invariable hues. Four colours were said to retain their hue until no longer detectable in the outer field. Using these, the 'colour zones' were mapped; yellow and blue zones were found more extensive than red and green ones. However, these studies lacked careful control of the experimental conditions, and first the works of Ferree & Rand (24) and Wentworth (104) were made with sufficient precision. These studies showed that the chromatic threshold increases with eccentricity; the increment slope, however, varies with both hue and meridian (Fig. 6). Equal-energy stimuli of different hue give non-identical colour fields. There are no 'invariable' hues. With a given stimulus brightness and retinal location, there exists a certain order of detectability, but this order may be reversed under other conditions. The form of the colour isopter thus varies with stimulus brightness. With sufficient target intensity, colour isopters reach out to the outer limit of the visual field. Colour zones contract with decreasing target size and under dark adaptation. In the latter condition, there is also a central depression for all colours.

Influence of target saturation on isopter size was more recently demonstrated by Carlow, Flynn & Shipley (8).

These studies show that it is futile to compare normal and pathological fields unless the testing conditions are identical. Ferree & Rand (24) standardized their test conditions and chose equal target/background lightness. This way, the subject's task was made easier, viz., only to signal target detection which on an equal lightness background must mean chromatic perception. Engelking & Eckstein's (21) test plates work on a similar basis. The equal lightness colour plate is selected and can then be used to show red-green or yellow-blue isopter contraction in acquired colour vision deficiencies.

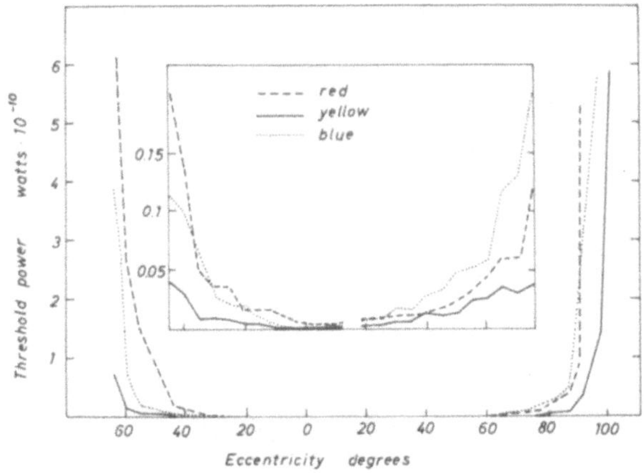

Fig. 6. Chromatic thresholds to red, yellow and blue stimuli on the horizontal meridian under light adaptation. Inset shows the central field expanded. (From Wentworth, 1930).

The peripheral colour zone irregularities were confirmed by colour-identification studies which demonstrated significant fluctuations in the peripheral cutoffs (12, 13). Irregular curves and desaturation were shown by Boynton, Schafer & Neun (7) by a colour-naming procedure. Reduced colour discrimination mimicking a red-green colour deficiency was found, as recently confirmed by Graham (34). With small targets, peripheral desaturation and uncertain hue responses were shown by Gordon & Abramov (30) at 45°. Their findings, however, pointed at a tritan type of peripheral deficiency.

Wavelength discrimination in the periphery

The deterioration found in colour-naming procedures has been quantified in studies of wavelength discrimination thresholds and by colour matching.

Weale (102) and Moreland (62) showed impaired wavelength discrimination towards the periphery, most evident in the medium spectral region at about 520 nm (Fig. 7). Recently it was shown, however, that this deterioration first appeared under dark adaptation, whereby rods were supposed to cause the effect (77).

By colour matching, a progressive, brightness dependent, reduction of the spectrum locus with increasing distance from the fixation point has been shown (Fig. 8; 10, 11, 63). The impairment was compatible with a gradual deterioration of colour vision almost to monochromacy at 40–50°. The findings could be explained by postulating either an increasing influence of neural links or rod intrusion towards the periphery. Recent measurements were performed at the cone plateau (73–75). In the periphery, hue shifts of red and green towards yellow and from violet towards blue were found.

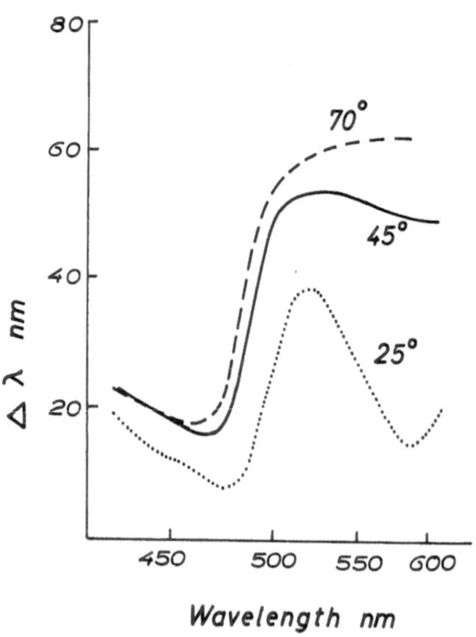

Fig. 7. Wavelength discrimination thresholds at different locations with a low luminance target. Individual data points of the original graph have been omitted. (From Weale, 1953).

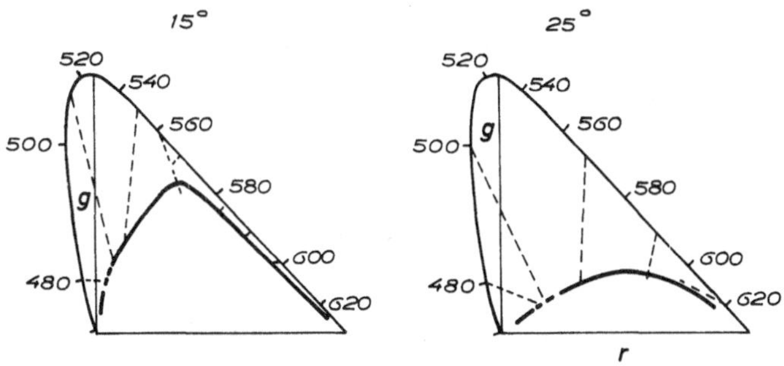

Fig. 8. Asymmetric colour matches between a 15° (left) and a 25° (right) test stimulus and a R + G + B foveal comparison field. Data are plotted in the WDW chromaticity chart; r and g are the relative admixtures of the red and green primary stimuli. The thick line is the extrafoveal spectrum locus. For reference, the thin line shows the subject's foveal spectrum locus. Dashed lines show examples of how spectral stimuli change localization with eccentricity. (From Moreland, 1972).

Suggested reasons were broader cone absorption curves, changes in the relative contribution of the cone mechanisms or neural pathway fusion. After completed dark adaptation, the changes were similar but more extensive and supposed to depend also upon rod intrusion.

Saturation thresholds

Verduyn Lunel & Crone (81) measured the saturation thresholds for colours of different hue in different locations of the visual field. They showed that thresholds increased along the temporal meridian for all hues; yellow-green was most desaturated, blue-green and red least. In a later modification of the apparatus (82), the background luminance was raised to 900 cd. m^{-2} in order further to suppress rod activity. Using 16 wavelengths, spectral sensitivity and saturation thresholds were measured. Normals showed outside 20° a distinct impairment of saturation sensitivity with a neutral zone around 550 nm, i.e., a tritan type of colour vision (Fig. 9).

Arizaga & Mattiello (4) measured the foveal and 20° magnitude of saturation. Low stimulus brightness was accompanied by reduced saturation sensation. In the periphery, red and green stimuli retained their magnitude better than yellow and blue stimuli.

Rod intrusion

It has been pointed out above that rods may influence spectral sensitivity and colour discrimination in the periphery. It has also been shown that chromatic thresholds increase after the cone-rod break in dark adaptation. The effect is most pronounced for medium wavelengths, and the sensitivity loss can be explained by an achromatic desaturant added by rods (3, 74, 106). Evidence for a common rod and B cone pathway has been presented by Trezona (79, 80).

Rods are supposed to saturate at a luminance level of 120–300 cd. m^{-2}

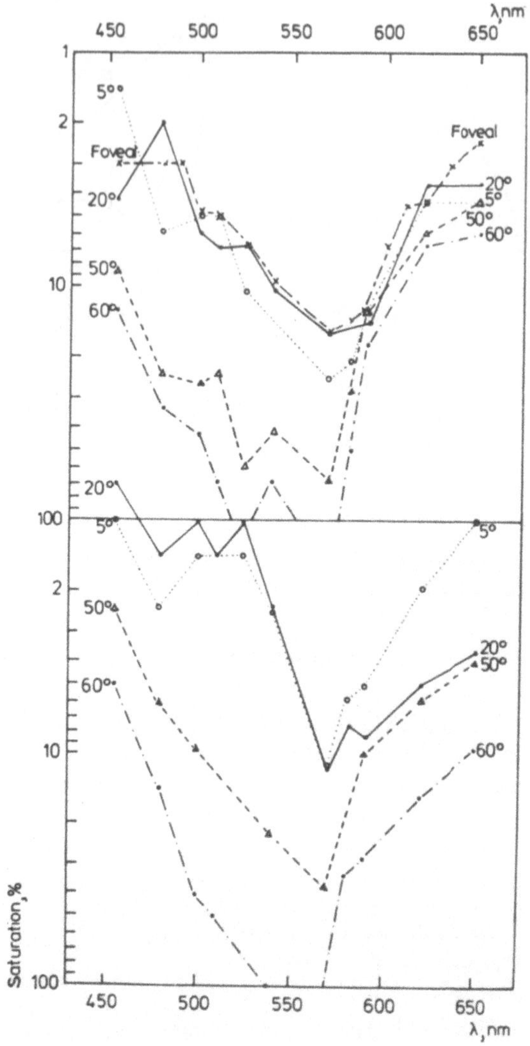

Fig. 9. Saturation thresholds at different eccentricities and for different wavelengths; two normal observers. Ordinate shows percentage of spectral light necessary for colour perception. (From Verduyn Lunel & Crone, 1978)

(78) which means that rod activity cannot be excluded in many of our routine examinations.

CLINICAL COLOUR PERIMETRY

Thresholds and clinical potentials

In clinical colour perimetry, the end-points most frequently used are the achromatic and the chromatic threshold. The former only demands mere detection of the stimulus, and variability is not much greater than in white light perimetry (53, 87). When measuring the chromatic thresholds, however, the subject is faced with a much more difficult task, viz., to signal when he perceives a chromatic component in the stimulus. This does not mean the same to all subjects, and variability is further exaggerated by the irregular borders of the colour zones. Even worse is the situation when the subject is asked to recognize a given colour (5, 43). Great testing difficulties arise even with trained subjects (6).

Under certain adaptation conditions and with certain stimulus hues, the threshold for light perception is lowest for rods *or* cones. Under photopic conditions and with certain target/background characteristics, the spectral response is dominated by colour-opponent mechanisms. When measuring the photo-chromatic interval, wavelength discrimination limens or saturation thresholds, the colour-opponent mechanisms also determine the results obtained. With chromatic backgrounds, single cone classes can be studied more or less isolated.

Thus, using coloured targets and with an appropriate selection of test conditions it should be possible to disclose

1. cone or rod dysfunction
2. dysfunction of isolated cone classes
3. colour-opponent damage

Diseases possibly giving rise to these defects would include retinal dystrophies or inflammatory conditions, optic nerve diseases etc.

Early colour perimetry

Coloured pigment stimuli were used already by Köllner (51) to demonstrate peripheral acquired colour vision defects. He measured chromatic thresholds and showed that the blue isopter is contracted in chorioretinal disorders while in optic nerve diseases the red and green isopters are reduced. Wilbrand & Sänger (105) showed that the photochromatic interval is increased in optic nerve disorders.

These studies lacked careful control of the test conditions. The first clinical study where the problems were considered is that of Zanen (110). He used monochromatic stimuli and measured the static foveal achromatic and chromatic thresholds in various diseases and confirmed some of the results above.

Achromatic colour perimetry with red objects was earlier used to reveal conduction defects and it was claimed that red fields might be disturbed when corresponding white fields are not. In later studies, it has not been possible to verify differences between white and coloured fields in conduction disorders (16, 22). Colour can be used to reduce stimulus brightness whereby a greater size target can substitute a small white one. These targets are less sensitive to ametropia and possibly easier to work with. Even within liberal definitions, this is not *colour* perimetry, however.

In order to disclose cone or rod dysfunction, red and blue objects have been used. Red and blue achromatic threshold profiles were recorded in Goldmann-Weekers' adaptometer and the Tübinger perimeter and revealed specific disturbances in diseases affecting the rod and cone systems (37, 113).

Sloan & Feiock (68) showed that the white light increment thresholds for normal rods and cones are about equal at a luminance level similar to that of the Tübinger perimeter ($3\,cd.m^{-2}$). With a red object, the achromatic rod threshold was raised almost 20 dB whereby cone thresholds could be selectively studied in cases of cone degeneration. Recently, Massof & Finkelstein (60) used red and blue-green targets in the Tübinger perimeter to map the extension of rod and cone dysfunction in various forms of retinitis pigmentosa.

Colour thresholds in the Goldmann and Tübinger perimeters

It was earlier stressed that colour perimetry demands careful control of the experimental conditions. The two common apparatuses for clinical perimetry provide neutral stable backgrounds and certain colour stimuli. In several studies, thresholds to chromatic stimuli have been recorded using these two perimeters.

Verriest (83, 84) used the Goldmann perimeter and showed that kinetic achromatic and chromatic colour isopters were abnormal in some eye disorders. Verriest & Israel (88) calibrated the targets and background of the Goldmann perimeter. They then measured the static achromatic thresholds to white, red, green, and blue objects at 0–50° in normals and subjects with congenital colour vision deficiencies. In the periphery, a relative increase in blue sensitivity was found. Findings in the deficient subjects were in the expected directions, i.e., reduced red sensitivity in protans etc. The differences were not, however, fully explained by assuming a luminous sensitivity shift equal to that of the fovea.

François, Verriest & Israel (25) used the same equipment to study acquired visual deficiencies. Wavelength specific sensitivity reductions were found in yellow/blue and type I red/green deficiencies; only minor abnormalities in red/green type II deficiencies, however. The results of this kind of perimetry was held to be easier to interpret than those of foveal pigment tests like pseudo-isochromatic charts. Maione & Carta (53) using kinetic Goldmann perimetry confirmed the early findings of contracted red and green isopters in retrobulbar neuritis.

Recently, the Goldmann perimeter has been modified to provide stimuli and backgrounds of high luminance (52). Preliminary studies of static achromatic thresholds to white and coloured stimuli showed selective sensitivity losses in a few subjects with colour vision deficiencies.

The Tübinger perimeter makes possible a greater selection of stimulus hues and easier static measurements. With this perimeter, Nolte (66) measured retinal profiles in normal eyes. Calibrations of stimuli and backgrounds were performed by Verriest, Padmos & Greve (91) and Kitahara & Ichikawa (49). Verriest & Kandemir (89) measured the static achromatic increment thresholds to nine wavelengths on backgrounds of different luminance. Mesopic trends were evident with a background luminance equal to or less than $3.15\,cd.m^{-2}$. Additional data were collected using 3.15 and $10\,cd.m^{-2}$ backgrounds, the latter giving responses of photopic character. Increment threshold spectral sensitivity curves at different locations were not smooth but multihumped with maxima for the filters 451, 528 and 600 nm. These humps were supposed to reflect activity in chromatic mechanisms, which is reasonable considering the test conditions: large stimuli of long duration (44–116′, 500 ms) and rather high background luminance. Towards the periphery, the red and green humps were less clearly separated (Fig. 3).

The achromatic thresholds were shown to depend to a high degree on the subject's age. Subjects with congenital colour vision deficiencies not only lacked one hump, but their thresholds were overall higher than those of normals (92).

120 pathological eyes were also studied (93). In general, the results were similar to those of the earlier study with the Goldmann perimeter. Abnormality was either wavelength specific or covered the whole spectrum (Fig. 10). Some subjects with optic neuritis showed increased short wavelength sensitivity. Peripheral abnormality was found in some diseases seemingly restricted to the fovea. Colour perimetry was sensitive also in cases with normal white light perimetry and normal visual acuity. It was further found that colour perimetry in the fovea was more sensitive than a battery of traditional colour vision tests. In a similar way, Marmion (56) showed that static colour perimetry was more sensitive than the 100-hue test in exudative diabetic retinopathy.

Colour thresholds in other perimeters

Nemtseev (65) used yellow and red stimuli in a bowl perimeter to detect nasal steps in glaucoma. Defects were evident both by achromatic and chromatic thresholds. Superiority to white objects was, however, not discussed. Friedmann (26) tested subjects with open angle glaucoma and optic nerve disease with coloured targets in the visual field analyser. In the few cases studied, scotomas were deeper and more extensive with coloured filters.

Perimetry with chromatic backgrounds

As discussed earlier, selective suppression of one or two cone classes can be achieved using a chromatic background of sufficient intensity. Most often, a yellow background is used to isolate the B cones, a purple for the G cones, and a blue for the R cones. This way, valuable information of the foveal colour vision has been obtained both in normals and subjects with various eye disorders (58). The same principle has also come to use in perimetry. It demands, however, high background and target luminance and careful calibration of the apparatus. Recent reports show that these problems can be solved (39, 50, 52). Due consideration must be paid to the normal variation of the cone mechanisms with eccentricity (57, 108).

Using this principle, it was shown that static measures of the blue thresholds on a yellow background was a sensitive test in cases with macular edema (36). Hansen (39) modified and calibrated the Goldmann perimeter to provide backgrounds of three colours and test stimuli of nine wavelengths. By measuring the static achromatic thresholds at different locations, profiles along meridians and spectral sensitivity curves were obtained (Fig. 11). Among the results were selective depressions of rods or certain cone classes

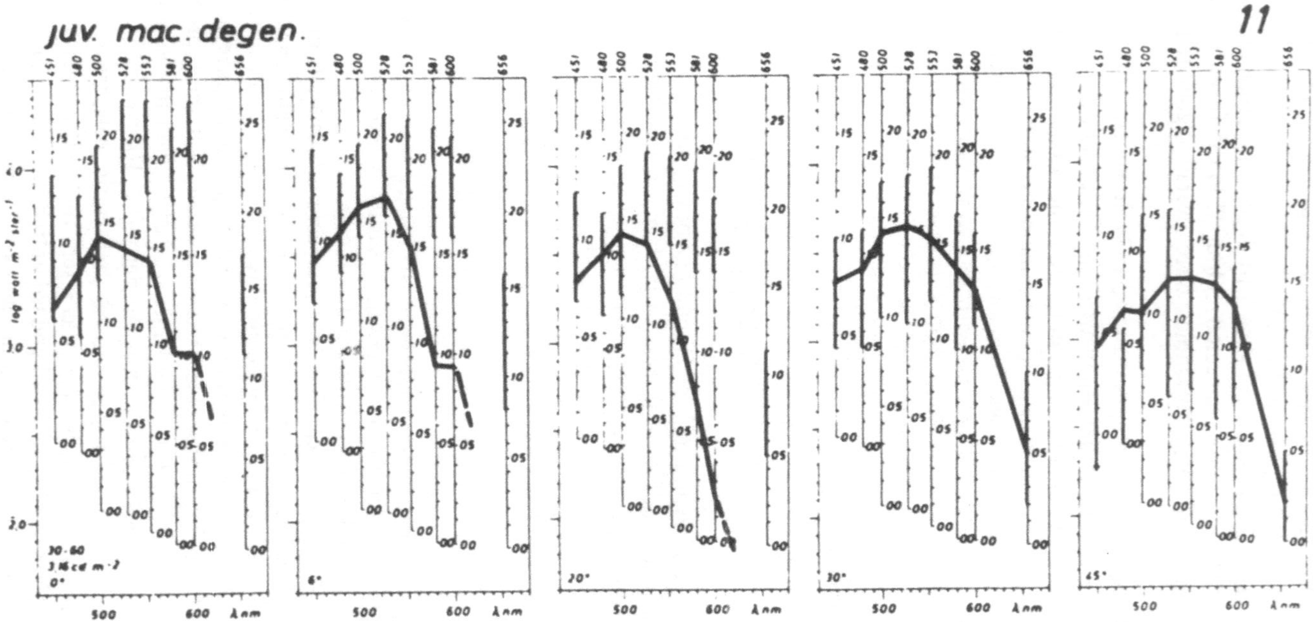

Fig. 10. Achromatic thresholds measured in the Tübinger perimeter in a case of juvenile macular degeneration (*cf.* normal spectral sensitivity in Fig. 3). Thick vertical lines show normal ranges. At 0–20° long wavelength sensitivity is reduced making the curves similar to scotopic sensitivity curves. (From Verriest & Uvijls, 1977b)

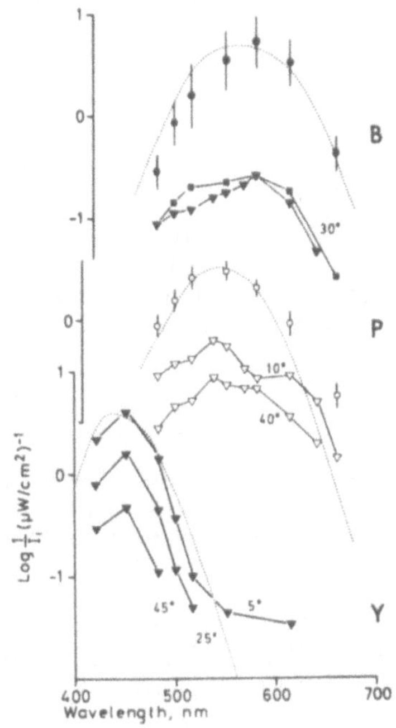

Fig. 11. Spectral sensitivity curves of normals measured in the Goldmann perimeter with coloured backgrounds; B = blue background, P = purple background, and Y = yellow background. Circles show foveal registrations; the others are eccentric according to the graph. Dotted lines show the red, green, and blue primaries of Walraven, 1974. (From Hansen, 1979)

in chloroquine retinopathy, cone dystrophies and retinitis pigmentosa (Fig. 12). Some of the subjects, as well as others with cerebromacular degeneration, amblyopia, or Refsum's disease, showed selective depression of one or several cone classes in restricted visual field areas. The method thus enabled detection and mapping of areas with impaired receptor function. Another study showed that the method can be used to differentiate between blue cone monochromacy and rod monochromacy.

Maione and coll. (54, 64) have used the Goldmann perimeter equipped with filters to provide coloured backgrounds of moderate brightness. Six or seven test colours were used. In the latter paper, the spectral sensitivity curves in the fovea and at 20° showed several humps attributed to some of Stiles' mechanisms. In optic neuritis and macular degeneration, selective sensitivity reductions were found; the peripheral data, however, not giving any information over the foveal.

Vola and coll. (95) recorded in the Tübinger perimeter the foveal thresholds for red and green stimuli on a red background. The threshold versus intensity curves showed several discontinuities similar to those of Stiles' original data. Some patients with congenital colour vision deficiencies or optic neuritis differed from the normals.

Promising results were recently published by Marré, Marré & Schreiber

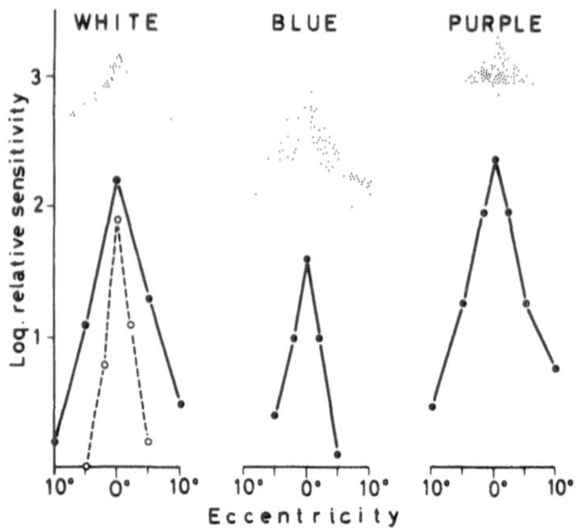

Fig. 12. Static achromatic thresholds at various eccentricities measured in the Goldmann perimeter with white and coloured backgrounds. Dotted areas: ranges of normal variation. Curves are from a case of retinitis pigmentosa. The stimuli were for the blue background 617.5 nm and for the purple background 562.5 nm. (From Hansen, 1979)

(57). They recorded the achromatic kinetic thresholds for a blue stimulus on a yellow background of 38 $cd.m^{-2}$. Out of 104 subjects with open angle glaucoma and normal white light perimetry, 57% showed arcuate scotomas or nasal steps with colour perimetry. A possible reason for these findings is an early yellow-blue opponent cell damage. B cones mediate brightness to a very small extent and the supposed dysfunction if therefore concealed when white stimuli are used.

Other methods

Yokoi (109) measured the critical fusion frequency with white and coloured stimuli in the Tübinger perimeter. This way retinal diseases were differentiated from optic nerve disease. Matsuo (61) showed that, in patients with glaucoma, the critical fusion frequency for red but not white objects was reduced in Bjerrum's area.

Spatial summation and early adaptation has also been studied with the aid of coloured targets in the Tübinger perimeter (14, 15).

Supra-threshold saturation studies

Desaturation is a feature of certain eye disorders that has been used to reveal visual field defects. Chamlin (9) presented a red object on both sides of the vertical meridian; relative visual field defects were characterized by a colour shift to pink or white. Frisén (27) used a self-luminous red or green object which was moved in a circle 10–20° from the visual axis. This test proved to be highly sensitive in subtle conduction defects. Defects showed up by a desaturation from red to orange, yellow or white; the green object looked pale blue or white. Thanks to the circular movement, peripheral hue shifts and local adaptation bias were avoided.

Supra-threshold moving stimuli have also been used in the perimeter (17).

In early chiasmal lesions, this technique was more sensitive than static or kinetic threshold perimetry. Coloured stimuli were superior to white, and among hues, red gave most positive results. Confrontation testing with suprathreshold pigment tests were frequently falsely negative. Another suprathreshold saturation test comprises simultaneous presentation of two identical coloured objects in the Goldmann perimeter (23). The stimuli were produced by the addition of prisms to the original projection system.

CONCLUSIONS

In this paper we have seen that colour vision deteriorates with increasing eccentricity in the visual field: hue-identification grows worse, wavelength discrimination thresholds rise, and the whole gamut of colours shrinks. Chromatic thresholds rise in an irregular manner depending on the test conditions. Spectral sensitivity is locus-specific and changes with retinal adaptation and recording procedure. Reasons for these findings are evident in the basic physiology.

We can easily see that strict demands must be made on experimental conditions if clinical tests of peripheral colour vision should express anything but the peculiar behaviour of the normal eye. In threshold studies, background luminance and colour, and test object intensity, chromaticity, size, and duration must be carefully controlled. It is better to use monochromatic stimuli, because their spectral distribution is not influenced by changes in the ocular media. Also, for the assessment of spectral sensitivity curves and of Stiles-Wald mechanisms, the object intensities have to be known in radiances.

It is evident that colour perimetry can be performed in a number of different ways. All comprise the use of colour stimuli, but these may be presented in dark adaptation, on white or coloured backgrounds of different intensities, kinetic or static etc. Quantitative data or qualitative attributes may be recorded. Foveal measurements are possible but colour *perimetry* demands that also the extrafoveal visual field can be studied. This is self-evident when the measurements are performed using a perimeter.

Many of the studies reviewed have proven that colour perimetry has given unique information of definite clinical value. Disorders dominated by impairment of rods or cones have been diagnosed with stimuli to which one or the other of the two receptor classes is much more sensitive (37, 68). Dysfunction of isolated cone mechanisms has been shown with two-colour methods and in records of the spectral sensitivity where chromatic mechanisms are dominating. The works of a.o. Verriest and Hansen have demonstrated the character and extent of cone damage in a number of eye diseases. Of special interest are the facts that peripheral abnormality can be evidenced in so-called macular disorders and that colour perimetry often is more sensitive than ordinary clinical tests of the foveal visual capacity.

In the recent studies by Marré *et al.* (57) and Friedmann (26), colour perimetry proved especially valuable. Glaucomatous visual field defects were *only* revealed by colour perimetry or were more extensive than with white objects. Importance is evident, since we know that white light perimetry is abnormal first when a large number of nerve fibers are damaged.

The special characteristics of the colour-opponent cells make them possibly more easily damaged in conduction defects or retinal disorders. A pure colour-opponent damage may show up by a smoothing out of the spectral sensitivity curve. For the fovea, this alteration has been shown in a few subjects (42, 46, 111). Also the contrary may be seen, i.e., an increased cone mechanism interaction (71, 93). It remains to be proven, however, that these abnormalities are of significance in the extrafoveal visual field.

Another manifestation of colour-opponent damage is impaired wavelength discrimination and desaturation. Wavelength discrimination is difficult to measure, especially in the periphery, and thus so far outside clinical interest. Threshold and supra-threshold saturation studies can, however, be performed with reasonable demands on the observer, as shown by Dannheim (16), Frisén (27) and Verduyn-Lunel & Crone (81, 82). With supra-threshold saturation tests, information of great clinical importance have been obtained.

With colour perimetry, it may be easier to disclose abnormal spectral sensitivity than using other tests. Foveal spectral sensitivity measurements are not possible with routine instruments; the reduced sensitivity may be easily revealed by a contracted colour isopter, however.

In several studies, colour perimetry has shown discrepancies from normality in eye disorders with other evident clinical characteristics. The *clinical* interest of colour perimetry is naturally restricted in, e.g., cases of retinitis pigmentosa with the eyeground mottled with pigmentations. Scientifically it may be of interest, however, to characterize and map the extent of the defect in these cases.

In some studies showing abnormal colour perimetry, superiority over other tests has not been proven. Further research may show this to be the case, however.

In summary, colour perimetry demands careful consideration of the test conditions in order to be meaningful. Calibrated apparatuses with specifications superior to those today available for clinical studies are necessary (see Appendix). When performed adequately, the method has already provided information of high interest. Therefore, clinical colour perimetry *is* useful.

APPENDIX

As chairman of the IPS research group on colour perimetry, G. Verriest has presented a report on the results of a questionary concerning the technical demands on colour perimeters. The following is the conclusion of that report:

In view of the further development of research in increment threshold colour perimetry and in view of its clinical application, it is desired that commercially available perimeters could be adapted and/or completed as follows:

1. The actual incandescence lamp could be replaced by a light source of higher intensity, as a halogen lamp, with control of its voltage and intensity; it

should be beneficial (but not necessary) that its correlated colour temperature should be higher than that of the CIE standard illuminant A.

2. The white background luminance could be augmented gradually or in steps to $\log_{10}$ cd. m^{-2} = 1.5, this is to 31.62 cd. m^{-2} (= 99.34 asb) in the full bowl extent.
3. A moveable fixation mark and a supplementary restricted fixed background field of at least 11° extent should be available; the maximal unfiltered luminance of this supplementary restricted background should reach gradually or in steps to 2000 cd. m^{-2} (= 6282 asb).
4. The white object luminance could be augmented in the usual 1 dB (= 0.1 $\log_{10}$ un.) steps to $\log_{10}$ cd. m^{-2} = 3.5, this is to 3162 cd. m^{-2} (= 9934 asb) or, still better and if possible, to 10000 cd. m^{-2} (= 31416 asb) or more, the range of attenuation by neutral density filters being extended, in view of perimetry with white lights, in proportion to the extension of the range between the background and target maximal luminance.
5. The object light could be filtered by narrow band (half height width ⩽ 20 nm) interference filters (when necessary combined with blocking filters), and of which the spectral transmittance curves peak either all 20 nm from 420 to 660 nm, or (when the number of filters is limited to 9) at 440, 470, 500, 525, 555, 570, 585, 600 and 640 nm.
6. The supplementary restricted background light could be filtered by broad band filters either to the same dominant wavelengths as that used for the object, or to yellow, blue, and purple lights (as specified in the answer in question 16 of the questionary).
7. The selective filters could be easily removed and replaced.
8. The constructor has to measure and to supply all relevant data concerning the intensity and spectral distribution of the light source, the spectral reflectance of the bowl, the spectral transmittance of all filters, the maximal radiances of all (nearly) monochromatic lights; the constructor has also to deliver a calibrated luxmeter and a standard light source in order that the user could check (but not measure) the luminances and radiances.
9. It is stressed that these recommendations do not include the least idea of setting standards for white or colour perimetry.

REFERENCES

1. Abramov, I. Retinal mechanisms of colour vision. In: Physiology of photoreceptor organs (M. G. F. Fuortes, ed.), 567–607 (1972).
2. Abramov, I. & J. Gordon. Color vision in the peripheral retina. I. Spectral sensitivity. J. Opt. Soc. Am. 67: 195–201 (1977).
3. Ambler, B. A. Hue discrimination in peripheral vision under conditions of dark and light adaptation. Percep. Psychophys. 15: 568–590 (1974).
4. Arizaga, R. A. & M. L. F. Mattiello. Influence of retinal locus on the discrimination of colorimetric purity. In: Color Vision Deficiencies V, Bristol, Adam Hilger (1980), pp. 207–210.
5. Aulhorn, E. & H. Harms. Visual perimetry. Handbook of sensory physiology VII/4: 102–145 (1972).
6. Barca, L. & G. Vaccari. Some remarks on the estimate of photochromatic interval in peripheral vision. Atti Fond. G. Ronchi 32: 859–873 (1977).

7. Boynton, R. M., W. Schaefer & M. E. Neun. Hue-wavelength relation by color-naming method for three retinal locations. Science 146: 666–668 (1964).
8. Carlow, T. J., J. T. Flynn & T. Shipley. Color perimetry parameters. Doc. Ophthalmol. Proc. Ser. 14: 427–429 (1977).
9. Chamlin, M. Minimal defects in visual field studies. Arch. Ophthalmol. 42: 126–139 (1949).
10. Clarke, F. J. J. Extra-foveal colour metrics. Optica Acta 7: 355–384 (1960).
11. Clarke, F. J. J. Further studies of extra-foveal colour metrics. Optica Acta 10: 257–284 (1963).
12. Connors, M. M. & P. A. Kelsey. Shape of red and green colour zone gradients. J. Opt. Soc. Am. 51: 874–877 (1961).
13. Connors, M. M. & J. A. Kinney. Relative red-green sensitivity as a function of retinal position. J. Opt. Soc. Am. 52: 81–84 (1962).
14. Conreur, L. & G. Meur. Influence de la longueur d'onde du stimulus lumineux dans les phénomènes de sommation spatiale rétinienne. Bull. Soc. Belge Ophthalmol. 143: 532–541 (1966).
15. Conreur, L., G. Meur & A. Zanen. Utilisation de stimuli colorés dans l'étude de l'adaptation locale précoce (Note préliminaire). Bull. Soc. Belge Ophthalmol. 143: 542–547 (1966).
16. Dannheim, F. Kinetic perimetry with supra-threshold stimuli. Doc. Ophthalmol. Proc. Ser. 14: 385–388 (1977).
17. Dannheim, F. Color perimetry in chiasmal lesions. Doc. Ophthalmol. Proc. Ser. 14: 449–455 (1977).
18. Daw, N. Neurophysiology of color vision. Physiol. Rev. 53: 571–611 (1973).
19. De Valois, R. L. Physiological basis of color vision. Die Farbe 20: 151–169 (1971).
20. De Valois, R. L. Processing of intensity and wavelength information by the visual system. Invest. Ophthalmol. 11: 417–427 (1972).
21. Engelking, E. & A. Eckstein. Physiologische Bestimmung der Musterfarben für die klinische Perimetrie. Klin. Monatsbl. Augenheilkd. 64: 88 (1920).
22. Enoksson, P. Perimetry in neuro-ophthalmological diagnosis. Acta Ophthalmol. (Kbh) Suppl. 82 (1965).
23. Enoksson, P. & B. Friström. Double point test with the Goldmann perimeter. Acta Ophthalmol. (Kbh) 53: 834–838 (1975).
24. Ferree, C. E. & G. Rand. Effect of brightness of preexposure and surrounding field on breadth and shape of the color fields for stimuli of different sizes. Am. J. Ophthalmol. 7: 843 (1924).
25. François, J., G. Verriest & A. Israel. Périmétrie statique colorée effectuée à l'aide de l'appareil de Goldmann. Résultats obtenus en pathologie oculaire. Ann. Ocul. (Paris) 199: 113–154 (1966).
26. Friedmann, A. I. A preliminary report on the use of colour filters in the Mark II visual field analyser. In: Colour Vision Deficiencies V, Bristol, Adam Hilger (1980), pp. 221–225.
27. Frisén, L. A versatile color confrontation test for the central visual field. Arch. Ophthalmol. 89: 3–9 (1973).
28. Frisén, L. & Frisén M. A simple relationship between the probability distribution of visual acuity and the density of retinal output channels. Acta Ophthalmol. (Kbh) 54: 437–444 (1976).
29. Gast, T. J. & S. A. Burns. Detection threshold for lights of varying purity. J. Opt. Soc. Am. 69: 632–633 (1979).
30. Gordon, J. & I. Abramov. Color vision in the peripheral retina. II. Hue and saturation. J. Opt. Soc. Am. 67: 202–207 (1977).
31. Gouras, P. Trichromatic mechanisms in single cortical neurons. Science 168: 489–492 (1970).
32. Gouras, P. Color opponency from fovea to striate cortex. Invest. Ophthalmol. 11: 427–434 (1972).
33. Gouras, P. & E. Zrenner. Enhancement of luminance flicker by color-opponent mechanisms. Science 205: 587–589 (1979).
34. Graham, B. V. Mechanisms of peripheral color vision. Mod. Probl. Ophthalmol. 17: 71–74 (1976).

35. Graham, B. V., R. Holland & D. L. Sparks. Relative spectral sensitivity to short wavelength light in the peripheral visual field. Vision Res. 15: 313–316 (1975).
36. Greve, E. L., W. M. Verduin & M. Ledeboer. Two-colour threshold in static perimetry. Mod. Probl. Ophthalmol. 13: 113–118.
37. Gunkel, R. D. Retinal profiles. Arch. Ophthalmol. 77: 22–25 (1967).
38. Guth, S. L., N. J. Donley & R. T. Marrocco. On luminance additivity and related topics. Vision Res. 9: 537–575 (1969).
39. Hansen, E. Selective chromatic adaptation studies with special reference to a method combining Stiles' two-colour threshold technique and static colour perimetry. Thesis, Oslo (1979).
40. Hedin, A. Pupillomotor spectral sensitivity in normals and colour defectives. Acta Ophthalmol. (Kbh) Suppl. 137 (1978).
41. Hedin, A. Color in peripheral vision. In: Topics in neuro-ophthalmology (H. S. Thompson, ed.), Baltimore, Williams & Wilkins (1979).
42. Ichikawa, H., T. Yasuma & S. Tanabe. Studies of color perceptive information processing in retinal-brain system. (1) Time duration effects of colored stimuli on a spectral sensitivity curve. Acta Soc. Ophthalmol. Jap. 81: 1563–1571 (1977).
43. Israel, A. & G. Verriest. Normal results of kinetic colour perimetry by means of the Goldmann apparatus. Doc. Ophthalmol. Proc. Ser. 14: 435–439 (1977).
44. Jacobs, G. H. Color vision. Ann. Rev. Psychol. 27: 63–89 (1976).
45. King-Smith, P. E. & D. Carden. Luminance and opponent-colour contributions to visual detection and adaptation and to temporal and spatial integration. J. Opt. Soc. Am. 66: 709–717 (1976).
46. King-Smith, P. E., K. Kranda & I. C. J. Wood. An acquired color defect of the opponent-color system. Invest. Ophthalmol. 15: 584–587 (1976).
47. Kinney, J. A. Comparison of scotopic, mesopic and photopic spectral sensitivity curves. J. Opt. Soc. Am. 48: 185–190 (1958).
48. Kinney, J. A. Light as a true visual quantity: principles of measurement. CIE publication No. 41 (TC-1.4) (1978).
49. Kitahara, K. & H. Ichikawa. An approach to equalizing the energy and the number of photons of chromatic lights of the Tübinger perimeter. Acta Soc. Ophthalmol. Jap. 79: 59–66 (1975).
50. Kitahara, K., K. Kitahara & H. Matsuzaki. Trial of color perimeter. 3rd Int. IPS symposium, Tokyo 1978.
51. Köllner, H. Die Störungen des Farbensinnes; ihre klinische Bedeutung und ihre Diagnose. Berlin, Karger (1912).
52. Lakowski, R., W. D. Wright & K. Oliver. A Goldmann perimeter with high luminance chromatic targets. Can. J. Ophthalmol. 12: 203–210 (1977).
53. Maione, M. & F. Carta. The visibility of the Goldmann's perimeter coloured targets in the ageing and in retrobulbar neuritis. Mod. Probl. Ophthalmol. 11: 72–75 (1972).
54. Maione, M., F. Carta, E. Barberini & L. Scoccianti. Achromatic isopters on coloured background in some acquired color vision deficiencies. Mod. Probl. Ophthalmol. 17: 85–93 (1976).
55. Marc, R. E. & H. G. Sperling. Chromatic organization of primate cones. Science 196: 454–456 (1977).
56. Marmion, V. J. The results of a comparison between the hundred hue test and static colour perimetry. Doc. Ophthalmol. Proc. Ser. 14: 473–474 (1977).
57. Marré, E., M. Marré & E. Schreiber. Detection of early visual field defects in open angle glaucoma by kinetic perimetry of the blue color mechanism. Regional Symposium of the IRGCVD, Dresden 1978.
58. Marré, M. Investigation of acquired color vision deficiencies. In: Colour 73, London, Hilger (1977), pp. 99–135.
59. Marré, M. & E. Marré. Different types of acquired colour vision deficiencies on the base of CVM patterns in dependence upon the fixation mode of the diseased eye. Mod. Probl. Ophthalmol. 19: 248–252.
60. Massof, R. W. & D. Finkelstein. Rod sensitivity relative to cone sensitivity in retinitis pigmentosa. Invest. Ophthalmol. Visual Sci. 18: 263–272 (1979).

61. Matsuo, H. Studies on the visual field. Acta Soc. Ophthalmol. Jap. 83: 1815–1854 (1979).
62. Moreland, J. D. Peripheral colour vision. Handbook of sensory physiology VII/4: 517–536 (1972).
63. Moreland, J. D. & A. C. Cruz. Colour perception with the peripheral retina. Optica Acta 6: 117–151 (1958).
64. Moreland, J. D., M. Maione, F. Carta, E. Barberini, L. Scoccianti & S. Lettieri. The clinical assessment of the chromatic mechanisms of the retinal periphery. Doc. Ophthalmol. Proc. Ser. 14: 413–421 (1977).
65. Nemtseev, H. J. Color static perimetry in early glaucoma. Regional Symposium of the IRGCVD, Dresden 1978.
66. Nolte, W. Bestimmung achromatischer Schwellen für verschiedene Spektrallichter. Inaugural-Dissertation, Tübingen (1962).
67. Obstfeld, H. Human colour vision mechanisms along four cardinal meridians. In: Colour Vision Deficiencies V, Bristol, Adam Hilger (1980), pp. 211–216.
68. Sloan, L. L. & K. Feiock. Selective impairment of cone function. Mod. Probl. Ophthalmol. 11: 50–62 (1972).
69. Sperling, H. G. & R. S. Harwerth. Red-green cone interactions in the increment-threshold spectral sensitivity of primates. Science 172: 180–184 (1971).
70. Sperling, H. G. & Y. Hsia. Some comparisons among spectral sensitivity data obtained in different retinal locations and with two sizes of foveal stimulus. J. Opt. Soc. Am. 47: 707–713 (1957).
71. Sperling, H. G., T. P. Piantanida & D. S. Garrett. An atypical color deficiency with extreme loss of sensitivity in the yellow region of the spectrum. Mod. Probl. Ophthalmol. 17: 338–344 (1976).
72. Spillmann, L. & S. Seneff. Photochromatic intervals as a function of retinal eccentricity for stimuli of different size. J. Opt. Soc. Am. 61: 267–270 (1971).
73. Stabell, B. & U. Stabell. Rod and cone contributions to peripheral colour vision. Vision Res. 16: 1099–1104 (1976a).
74. Stabell, B. & U. Stabell. Effects of rod activity on color threshold. Vision Res. 16: 1105–1110 (1976b).
75. Stabell, U. & B. Stabell. Absence of rod activity from peripheral vision. Vision Res. 16: 1433–1437 (1976c).
76. Stabell, U. & B. Stabell. Wavelength discrimination of peripheral cones and its change with rod intrusion. Vision Res. 17: 432–426 (1977).
77. Stiles, W. S. & B. H. Crawford. The liminal brightness increment as a function of wave-length for different conditions of the foveal and parafoveal retina. Proc. R. Soc. Lond. Biol. 113: 496–530 (1934).
78. Stiles, W. S. & G. Wyszecki. Rod intrusion in large-field color matching. Acta chromatica 2: 155–163 (1973).
79. Trezona, P. W. Rod participation in the "blue" mechanism and its effect on colour matching. Vision Res. 10: 317–332 (1970).
80. Trezona, P. W. Aspects of peripheral colour vision. Mod. Probl. Ophthalmol. 17: 52–70 (1976).
81. Verduyn Lunel, H. F. E. & R. A. Crone. Static perimetry with purely chromatic stimuli. Mod. Probl. Ophthalmol. 13: 103–108 (1974).
82. Verduyn Lunel, H. F. E. & R. A. Crone. Determination of peripheral spectral sensitivity and saturation discrimination characteristics with a modified Goldmann perimeter. Mod. Probl. Ophthalmol. 19: 181–186 (1978).
83. Verriest, G. Studie over de achromatische gezichtsfuncties in de congenitale sensoriële anomalieën van het menselijk oog en bij sommige Amphibia en Reptilia. Junk, The Hague (1960).
84. Verriest, G. Further studies on acquired deficiency of color discrimination. J. Opt. Soc. Am. 53: 185–195 (1963).
85. Verriest, G. La périmétrie colorée hier et aujourd'hui. Ann. Ottalmol. Clin. Ocul. 105: 1–22 (1979).
86. Verriest, G. Color perimetry. In: Congenital and acquired color vision defects (J. Pokorny, V. C. Smith, G. Verriest, A. J. L. G. Pinckers, eds.), New York, Grune & Stratton (1979), pp. 174–181.

87. Verriest, G. & A. Israel. Application du périmètre statique de Goldmann au relevé topographique dues seuils différentiels de luminance pour de petits objets colorés projetés sur un fond blanc. I – Principes, calibrage de l'appareil et étude comparative de groupes de sujets normaux d'âges différents. Vision Res. 5: 151–174 (1965).
88. Verriest, G. & A. Israel. Idem. II – Etude comparative de sujets atteints de déficiences congénitales de la vision des couleurs et d'un groupe de sujets normaux. Vision Res. 5: 341–359 (1965).
89. Verriest, G. & H. Kandemir. Normal spectral increment thresholds on a white background. Die Farbe 23: 3–16 (1974).
90. Verriest, G. & P. Metsälä. Résultats en vision latérale de quelques tests de la discrimination chromatique maculaire. Rev. Opt. (Paris) 42: 391–400 (1963).
91. Verriest, G., P. Padmos & E. L. Greve. Calibration of the Tübinger perimeter for colour perimetry. Mod. Probl. Ophthalmol. 13: 109–112 (1974).
92. Verriest, G. & A. Uvijls. Central and peripheral increment thresholds for white and spectral lights on a white background in different kinds of congenitally defective colour vision. Atti Fond. G. Ronchi 32: 213–254 (1977a).
93. Verriest, G. & A. Uvijls. Spectral increment thresholds on a white background in different age groups of normal subjects and in acquired ocular diseases. Doc. Ophthalmol. 43: 217–248 (1977b).
94. Voke, J. Factors affecting the detection of simple coloured stimuli. A review of psychophysical research. The Ophthalmic Optician 1979 (July), pp. 526–528.
95. Vola, J., G. Leprince, D. Langle, L. Cornu & J. B. Saracco. Preliminary results on the clinical interpretation of Stiles two-colour threshold method. Mod. Probl. Ophthalmol. 19: 266–269 (1978).
96. Wagner, G. & R. M. Boynton. Comparison of four methods of heterochromatic photometry. J. Opt. Soc. Am. 62: 1508–1515 (1972).
97. Wald, G. Human vision and the spectrum. Science 101: 653–658 (1945).
98. Wald, G. The receptors of human color vision. Science 145: 1007–1016 (1964).
99. Wald, G. Blue-blindness in the normal fovea. J. Opt. Soc. Am. 57: 1289–1303 (1967).
100. Walters, H. V. & W. D. Wright. The spectral sensitivity of the fovea and extrafovea in the Purkinje range. Proc. R. Soc. Lond. Biol. 131: 340–361 (1943).
101. Weale, R. A. The foveal and para-central spectral sensitivities in man. J. Physiol. 114: 435–446 (1951).
102. Weale, R. A. Spectral sensitivity and wave-length discrimination of the peripheral retina. J. Physiol. 119: 170–190 (1953).
103. Weale, R. A. Problems of peripheral vision. Br. J. Ophthalmol. 40: 392–415 (1956).
104. Wentworth, H. A. Quantitative study of achromatic and chromatic sensitivity from center to periphery of the visual field. Psy. Monog. 40: 183–375 (1930).
105. Wilbrand, H. & A. Sänger. Die Neurologie des Auges. Wiesbaden, J. G. Bergmann (1913).
106. Wooten, B. R. & T. W. Butler. Possible rod-cone interaction in dark adaptation. J. Opt. Soc. Am. 66: 1429–1430 (1976).
107. Wooten, B. R., K. Fuld & L. Spillmann. Photopic spectral sensitivity of the peripheral retina. J. Opt. Soc. Am. 65: 334–342 (1975).
108. Wooten, B. R. & G. Wald. Color-vision mechanisms in the peripheral retinas of normal and dichromatic observers. J. Gen. Physiol. 61: 125–145 (1973).
109. Yokoi, T. Color critical fusion frequency in the Bjerrum area. Acta Soc. Ophthalmol. Jap. 75: 2243–2248 (1972).
110. Zanen, J. Introduction à l'étude des dyschromatopisies rétiennes centrales acquises. Bull. Soc. Belge Ophtalmol. 103: 7–148 (1953).
111. Zisman, F., P. E. King-Smith & S. K. Bhargava. Spectral sensitivities of acquired defects analyzed in terms of color opponent theory. Mod. Probl. Ophthalmol. 19: 254–257 (1978).
112. Zrenner, E. Influence of stimulus duration and area on the spectral luminosity function as determined by sensory and VECP measurements. Doc. Ophthalmol. Proc. Ser. 13: 21–30 (1977).
113. Zweifach, P. H. & E. Wolf. Acquired cone dysfunction and other photopic system diseases. Arch. Ophthalmol. 79: 18–21 (1968).

Authors' addresses:

Anders Hedin
Dept. of Ophthalmology
Karolinska sjukhuset
Stockholm
Sweden

Guy Verriest
Dept. of Ophthalmology
Akademisch Ziekenhuis
Ghent
Belgium

EXTRAFOVEAL STILES' π_5 – MECHANISM

HIROSHI KITAHARA, KENJI KITAHARA, JUNJI IRIE,
AKITO SHIRAKAWA & HIROSHI MATSUZAKI

(Tokyo, Japan/Ann Arbor, MI, U.S.A.)

ABSTRACT

The field sensitivity of Stiles' long wavelength sensitive mechanism $\pi_{5\,(\mu)}$ was measured at the fovea and at 10° and 20° extrafoveally using a Maxwellian view optical system.

The fact that the field displacement law proved to hold good extrafoveally even for test durations of 200 msec suggests a difference in temporal integration property between the fovea and other regions.

Compared with the foveal measurements, the extrafoveal field sensitivity action spectra of $\pi_{5\,(\mu)}$ were higher in the short wavelength regions and lower on the long wavelength side with a tendency for the curve to fall off with a somewhat steeper slope.

INTRODUCTION

In order to make clinical use of color perimetry and to investigate the processing of color information in ocular disease, it is first necessary to obtain accurate knowledge of the color mechanisms measured at various retinal eccentricities in the normal eye.

Wooten and Wald (7) have shown that three color mechanisms can be separated even at a retinal eccentricity of 80° by the selective adaptation technique. In earlier studies, we have also successfully separated three color mechanisms at retinal eccentricities of up to 20° [Kitahara (1); Kitahara, Kitahara and Matsuzaki (2)]. The exact shape of the action spectra seemed to depend on the intensity and spectral characteristics of the background, a fact which we attributed to the difficulties involved in obtaining high intensity fields.

In the present experiments, an attempt was made to measure the field sensitivity of Stiles' long-wavelength sensitive mechanism at the fovea and at 10° and 20° of visual angle eccentric to the fovea. These detailed measurements were made to lay the groundwork for theoretically sound color perimetry.

METHOD

The apparatus used in this study was a Maxwellian view optical system with 3 channels. The light source was a 500 W Xenon arc lamp. The test flash was round and it subtended 1° of visual angle. It was presented for 200 msec at the center of a continuously illuminated, round background field with a visual angle of 35°. A red fixation target was introduced in the visual field from an accessory system. For extrafoveal measurements, the observer was instructed to fixate this red target which was placed at angles of 10° or 20° on the visual field meridian of 225°. The biting board was adjusted so as to allow the test flash and the main field light to pass through the center of the pupil, when the eye fixed each eccentric position in turn.

Two male observers with normal color vision were used in this study. Prior to the experiment tropicamide was administered topically to the right eye of each observer to produce maximal mydriasis with a pupil diameter of approximately 8 mm. The observer was dark-adapted for 30 min at the beginning of each session and was adapted to each background light for 3 min before threshold measurement began. Detection threshold for the test flash was measured five times for each background condition by the method of adjustment. The subject adjusted the position of the N.D. wedge in the test beam until the test was just detectable. The measurements were calibrated with a Sanso Manufacturing Co. radiometer at each experiment.

RESULTS

The threshold versus intensity (t.v.i.) curve

A study was made on the threshold versus intensity (t.v.i.) curve at different positions on the retina using a short (430 nm), middle (530 nm) and long wavelength (650 nm) background in the main field, while the test color light had a wavelength of 650 nm. Fig. 1 shows the t.v.i. curves at the fovea. The solid line indicates the standard increment threshold function of Stiles (6). The curves were prepared from the data for observers H.K. and J.I. All the data and the curve for observer J.I. are transposed vertically by 3 log units. While the curves of both observers for $\lambda = \mu = 650$ nm (○) well fitted Stiles' template curve, curves for $\mu = 430$ nm (△) and 530 nm (●) failed to conform to the field displacement law as the background light became intense, and thus the presence of another branch or π_5'-mechanism had to be taken into account.

Figs. 2 and 3 show the t.v.i. curves at 10° and 20° temporal locations. Apparently, the curve consists of two branches i.e., the lower branch corresponding to rod or $\pi_{0(\mu)}$and the upper one corresponding to the long wavelength sensitive mechanism or $\pi_{5(\mu)}$. The solid line represents the Stiles' template curve.

Field sensitivity action spectrum of $\pi_{5(\mu)}$

Field sensitivity action spectra of $\pi_{5(\mu)}$ at the fovea of observers H.K. and J.I. are shown in Fig. 4. Measurement was made of the t.v.i. curve for each background with the test light (λ) fixed at 650 nm and the main field (μ) varying from 400 nm to 700 nm to determine field sensitivity according to Stiles'

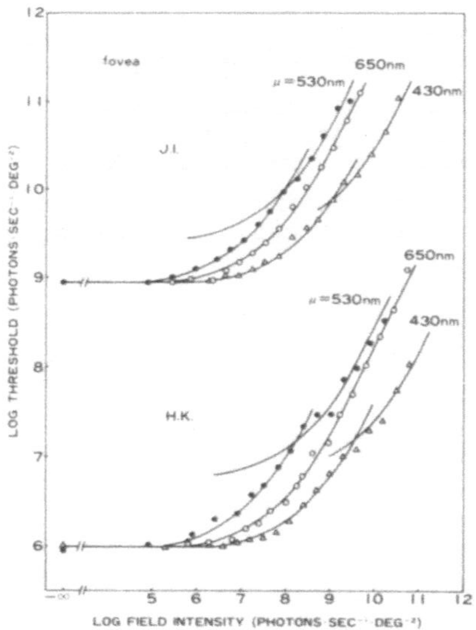

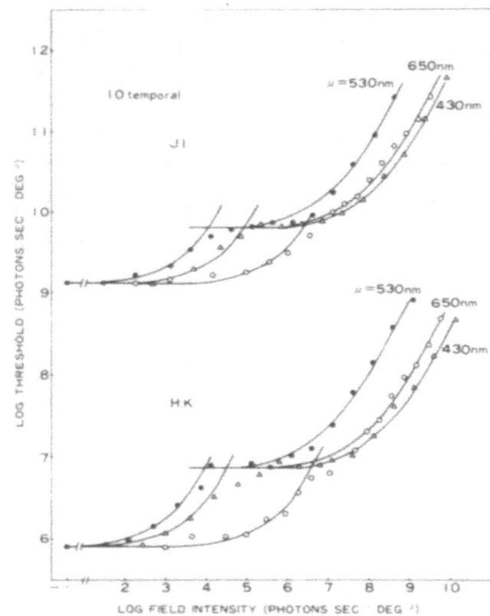

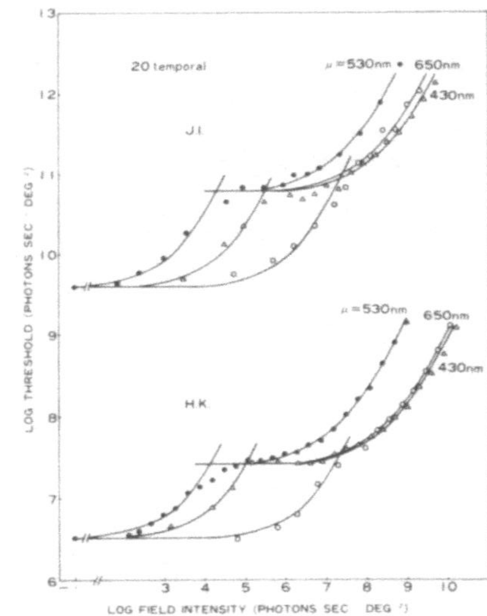

Fig. 1. The foveal threshold versus intensity (t.v.i.) curves of the two observers. The solid line indicates Stiles' standard increment threshold function. All the data and curve for J.I. have been slid up 3 log units. The test flash was fixed at 650 nm. The triangles show the means of 5 repetitions when the background was 430 nm, the filled circles show the mean when the background was 530 nm and the open circles show the means for the 650 nm background.

Fig. 2. The t.v.i. curves at 10° temporal retina. Symbols as in Fig. 1. The solid line indicates Stiles' standard increment threshold function. The curve consists of two branches i.e., the lower branch corresponding to $\pi_0(\mu)$ and the upper one corresponding to $\pi_5(\mu)$. The upper branches had no component corresponding to π'_5 operating at high level of brightness even in the middle and short wavelength spectral range of background lights.

Fig. 3. The t.v.i. curves at 20° temporal retina. The curve consists of two branches as in Fig. 2.

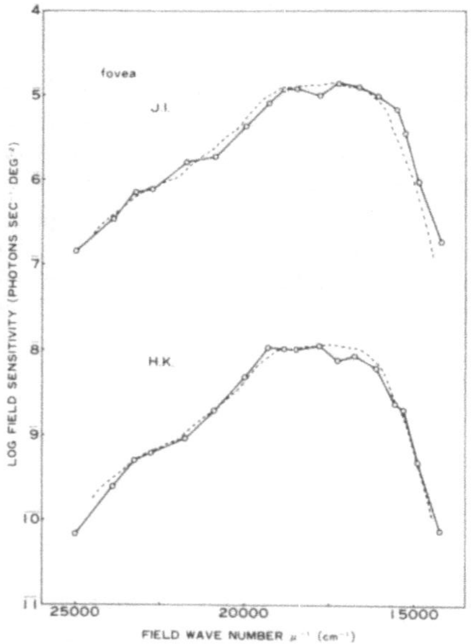

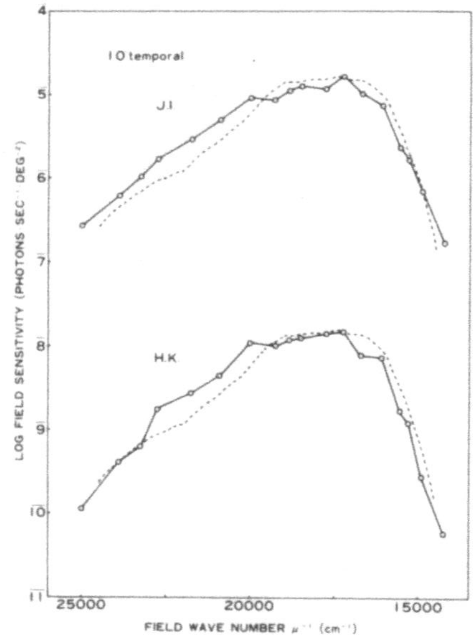

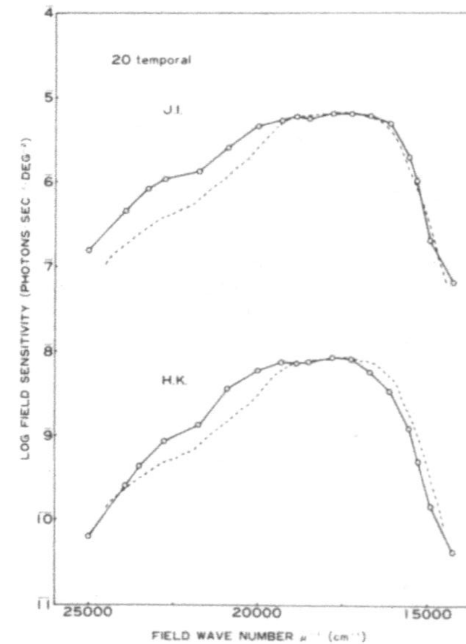

Fig. 4. The foveal field sensitivity action spectra of π_5 for observers H.K. (below) and J.I. (above). The data and curve for observer J.I. are slid up 3 log units. The pattern obtained closely resembled Stiles' $\pi_5(\mu)$ (broken line), slid up about 0.1 log unit for H.K. and about 0.2 log unit for J.I.

Fig. 5. The field sensitivity action spectra for π_5 at 10° temporal retina. The field sensitivity of the upper branch was determined by the auxiliary field method with a wavelength of 430 nm. The brightness of the auxiliary field was set so as the π_5 mechanism determined threshold. The pattern has a relatively wide peak in long wavelength range, as the $\pi_5(\mu)$ at the fovea.

Fig. 6. The field sensitivity action spectra of π_5 at 20° temporal retina. Much the same tendency is observed as at a 10° temporal retina. In each experiment the auxiliary field of 430 nm was added as in the experiment at 10° temporal retina.

criteria. The abscissa indicates wave numbers. The pattern obtained closely resembled Stiles' $\pi_{5(\mu)}$, indicated by the dotted line, having a relatively extended peak ranging from 520 nm to 580 nm. The field sensitivity of the observer J.I. was clearly higher in the long wavelength ranges than that of Stiles' curve.

The field sensitivity of the upper branch at the extrafoveal retina was determined by the auxiliary field method of Stiles (4) with an auxiliary field wavelength of 430 nm. The light intensity of the auxiliary field was set so that test threshold was always on π_5 rather than on π_0. Field sensitivity curves are shown in Figs. 5 and 6 for 10° and 20° temporal retina of observers H.K. and J.I. The action spectrum has a relatively wide peak in long wavelength range, just like $\pi_{5(\mu)}$ at the fovea. On its long wavelength side, the sensitivity was lower than at the fovea, giving a steep curve, whereas on the short wavelength side, its sensitivity was rather higher than at the fovea, giving a slowly declining curve. The broken line indicates Stiles' π_5-mechanism, the peak value of which has been arranged to the same height as ours.

DISCUSSION

t.v.i. curve

The t.v.i. curve at the central fovea, when both the test and the background light had the same wavelength of 650 nm ($\lambda = \mu = 650$ nm) were well fit by the template curve of Stiles. When the background field had a middle to long wavelength, by contrast, the t.v.i. curve was shallow, keeping the field displacement law from holding good. In subject J.I., in particular, the segment of the curve starting at about 0.5 log unit from the absolute threshold suggested the necessity of postulating the presence of another mechanism, namely π_5' (Fig. 1).

Conversely, the t.v.i. curves at extrafoveal retina comprised 2 distinct branches: The field sensitivity action spectrum of the lower branch (not shown) exhibited the characteristics of the rod or $\pi_{0(\mu)}$, while that of the upper branch showed the pattern of the long wavelength sensitive mechanism or $\pi_{5(\mu)}$. Here the upper branch had no component corresponding to π_5' operating at high level of brightness. t.v.i. curves measured on middle to short wavelengths background are well fit by the Stiles' template curve even up to 1.5 log units from the absolute threshold for $\pi_{5(\mu)}$. Moreover, these curves conform to the field displacement law. Pugh and Wandell (3) explained π_5' mechanism by the two-pathway hypothesis. They argue that the t.v.i. curve for the long wavelength sensitive mechanism conforms to the field displacement law and the principle of field addilivity for a short (10 msec) test flash duration. The fact that in our present study the field displacement law proved to hold good in the extrafoveal retina even for a duration of 200 msec suggests a difference in temporal integration time between the central fovea and other regions. The Fechner fractions of the π_5 mechanism are as follows:

Subject	Fovea	10°	20°
H.K.	0.019	0.091	0.130
J.I.	0.032	0.109	0.676

$\pi_{5(\mu)}$ *field sensitivity action spectrum*

The difference in the slope of the field sensitivity action spectrum of π_5 between the fovea and 10° and 20° temporal retina was examined. Especially for wavelengths shorter than 500 nm, the sensitivity was higher in the extra-foveal retina than at the fovea. On the other hand, the sensitivity was lower on the long wavelength side with a tendency for the curve to be steep. The sensitivity difference in the short-wavelength end of the spectrum is probably due to macular pigmentation. The logarithm of the ratio between the sensitivities measured at the fovea and 10° in the temporal retina is shown as a function of wavenumber in Fig. 7. A smooth curve representing the absorption spectrum of human macular pigment (6) is fit to these data. It would, of course, be preferable to use the absorption spectrum of the macular pigment of a Japanese eye measured by other methods, as the macular pigment of Japanese people may differ from Caucasian macular pigment in density and perhaps in other ways as well. Even after the absorption by macular pigment is taken into account, the long-wavelength part of the 10° curve falls off more steeply than the corresponding part of the foveal curve; this is shown by the fact that in the long-wavelength end, the data in Fig. 7 fall below zero. Differences in self-screening between the longer foveal cones and the shorter extra-foveal cones may be partly responsible for this remaining discrepancy. The logarithm of the ratio between the 10° and 20° field sensitivities is plotted as a function of wavenumber in Fig. 8. The data shows some scatter, but there is no systematic change in this ratio with field wavelength.

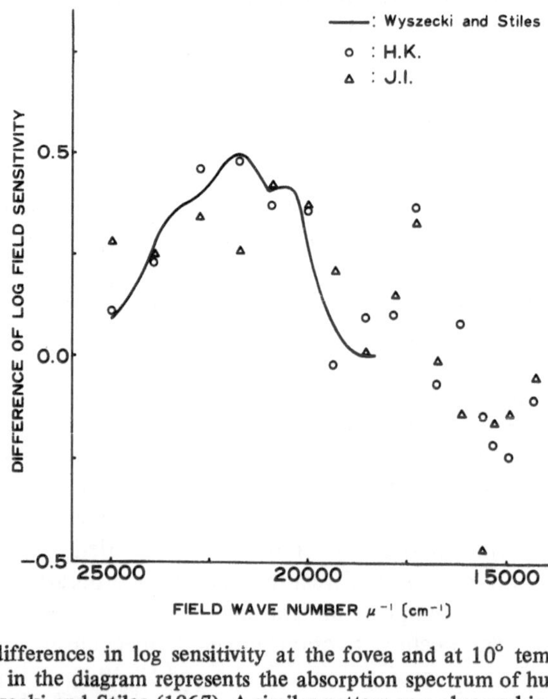

Fig. 7. The differences in log sensitivity at the fovea and at 10° temporal retina. The smooth curve in the diagram represents the absorption spectrum of human macular pigment by Wyszecki and Stiles (1967). A similar pattern was observed in H.K. particularly in the short wavelength ranges.

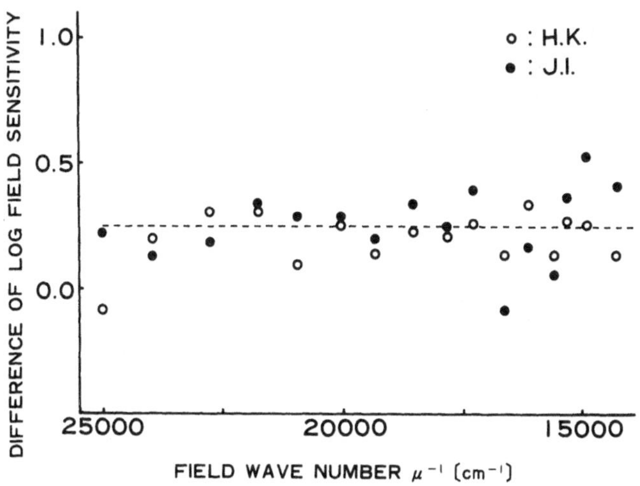

Fig. 8. The differences in log sensitivity to 10° temporal retina and 20°. This difference seemed to be essentially independent of wavelength.

ACKNOWLEDGEMENT

The authors deeply appreciate Prof. Tomoya Funahashi's guidance in our study and his reviewing of it.

REFERENCES

1. Kitahara K. Measurement of spectral sensitivity of retinal receptors. Acta Soc. Ophthal. Jap. 81(10): 1549–1562 (1977).
2. Kitahara, H., K. Kitahara & H. Matsuzaki. Trial of a color perimeter. Docum. Ophthal. Proc. Series, 19: 439 (1979).
3. Pugh, Jr., E. N. & B. A. Wandell. Stiles' π_5' color mechanism. ARVO meeting, (1979).
4. Stiles, W. S. Further studies of visual mecahnisms by the two-color threshold method. In 'Coloquio sobre problemas opticos de la vision' (Madrid), Vol. I: 65–103 (1953).
5. Stiles, W. S. Color vision: The approach through increment threshold sensitivity. Proc. Nat. Acad. Sci. (Wash.) 45: 100–114 (1959).
6. Wyszecki, G. W. & W. S. Stiles. Color science: Concepts and methods, quantitative data and formulas. New York: Wiley (1967).
7. Wooten, B. R. & G. Wald. Color-vision mechanisms in the peripheral retinas of normal and dichromatic observers. J. Gen. Physiol. 61: 125 (1973).

Authors' address:
Hiroshi Kitahara
Department of Ophthalmology
The Jikei University School of Medicine
19-18 Nishi-Shinbashi 3-chome, Minato-ku
Tokyo
Japan

Kenji Kitahara
Ann Arbor, MI, U.S.A.

AN INSTRUMENT FOR THE ESTABLISHMENT OF CHROMATIC PERIMETRY NORMS

R. LAKOWSKI & P. M. DUNN

(*Vancouver, Canada*)

ABSTRACT

A perimeter has been developed which represents a unique solution to requirements set out by the I.P.S. Perimetric Standards (1978). Extensive modification of a Goldmann perimeter has made possible high-luminance chromatic perimetry under fully-photopic and -scotopic conditions. An electronically-controlled shutter mechanism permits precise control of interstimulus interval (0.5 to 6.5 sec) and stimulus duration (50 to 1000 msec). The use of Xenon-arc lamps for projection of stimuli and background provides high luminance chromatic stimuli and a high-luminance background approximating Illuminant 'C'. This instrument has been used to establish static chromatic perimetry norms under fully-photopic (250 cd.m^{-2}) and -scotopic conditions. Achromatic thresholds are shown for a 17-year-old emmetropic, normal trichromat for 6.8′ stimuli of $\lambda_D = 474$, 535, and 617 nm, as well as an achromatic stimulus.

INTRODUCTION

The recent upsurge of interest in perimetric research has brought to attention the need for a set of standards to be applied to all research in this field. Accordingly the International Perimetric Society (I.P.S.) has published 'Perimetric Standards' (2). These standards specify certain requirements for a modern perimeter which are met by the modified Goldmann perimeter in use in the Visual Laboratory in the Department of Psychology, University of British Columbia.

Of specific interest was the development of a chromatic perimeter capable of functioning over a wide range of adaptation luminances. Although the past 15 years has seen a dramatic increase in the number and scope of chromatic perimetric studies, the majority of these studies have been carried out under mesopic adaptation conditions (usually 10 cd.m^{-2}) (6, 7), though some fully-scotopic results have been reported (5, 8). The modifications to the Goldmann Projection Perimeter reported here and in earlier papers (3, 4) have been directed at overcoming the technical and methodological difficulties associated with extremes of adaptation luminance. In addition, precise control of the temporal aspects of stimulus presentation has been implemented. As a result, the modified instrument is capable of exploring the visual field under extreme adaptation conditions, using stimuli which are precisely specified in terms of temporal as well as chromatic and spatial characteristics.

PRESENT MODIFICATIONS

To allow assessment of perimetric thresholds under fully-photopic conditions, higher luminance was required for both the stimulus and background sources.

Target luminance. To achieve the high target luminance required a Leitz XBO 75W Xenon-arc lamp was installed for stimulus projection. The 75-watt lamp has a smaller, brigher arc than the 150-watt, yielding approximately a 3-fold increase in luminance at the bowl surface. The light-path of the stimulus light was shortened by 30% and the components made more rigid. The result of these modifications to the projection system is a stable, uniform light stimulus of approximately 8000 $cd.m^{-2}$, measured at the adaption bowl surface.

This increase in luminance necessitated the addition of two neutral-density filters in the stimulus light-path. Thus with the neutral filters built into the instrument, the two neutral filter caps supplied with the instrument, and the two additional filters, stimulus luminance is variable in 0.1 log-unit steps over a range of ten log-units.

Background luminance. Here the increase in luminance was achieved through the use of the Leitz XBO 150W Xenon-arc lamp, where the luminous output is directed via a front-surface mirror to the top of the adaptation bowl whence it is diffused throughout the bowl according to the Ulbrich sphere principle. In addition the adaptation bowl was painted with Kodak Eastman White Reflectance Paint, which yielded 98% reflectance across the visible spectrum. These modifications resulted in a maximum adaptation luminance of 300 $cd.m^{-2}$, well above that required for saturation of the rod mechanism (Aguilar & Stiles, 1954) and thus fully-photopic adaptation. In addition the background and stimulus sources have the same spectral energy distribution, thus eliminating simultaneous contrast effects with the use of the achromatic stimulus. The xenon-arc lamps have a spectral distribution approximating C.I.E. Illuminant 'C', thus yielding high energy across the entire visible spectrum.

Temporal aspects. The manual interrupter-system was replaced by electronically-controlled 5-blade shutter mechanism with a feedback switch, mounted close to the focal point of the light source with resulting fast edge movement. The shutter speed is continuously variable from 50 to 1000 msec, and the inter-stimulus interval is variable from 0.5 to 6.5 sec. As a result, stimulus duration and interstimulus interval can be precisely specified.

Finally complete photometric specification of all stimuli and the adaptation background have been done and can be routinely monitored. The Spectra Pritchard Photometer (Model 1980A-PL) using a narrow angle of acceptance (6′) has a response curve closely approximating $V(\lambda)$, and gives measurements in metric luminance units at the adaptation bowl surface. Furthermore, this instrument is capable of making scotopic and pulse measurements. Radiometric measurements were made at the bowl's surface by means of the Gamma Scientific Telespectro-radiometer (Model 2000-F).

METHODS AND RESULTS

The flexibility of this instrument is illustrated by the following sample results which were obtained from one emmetropic normal trichromat, whose colour vision was assessed with a Pickford-Nicolson Anomaloscope. Subject and stimulus and adaptation specifications are given in Table 1. A modified ascending method of limits was used to obtain achromatic thresholds, wherein stimulus luminance was increased in 0.1 log-unit steps from sub-threshold until a threshold response was elicited, whereupon the luminance was decreased to a subthreshold level and again increased. A threshold was generally determined by two or three consistent responses at the same luminance level.

Fig. 1 presents the fully-photopic, mesopic, and fully-scotopic threshold gradients obtained. The mesopic ($L = 10\,cd.m^{-2}$) results were obtained before the most recent modifications were completed, using the manual stimulus presentation method available in the original instrument; for these results the stimulus duration and interstimulus interval could only be estimated at one-half and one second respectively.

Several important trends are apparent in this data. Excluding the fovea, the differences among the gradients for the three chromatic and the achromatic stimuli increase as adaptation luminance is decreased. The separation among the gradients found with $L = 0$ reflects the Purkinje shift, the red stimulus yielding a gradient from 1 and 1/2 to 2 log-units below the others. At $L = 10\,cd.m^{-2}$ the gradients still show a separation among the colours, but when the background is increased to $250\,cd.m^{-2}$ the gradients are all very close together (excluding the fovea).

Table 1. Stimulus, adaptation, and subject specifications

Stimulus	Duration = 150 msec*		
	Interstimulus interval = 1.00 sec*		
	Angle subtended at eye = 6.8′**		
	Chromaticities:	achromatic (Tc = 6000 K)	
		blue λ_D 475 nm.	
		green λ_D 532 nm.	
		red λ_D 630 nm.	
	Chromatic stimuli photometrically equated at the fovea.		
Background	Colour temperature = 6000 K		
	Luminance:	$0\,cd.m^{-2}$	
		$10\,cd.m^{-2}$	
		$250\,cd.m^{-2}$	
Subject	One female:	Age – 18 years	
		Colour vision – normal	
		Acuity – +0.50 to 1.3	
Pre-adaptation	25 minutes for $L = 0\,cd.m^{-2}$		
	4 minutes for $L = 10\,cd.m^{-2}$ and $L = 250\,cd.m^{-2}$		

* These values apply only to the $L = 0$ and $L = 250\,cd.m^{-2}$ conditions; for $L = 10\,cd.m^{-2}$ duration was approximately 0.5 sec, and interstimulus interval was approximately 1 sec.

** Goldmann size I, according to Verriest and Israel (1965).

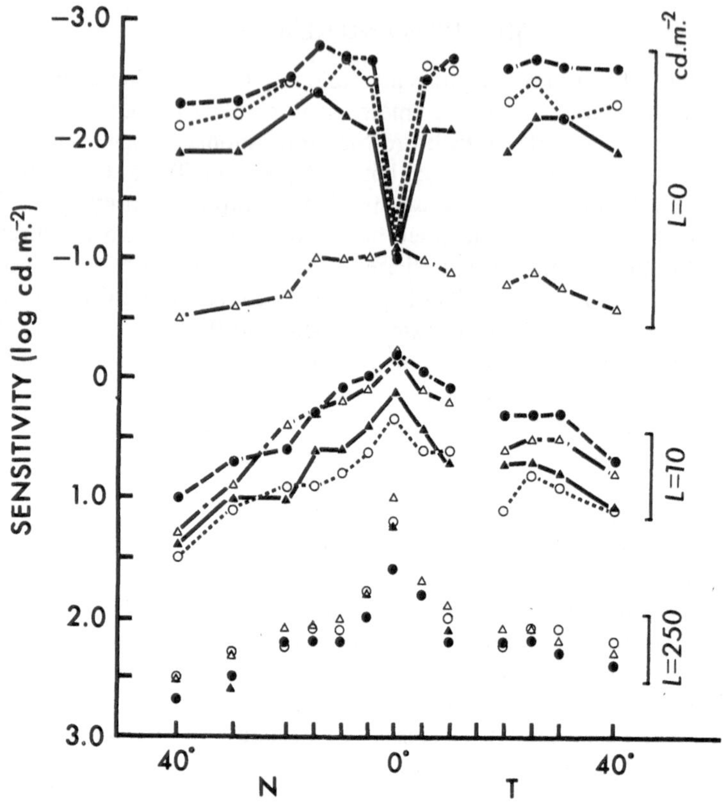

Fig. 1. Sensitivity gradients under fully-photopic (250 cd.m^{-2}), mesopic (10 cd.m^{-2}) and fully-scotopic conditions. Stimulus size = 6.8′ visual angle; stimuli were blue (●), green (○), red (△) and achromatic (▲).

The foveal results were excluded in the foregoing discussion, because fixation during foveal measurements cannot be monitored directly at present in this instrument. Unless it can be objectively determined where the eye is fixating when a measurement is taken, the threshold obtained cannot be verified as applying to the retinal position presumed. To circumvent this problem the present instrument is being fitted with an infra-red fixation monitoring device functioning under all adaptation levels.

In conclusion the Goldmann perimeter described here makes possible chromatic perimetric investigations under a wide range of adaptation conditions, with precise specification of relevant adaptation field and target parameters and as such meets the recommended requirements suggested by I.P.S.

REFERENCES

1. Aguilar, M. & W. S. Stiles. Saturation of the rod mechanism at high levels of stimulation. Optica Acta 1: 59–65 (1954).

2. Enoch, J. M. (Ed.) International Perimetric Society perimetric standards 1978. Dr. W. Junk bv Publishers, The Hague (1979).
3. Lakowski, R., W. D. Wright & K. Oliver. A Goldmann perimeter with high luminance chromatic targets. Canad. J. Ophthal. 12: 203–210 (1977a).
4. Lakowski, R., W. D. Wright & K. Oliver. High luminance chromatic Goldmann Perimeter. Docum. Opth. 14: 441–443 (1977b).
5. Nolte, W. Bestimmung achromatischer Schwellen für verschiedene Spektrallichter. Inaugural Dissertation, Tübingen, 1962.
6. Sloan, L. L. Instruments and technics for the clinical testing of light sense: III An apparatus for studying regional differences in light sense. Arch. Opth. 22: 233–251 (1939).
7. Verriest, G. & A. Israel. Application du périmètre statique de Goldmann au relevé topographique des seuils différentiels de luminance pour de petits objets colorés projetés sur un fond blanc. I. Principes, calibrage de l'appareil et étude comparative de groupes de sujets normaux d'âges différents. Vision Res. 5: 151–174 (1965).
8. Wentworth, H. A quantitative study of achromatic and chromatic sensitivity from center to periphery of the visual field. Psych. Monographs, 40, No. 183 (1930).

This work was supported by MRC Grant No. 4342 and 684304.

Authors' address:
Visual Laboratory
Department of Psychology
The University of British Columbia
2075 Wesbrook Place
Vancouver, B.C. V6T 1W5
Canada

FULLY-PHOTOPIC AND -SCOTOPIC SPATIAL SUMMATION IN CHROMATIC PERIMETRY

P. M. DUNN & R. LAKOWSKI

(*Vancouver, Canada*)

ABSTRACT

Chromatic static perimetry has in general been limited in the past to investigations involving one stimulus size only (13, 17) or different sizes for different chromatic stimuli (16) making the study of spatial summation impossible. In the present study a modified Goldmann perimeter has been used to study spatial summation for chromatic stimuli using Goldmann stimulus sizes I, II, III, and IV (6.8′, 13.6′, 27.2′ and 54.3′). Achromatic thresholds have been obtained for 5 emmetropic normal trichromats for an achromatic and three chromatic stimuli; results are presented here for stimuli of $\lambda_D = 474$ and 617 nm under fully-photopic (250 cd.m^{-2}) and -scotopic conditions. The obtained results are discussed with reference to the earlier work on summation for achromatic stimuli by Fankhauser and Schmidt (6, 7), Sloan (15), and Gougnard (10).

INTRODUCTION

Studies of spatial summation in perimetry have previously utilized only achromatic stimuli (2–10, 14, 15). Furthermore, in most a mesopic (10 cd.m^{-2}) adaptation luminance was used, although Fankhauser and Schmidt (7) investigated summation under a range of adaptation levels from 0.04 to 40 asb. This study differs in two respects: chromatic stimuli are used, and they are presented under two levels of adaptation – fully-photopic (250 cd.m^{-2}) and fully-scotopic. Although we have used red, green, and blue photometrically-equated stimuli as well as the traditional achromatic, for the sake of brevity only the results for the blue and red are discussed here.

Perimetric data obtained on spatial summation has generally been presented in three different ways: (1) a comparison of changes in sensitivity-gradient slopes with changes in stimulus size (e.g. 6, 7); (2) the calculation of the summation exponent 'K', calculated at individual field locations in static perimetery [$k = (\log L_1 - \log L_2)/(\log A_2 - \log A_1)$], (10); and from equivalent isopters in kinetic perimetry $\Phi = (A_1/A_2)^k$, (8); or (3) the plotting of summation graphs in which $\log \Delta L = -K \log A +$ constant (5, 14). While the summation exponent 'K' can be calculated for both moving (kinetic perimetry) and stationary (static perimetry) stimuli, the direct comparison of these statistics would seem inadvisable due to the variable influence of temporal summation factors in the kinetic data, as well as the fact that there can be no precise specification of the retinal area involved in response to a moving

Doc. Ophthal. Proc. Series, Vol. 26, ed. by E. L. Greve & G. Verriest

target, which yields 'successive lateral spatial summation' (11, p. 79). In the present study static presentation of stimuli was used, as this method allows precise control of the temporal and spatial characteristics of the stimulus.

METHOD

The modified Goldmann perimeter described elsewhere in this volume (12) was used to obtain static achromatic thresholds at 13 points on the horizontal (0°–180°) meridian for the dominant eye of five young (17–29 years), emmetropic (±1.25 to 1.33) normal trichromats. Two chromatic stimuli were used, $\lambda_D = 474$ nm (blue) and $\lambda_D = 617$ nm (red), and they were equated photometrically. Four Goldmann stimulus sizes were used, subtending 6.8 (size I), 13.6 (II), 27.2 (III), and 54.3 (IV) minutes of visual angle (subtenses after Verriest and Israel, 15). All stimuli were presented for 150 msec with a minimum of 1 second between presentations. A modified ascending method of limits was used, wherein stimulus luminance was increased in 0.1 log unit steps until the subject responded, whereupon the stimulus luminance was decreased to a sub-threshold level and again increased. This was repeated until the same threshold was obtained consistently. Fully-photopic testing was achieved using a 250 $cd.m^{-2}$ background (6000 K), a luminance well above the threshold for rod saturation determined by Aguilar and Stiles (1). Fully-scotopic testing was done by eliminating all light from the adaptation bowl except the stimulus and fixation lights. A pre-adaptation period of 4 minutes for the photopic and 25 minutes for the scotopic condition was used before testing commenced.

RESULTS

All three forms of data presentation discussed in the Introduction are used to illustrate the spatial summation characterizing the retina under the present experimental conditions: gradient-slope changes, summation exponents (K), and summation graphs (log ΔL plotted against log A). The summation graphs have been plotted for the fovea and nasal eccentricities only; similar results were obtained on the temporal meridian.

Fully-photopic adaptation. Here spatial summation for the two chromatic stimuli increased with eccentricity. In Fig. 1 we see a flattening of the gradients with increasing stimulus size, and in Fig. 2 we see the tendency for K to increase with eccentricity. In Fig. 3 the slope of the line defined by $\log \Delta L = k \log A +$ constant, that is (–)K, increases with eccentricity. There was no clear indication of a difference between the red and blue stimuli: in each case summation increased with eccentricity, though this trend was more consistent for the red.

The second major aspect of spatial summation found under fully-photopic conditions was its tendency to increase with decreasing stimulus size. Our results show this trend in the increasing difference between gradient slopes

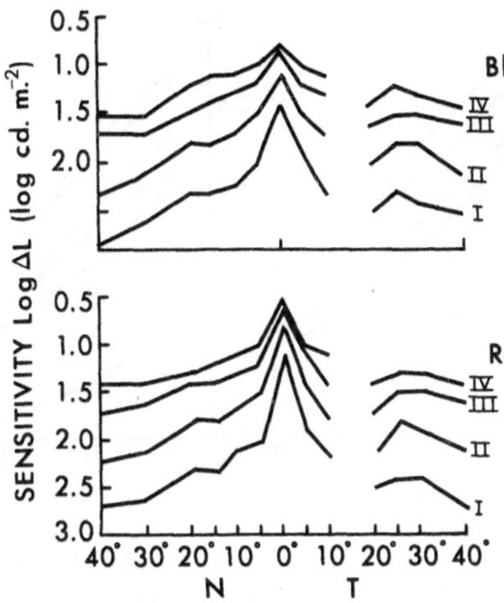

Fig. 1. Mean fully-photopic sensitivity gradients.

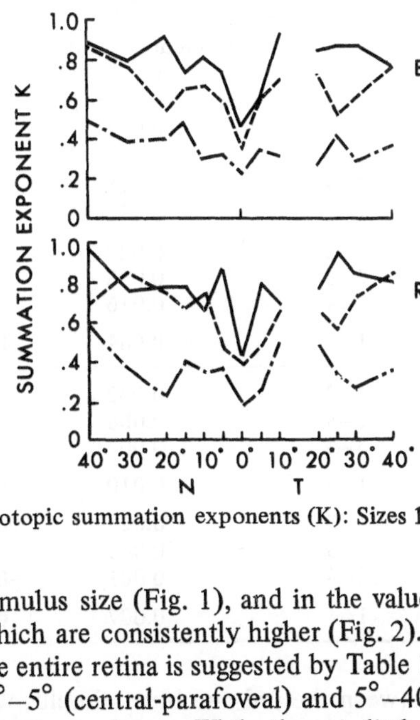

Fig. 2. Mean fully-photopic summation exponents (K): Sizes 1–2 (——), 2–3 (- - -), 3–4 (— -).

with decreasing stimulus size (Fig. 1), and in the values of K obtained with the smaller sizes which are consistently higher (Fig. 2). That this effect is not characteristic of the entire retina is suggested by Table 1, in which differences in slopes for the 0°–5° (central-parafoveal) and 5°–40° (parafoveal–peripheral) gradient segments are shown. While there is little change in the 5°–40° gradient slopes, the 0°–5° segments show slope differences which increase with decreasing size. In the summation graphs (Fig. 3) the increase in summation with decreasing stimulus size is indicated by decreasing slope of the graphs with increasing size. The fact that the 0° and 5° Nasal plots take the form of curves of decreasing slope illustrates the inverse relationship between stimulus size and summation at these locations. For the more extreme eccentricities, the straight-line plots for sizes I to III indicate constant summation for these sizes. From all three forms of data presentation there was again no

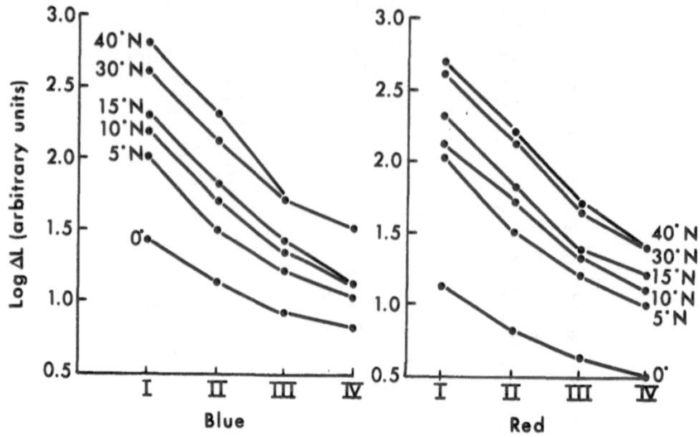

Fig. 3. Fully-photopic summation graphs for sizes I to IV. Calculated slopes for best-fit lines are −0.73, −0.73, −0.73, −0.93 (blue) and −0.66, −0.75, −0.83, −0.83 (red). Graphs have been shifted on the ordinate for clarity; slopes given for 10, 15, 30, 40° only.

Table 1. Differences between photopic sensitivity gradient segments

Gradient segment	Sizes	Difference between gradient slopes Blue	Red
5°N – 0°	1–2	0.032	0.052
	2–3	0.024	0.012
	3–4	0.016	0.020
	1–4	0.072	0.084
0° – 5°T	1–2	0.020	0.044
	2–3	0.028	0.012
	3–4	0.016	0.008
	1–4	0.064	0.064
40°N – 5°N	1–2	0.002	0.001
	2–3	0.006	0.004
	3–4	0.002	0.003
	1–4	0.010	0.008
5°T – 40°T	1–2	0.003	0
	2–3	0.003	0.016
	3–4	0.001	−0.008
	1–4	0.007	0.008

consistent difference between the red and blue stimulus with respect to this finding: for each colour, spatial summation increased with decreasing stimulus size in the central region only.

Fully-scotopic adaptation. The results obtained under scotopic conditions are presented in Figs. 4 to 6. Spatial summation at all non-foveal points was found to be greater under scotopic than photopic conditions. This is indicated by the higher K values in Figures 5 and 6 as opposed to those in Figures 3 and 4. In addition, spatial summation outside the fovea was not found to increase with eccentricity, as was the case under photopic conditions. This is indicated

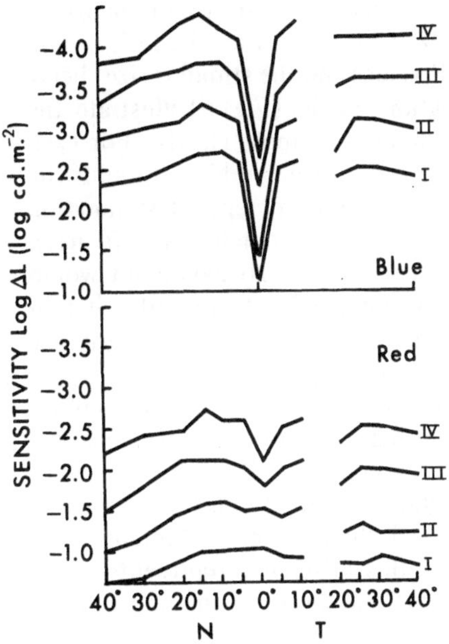

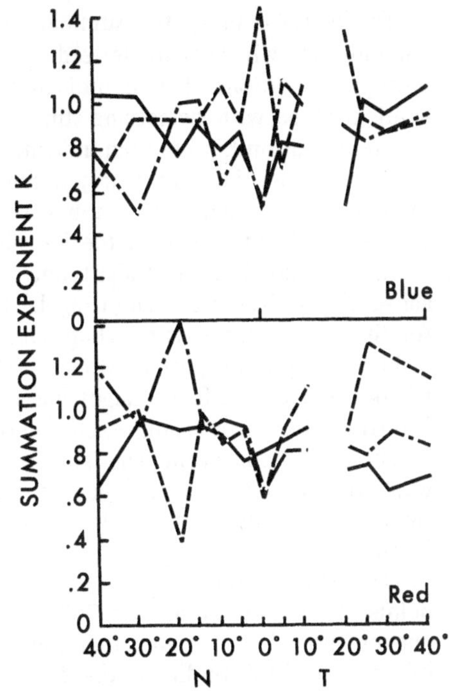

Fig. 4. (Left) Mean fully-scotopic sensitivity gradients.

Fig. 5. (Right) Mean fully-scotopic summation exponents (K): Sizes 1–2 (—), 2–3 (- - -), 3–4 (— -).

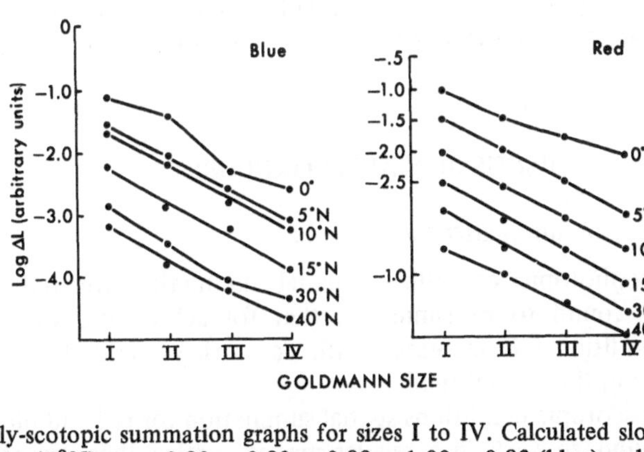

Fig. 6. Fully-scotopic summation graphs for sizes I to IV. Calculated slopes for best-fit lines (5°N to 40°N) are –0.83, –0.83, –0.89, –1.00, –0.83 (blue) and –0.91, –0.87, –0.94, –0.91, –0.89 (red). Graphs have been shifted on the ordinate for clarity.

by the lack of any consistent change of gradient slope with stimulus size (Fig. 4), and by the lack of a clear relationship between extra-foveal eccentricity and either individual K values (Fig. 5) or average K values from the summation graphs (Fig. 6). There is an indication in Figure 6 that for both the red and blue stimuli the highest value of K and thus the greatest spatial summation was at 15° nasal.

The increase in spatial summation in the central field with decreasing stimulus size which characterized the photopic results was not found under scotopic conditions. This is indicated by the lack of a consistent change of gradient slope with decreasing stimulus size (Fig. 4) and by the lack of any apparent relationship between individual K values and the stimulus sizes being compared (Fig. 5). The scotopic summation graphs (Fig. 6) illustrate the invariance of spatial summation with stimulus size most clearly. For each extra-foveal location except the 30° nasal position for the blue stimulus the summation graph is a straight line, implying constant spatial summation across the 4 sizes used. The irregularity in the results obtained at 30° nasal for the blue stimulus is puzzling: Omission of the size III data-point would yield a straight-line plot of slope $= -0.83$, comparable to the other eccentricities, but the perfect straight line of slope $= -1.0$ obtained from the size I to III points argues against exclusion of the size III point.

The results concerning spatial summation as a function of stimulus colour were to some extent contradictory: While there was no clear difference between the individual K values for the blue and red stimuli (Fig. 5), the average K values obtained from the summation graphs (Fig. 6) indicate that extra-foveally summation was greater for the red than the blue stimulus at all points except the anomalous 30° nasal. If this difference represents a real phenomenon, it is possible that the extreme variability in the individual K values masked this finding in Fig. 5.

Variability in the value of K was found to be of considerable magnitude under scotopic conditions, being greater than that under photopic conditions. This is apparent both in Fig. 5 and in the standard deviations for the mean K values, which ranged for the scotopic K's from zero to an extreme of 1.98, generally varying between 0.1 and 0.4. This variance in the value of K was found to be greatest in the fovea, but to show no consistent relationship with eccentricity.

DISCUSSION AND CONCLUSIONS

Our findings may be summarized as follows:

1. Under fully-photopic conditions, spatial summation for red and blue stimuli was found to be similar to that for achromatic stimuli under mesopic conditions: it increased with eccentricity, and decreased with stimulus size in the central field.
2. Under fully-scotopic conditions spatial summation for red and blue stimuli was not found to vary in a regular manner with either eccentricity or stimulus size, and was in fact remarkably constant over the 4 stimulus sizes used. In general fully-scotopic summation was higher than fully-photopic summation.
3. Only under scotopic conditions was spatial summation found to differ for the blue and red stimuli, being greater for the red. As these chromatic stimuli were equated photometrically, the difference between them found under scotopic conditions may reflect the fact that they were not equated scotopically.

4. Variance in the value of K was found to be considerable under scotopic conditions in particular.

The variance in the scotopic K values was in many cases of sufficient magnitude to suggest that caution be used in interpreting the mean values. Because of this high variability in the K values calculated at individual field positions between pairs of stimulus sizes, the summation graphs may be a preferable method of data presentation. In these graphs K is calculated from the slope of a line joining several area-luminance points, and thus represents an average value. Of course this method of calculating K can best be used when there is constant summation over several stimulus sizes.

The fovea was excluded from the descriptions of the scotopic results because of the particular uncertainties in scotopic foveal measurements resulting from methodological limitations. Because the foveal threshold cannot be measured by the same method as are the eccentric thresholds, there must always be uncertainty as to its comparability to non-foveal measurements. Under scotopic conditions, this problem is compounded by the lack of adequate monitoring of fixation and by the nature of the central retina's scotopic sensitivity gradient, which for all but some long-wavelength stimuli has a very steep slope down to the fovea.

The higher spatial summation found under scotopic as compared to photopic conditions is in concert with Fankhauser and Schmidt's (7) findings that over the range 40 to 0.04 asb spatial summation increased as the adaptation level decreased; our results represent the two extreme conditions of adaptation. The agreement of our fully-photopic, chromatic results with those obtained with achromatic stimuli under mesopic conditions (6, 10, 14) may seem surprising, especially as no differences were evident between the colours. However, the red and blue stimuli had been equated photometrically, and so were specifically chosen to have the same luminous effect on the visual system.

Little attention has been drawn to the actual magnitude of the K values obtained, in relation to the original 0.84 of Goldmann (8. 9) or the values found by others. Because of the wide variations in individual K's calculated for specific field locations and the multiple factors which vary from one experiment to another and which may well influence this measure, it seems advisable to restrict our attention to differences in the value of K under equivalent experimental conditions rather than to seek significance in its absolute value.

REFERENCES

1. Aguilar, M. & W. S. Stiles. Saturation of the rod mechanism at high levels of stimulation. Optica Acta 1: 59–65 (1954).
2. Aulhorn, E. Entwicklung und Fortschritt in der Augenheilkunde. Fortbildungskurs für Augenärtze. Hamburg (1962).
3. Aulhorn, E. Über die Beziehung zwischen Lichtsinn und Sehschärfe. Von Graefes Archiv für Ophthal. 167: 4–74 (1964).
4. Dubois-Poulson, A. Le champ visuel. Paris, Masson (1952).
5. Dubois-Poulson, A. & C. Magis. La notion de sommation spatiale en physiopathologie oculaire. Mod. Prob. Ophthal. 1: 218–238 (1957).

6. Fankhauser, F. Van & T. Schmidt. Die Untersuchung der räumlichen Summation mit stehender und bewegter Reizmarke nach der Methode der quantitativen Lichtsinnperimetrie. Ophthalmologica 135: 660–666 (1958).
7. Fankhauser, F. Van & T. Schmidt. Die optimalen Bedingungen für die Untersuchung der räumlichen Summation mit stehender Reizmarke nach der Methode der quantitativen Lichtsinnperimetrie. Ophthalmologica 139: 409–423 (1960).
8. Goldmann, H. Grundlagen exakter Perimetrie. Ophthalmologica 109: 57–70 (1945a).
9. Goldmann, H. Räumliche Reizsummation der helladaptierten Netzhaut. Experientia 1: 24 (1945b).
10. Gougnard, L. Etude des sommations spatiales chez le sujet normal par la périmétrie statique. Ophthalmologica 142: 469–486 (1961).
11. Greve, E. L. Single and multiple stimulus static perimetry in glaucoma: The two phases of perimetry. Thesis, Docum. Ophth. 36 (1973).
12. Lakowski, R. & P. M. Dunn. An instrument for the establishment of chromatic perimetry norms. In this volume (1980).
13. Nolte, W. Bestimmung achromatischer Schwellen für verschiedene Spektrallichter. Inaugural Dissertation, Tübingen, 1962.
14. Sloan, L. L. Area and luminance of test object as variables in examination of the visual field by projection perimetry. Vision Res. 1: 121–138 (1961).
15. Sloan, L. L. & D. J. Brown. Area and luminance of test object as variables in projection perimetry: Clinical studies of photometric dysharmony. Vision Res. 2: 527–541 (1962).
16. Verriest, G. & A. Israel. Application du périmètre statique de Goldmann au relevé topographique des seuils différentiels de luminance pour de petits objets colorés projetés sur un fond blanc: I. Principes, calibrage de l'appareil et étude comparative de groupes de sujets normaux d'âges différents. Vision Res. 5: 151–174 (1965).
17. Wentworth, H. A quantitative study of achromatic and chromatic sensitivity from center to periphery of the visual field. Psych. Monographs, 40, No. 183 (1930).

This work was supported by MRC grant no. 4342

Authors' address:
Visual Laboratory
Department of Psychology
The University of British Columbia
2075 Wesbrook Place
Vancouver, B.C. V6T 1W5
Canada

A COMPARISON BETWEEN WHITE LIGHT AND BLUE LIGHT ON ABOUT 70 EYES OF PATIENTS WITH EARLY GLAUCOMA USING THE MARK II VISUAL FIELD ANALYSER

C. GENIO & A. I. FRIEDMANN

(London, Great Britain)

INTRODUCTION

In doing perimetry, we aim for the earliest and most effective detection of visual field defects (9); with the introduction of new and standardized instruments, accuracy in the detection of visual field defects has increased.

The presence of early visual field defects in suspected cases may, in glaucoma, indicate the start of medical therapy. This is one of the reasons for the increasing number of papers done on the early perimetric defects of open angle glaucoma in recent years (1, 3, 9). Observations of patients at risk who developed visual field defects in a previously normal field confirmed old concepts about the mode of development of field defects in glaucoma (8, 10, 13). All of these works were done with white light. In glaucoma, few attempts have been made to carry out perimetry with colours. There have been numerous researches on colour vision disturbances in ocular hypertensive and glaucomatous patients, implicating the importance of colour vision tests in predicting the high risk patients (4, 5, 11).

In this paper, we aim to show that, where routine perimetric examinations with white light are inadequate, colour perimetry using blue light offers excellent means of obtaining early and detailed information concerning defects in the visual field in glaucoma cases.

MATERIALS AND METHODS

Seventy eyes of glaucoma and suspected glaucoma patients were included in this study, using the following criteria for admission:

1. Open angle.
2. Visual acuity adequate for fixation.
3. Definite or suspicious glaucomatous disc changes (but see below).
4. Raised intra ocular pressures on a number of occasions.
5. Absence of other pathology unrelated to glaucoma that could complicate the visual field.
6. Good witnesses.

All perimetric examinations were done with Friedmann's Visual Field Analyser Mark II with incandescent white background of 10.76 lux luminance.

Table 1. Clinical profile of 70 eyes included in study.

Name	No. of years follow-up	V.A.	Disc	No. of times IOP >21	≤21	IOP on exam.	Pupil size	Treatment	White	Blue
1. JS	9	6/6 L	Deep cup	11	30	18	Miosed	Pilo 4%	–	±
GC 308								Epinal 1%		
2. SS	13	6/4 L	(+) tissue loss	21	27	38	Normal	–	–	±
66 4334										
3. FD	1	6/6 R	? cupped	3	4	25	Miosed	Pilo 2%	–	±
78 1109		6/12 L	? cupped	3	4	22	Miosed	Epinal 1%	–	±
4. EG	2	6/9 L	Normal	4	2	22	Miosed	Pilo 2%	+	++
GC 620		6/6 R	Normal	0	6	21	miosed	Pilo 2%	–	±
5. FG	3	6/9 R	Normal	6	5	30	Normal	Timoptol	–	±
GC 567										
6. WW	2	6/6 L	(+) cupping	6	6	17	Miosed	Pilo 2%	+	++
GC 644		6/6 R	(+) cupping	6	6	16	Miosed	Pilo 2%	–	±
7. AA	1	6/5 R	Normal	3	1	16	Normal	–	–	±
79 2269		6/5 L	(+) tissue loss	3	1	29	Normal	–	–	–
8. ES	6	6/9 R	Slight cupping	1	24	12	Miosed	Pilo 2%	–	±
GC 401								Epinal 1%		
9. DE	4	6/4 R	(+) tissue loss	1	14	21	Miosed	Pilo 2%	–	±
GC 530										
10. IF	2	6/5 R	? normal	8	8	15	Miosed	Pilo 2%	–	±
77 38										
11. FL	2	6/9 R	(+) cupping	4	9	15	Miosed	Pilo 2%	–	±
GC 593								Epinal		
12. RE	5	6/5 R	(+) tissue loss	25	6	25	Miosed	Pilo 4%	±	++
74 3572		6/5 L	normal	21	10	29	Miosed	Pilo 4%	±	++
13. RL	2	6/4 R	(+) tissue loss	12	2	22	Normal	Timoptol	±	++
GC 614										
14. JL	12	6/12 R	early cupping	2	33	23	Miosed	Pilo 2%	±	++
GC 189										
15. AD	9/12	6/4 R	(+) tissue loss	4	2	28	Normal	–	±	++
64 193		6/4 L	(+) tissue loss	4	2	24	Normal	–	±	++
16. CB	14	6/5 R	(+) cupping	13	30	26	Miosed	Pilo 4%	±	++
GC 135								Simplene		
17. EM	1	6/6 L	(+) nasal cupping	0	6	12	Miosed	Ocusert	±	++
GC 688										
18. FC	4	6/18 R	cupped	0	17	12	Miosed	Pilo 4%	±	++
GC 535								Epinal		
19. JH	1/12	6/4 L	(+) tissue loss	2	0	32	Normal	–	±	++
MO										
20. MS	1	6/12 R	Early cupping	3	5	18	Miosed	Pilo 4%	±	++
79 1797										
21. JD	3	6/18 L	cupping	9	2	26	Normal	Timoptol	±	++
GC 591										
22. ED	2	6/6 R	Early cupping	7	2	24	Normal	Timoptol	±	++
GC 681										
23. WS	10/12	6/6 R	(+) tissue loss	6	0	26	Miosed	Pilo 4%	±	++
79 565		6/6 L	(+) tissue loss	0	6	18	Miosed	Pilo 4%	±	++
24. SW	6/12	6/9 R	(+) cupping	3	1	26	Normal	–	±	++
79 1732										
25. DP	10	6/9 R	(+) temporal pallor	0	19	16	Normal	Surgery	++	+++
GC 288		6/12 L	Normal	0	19	18	Normal	Surgery	±	++
26. WF	3	6/18 L	Normal	0	13	16	Miosed	Pilo 4%	±	++
GC 552								Ganda		
27. IG	6	6/5 R	(+) cupping	0	22	18	Miosed	Pilo 4%	±	++
GC 457										
28. MM	5	6/5 R	(+) tissue loss	0	11	12	Miosed	Pilo 4%	±	++
GC 456										
29. SH	5	6/18 L	Suspicious	6	15	30	Miosed	Pilo 4%	±	++
GC 412										
30. ES	1	6/6 L	Normal	2	2	25	Miosed	Pilo 4%	±	++
79 2161										

Table 1 (continued)

Name	No. of years follow-up	V.A.	Disc	No. of times IOP >21	≤21	IOP on exam.	Pupil size	Treatment	White	Blue
31. PM GC 425	5	6/6 R 6/5 L	? Cupping ? Cupping	4 2	3 5	16 18	Miosed Miosed	Pilo 4% Pilo 4%	++ ±	+++ ++
32. DG 79 2144	3/12	6/9 R 6/9 L	Normal Cupping	2 4	2 0	23 24	Miosed Miosed	Pilo 4% Pilo 4%	± ++	++ +++
33. FJ 78 1764	1	6/5 R	Normal	8	2	22	Miosed	Pilo 4%	±	++
34. CJ 79 1625	3/12	6/7 R	Cupping	2	3	18	Normal	Ismelin	++	+++
35. HT GC 416	11	6/5 R	(+) Cupping	6	42	14	Normal	Surgery	++	+++
36. EA 59 2687	20	6/5 L	(+) Cupping	9	29	21	Miosed	Pilo 4%	++	+++
37. PW GC 576	3	6/5 L	Normal	3	9	21	Miosed	Pilo 4% Epinal	++	+++
38. PB GC 564	3	6/9 R	Cupped	4	13	12	Normal	Timoptol	++	+++
39. JE GC 610	2	6/9 R	Early cupping	7	6	26	Miosed	Pilo 4% Epinal	++	+++
40. PW GC 698	1	6/4 L	Cupped	1	3	18	Miosed	Pilo 4% Epinal	++	+++
41. HR GC 664	2	6/12 L	? tissue loss	3	11	24	Miosed	Pilo 4% Diamox	++	+++
42. FS GC 598	2	6/9 L	Cupped	4	12	21	Miosed	Pilo 4% Epinal	++	+++
43. JG GC 414	5	6/9 L	Cupped	8	16	16	Miosed	Pilo 4% Epinal	++	+++
44. DH GC 634	2	6/12 R	(+) tissue loss	0	11	14	Normal	Surgery	++	+++
45. FB GC 109	14	6/6 L	(+) cupping	1	36	18	Miosed	Pilo 4%	++	+++
46. MB GC 687	2	6/9 L	(+) tissue loss	2	8	16	Miosed	Pilo 4% Epinal	++	+++
47. DS GC 440	5	6/5 R	(+) cupping	2	13	12	Miosed	Pilo 2%	++	+++
48. JC GC 732	2	6/4 L	(+) tissue loss	6	2	28	Normal	–	–	±
49. AE 79/763	1 1	6/4 L	(+) tissue loss	2	1	22	Normal	–	–	±
50. EB GC 421	9	6/9 L	(+) cupping	4	13	26	Miosed	Pilo 2%	±	++
51. IG GC 457	5	6/5 R	Cupped	0	20	18	Miosed	Pilo 2%	±	++
52. JM GC 456	5	6/5 R	Normal	0	11	12	Miosed	Pilo 2%	±	++
53. HT GC 416	7	6/5 L	Not done (+) cataract	1	28	10	Miosed	Pilo 4% Timoptol .25%	++	+++
54. SH GC 412	5	6/18 L	Media not clear for good evaluation	9	16	32	Miosed	Pilo 4% Epinal 1%	±	++
55. ED 73/3369	6	6/5 L	(+) cupping	5	4	23	Miosed	Pilo 2% Epinal 1%	±	++
56. MK 76/1136	3	6/5 L	Normal	15	10	28	Miosed	Pilo 2% Epinal 1%	±	++
57. RS 78/590	2	6/6 R 6/5 L	(+) cupping (+) cupping	1 1	10 10	16 18	Normal Normal	– –	– –	± ±
58. DP 79/1513	1	6/24 L	(+) tissue loss	4	1	28	Miosed	Pilo 2%	++	++

Key: – = No defect
± = Suspicious defect
++ = Definite defect
+++ = Much denser defect

For colour stimulus, a built in, deep blue Wratten filter No. 47B, transmitting wavelengths below 490 nm with 5,700 K was used. Perimetric examinations were done first with white light, then followed with blue light. Working thresholds were obtained separately for white and blue light, changing when necessary the luminance of the stimulus in steps of 0.2 log units from the given age densities, until the patient could see about half the total number of stimuli presented.

After the field examination, IOP with applanation tonometry, and pupillary size were checked, When possible, ophthalmoscopic examinations to evaluate any disc change, were done. Previous records of disc changes were noted.

Ten eyes (Table 1) with normal discs were included, but their respective contralateral eyes were being treated for chronic simple glaucoma. They had glaucomatous field defects and disc changes. Nine of these ten eyes had raised IOP's on several occasions. One patient (Case No. 25) had bilateral operations for glaucoma before she entered this study, her IOP's being controlled thereafter.

RESULTS

In the interpretation of the results, reductions of 0.6 log units or more from working threshold were considered a definite defect, whereas reductions of 0.4 log units were suspicious unless the field defect was typical of glaucoma. 0.2 log units reductions from working threshold were ignored, but were considered probably significant if they occurred in a typical glaucoma pattern or if they were found on repeated testing.

The patients fell into three groups of subjects (Table 2):

A. Group I (18 eyes – 25.7%) patients that showed normal field with white, but with slight though definite defect with blue filter.

Table 2. Distribution of 70 eyes according to the classification given.

Classification	No. of eyes	Percentage
Group I (–) → (+) white normal → blue (+) defect	18	25.7
Group II (+) → (++) white suspicious → blue a more definite defect	32	45.71
Group III (++) → (+++) white early definite defect → blue a more characteristic and clearly defined defect	20	28.58

B. Group II (32 eyes – 45.7%) patients that showed suspicious defect with white but with a more definite defect using blue filter.
C. Group III (20 eyes – 28.5%) patients that showed early definite defects with white, but with a more characteristic and clearly defined area of defect using blue filter.

A case typical of each group will now be shown.

Group 1 Case

Name: WW		Age: 68
Sex: M	No. of Years Follow-up: 2	GC No.: 644
	R.E.	L.E.
Visual acuity	6/9	6/6
Disc	cupped	cupped
Pupillary size	normal	normal
IOP after field examination	16	17
No. of times IOP < 21 mm Hg	6	6
No. of times IOP ⩾ 21 mm Hg	6	6

Case I

Fields (Fig. 1) points seen at 0.2 log units less were not marked to eliminate confusion, unless they showed some pattern.

R.E. White: Showed at one point a defect which is close to the blind spot, which is considered normal.

R.E. Blue: Showed a supero-temporal paracentral scotoma and an early arcuate scotoma inferiorally, joining the blind spot with a reduction of 0.6 log units from working threshold.

Group II Case

Name: EM		Age: 57
Sex: F	No. of Years Follow-up: 1	GC No.: 688
	R.E.	L.E.
Visual acuity	6/4	6/4
Disc	+ tissue loss	Nasal cupping
Pupillary size	miosed	miosed
IOP after field examination	12	12
No. of times IOP > 21 mm Hg	2	2
No. of times IOP ⩽ 21 mm Hg	2	2

Fields (Fig. 2)

L.E. White: Showed a reduction of 0.4–0.8 log units which is suspicious, especially in the nasal area, but does not show a definite field defect characteristic of glaucoma.

L.E. Blue: Showed a reduction of 0.4–1.0 log units showing a well defined inferior paracentral scotoma, extending to the nasal field area.

Name: FS		Age: 67
Sex: M	No. of Years Follow-up: 2	GC No.: 598
	R.E.	L.E.
Visual acuity	6/12	6/4
Disc	cupped	cupped
Pupillary size	miosed	miosed
IOP after field examination	20	21
No. of times IOP > 21 mm Hg	12	3
No. of times IOP ≤ 21 mm Hg	3	12

Fields (Fig. 3)

L.E. White: Showed 0.8–1.4 log units reduction, suggesting a supero-paracentral scotoma.

L.E. Blue: Showed in the same area a large dense arcuate scotoma.

DISCUSSION

Our results revealed that blue light compared to white light is more sensitive in detecting early visual field defects in glaucoma. Furthermore, the defect with blue light is larger and denser.

At the beginning of our study, we tried using red and green stimuli. With red light our results were no better than with white light in glaucoma patients. However, better results were shown with red light as compared with white light in patients with neurological pathology. On the other hand, with green

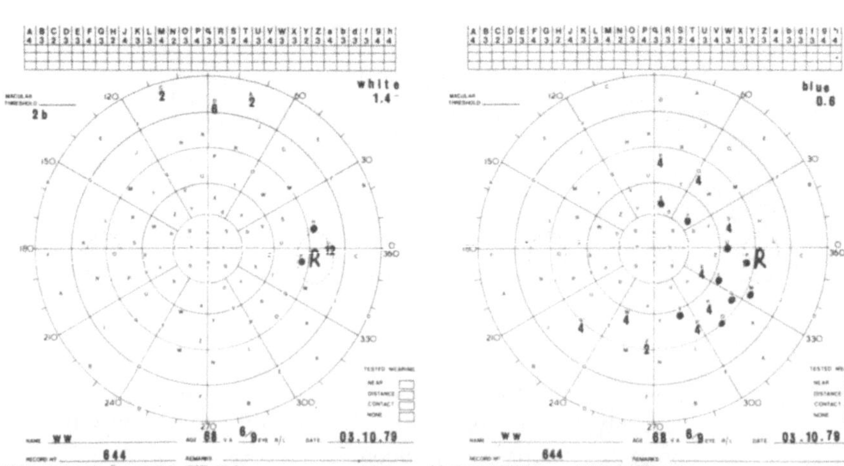

Fig. 1. Fields white and blue for Group I case.

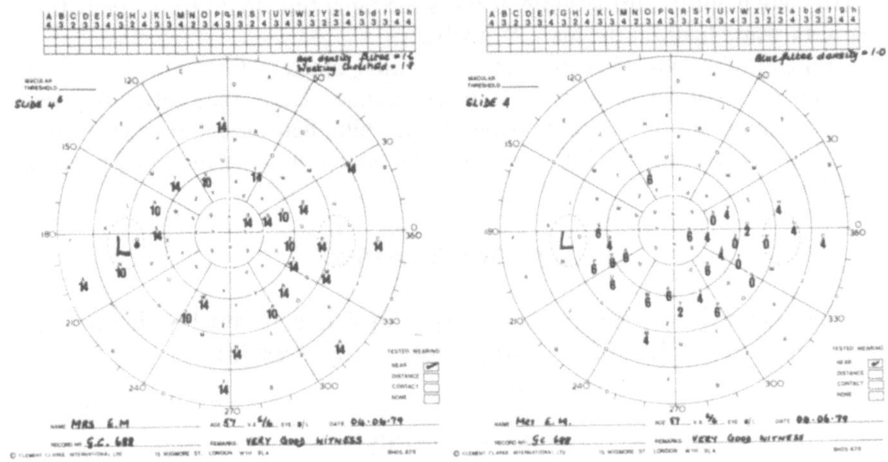

Fig. 2. Fields white and blue for Group II case.

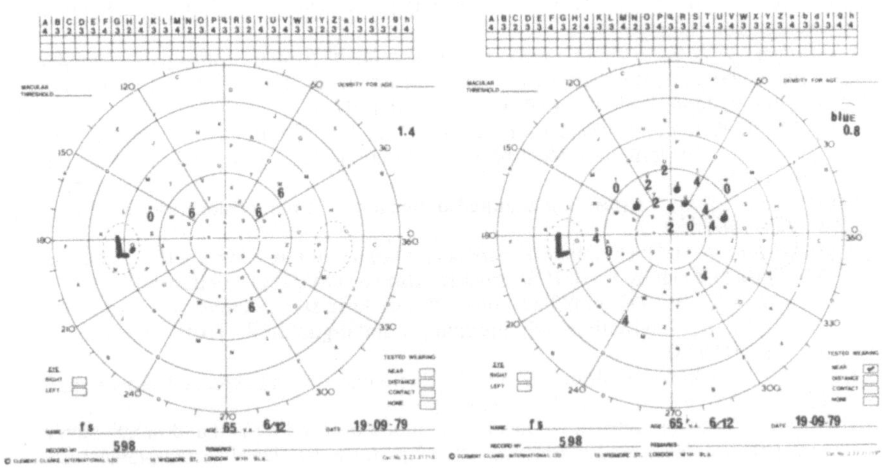

Fig. 3. Fields white and blue for Group III case.

light our results were as good as, but no better than white in both cases. We also tried using white light with dim background (to try and determine whether there is rod involvement); results however were not better than white with standard background illumination.

At this stage of our work we are unable to explain our results in terms of visual physiology. The possibility exists that 'blue receptors' are more vulnerable in glaucoma. Nevertheless, no pathological evidence exists at the moment to prove this hypothesis.

For clinical purposes, the detection of Type I patients ((−) defect in white, (+) in blue) and Type II patients ((±) in white, (+) in blue) using blue light is extremely helpful. Furthermore, it takes the same time to do the examination as with white light on the Mark II Analyser.

Finally, the typical, early cases presented indicate that our visual field studies were consistent with the clinical findings. These cases certainly prove that examination of glaucoma patients with blue light is not a useless effort, but may indeed provide an additional parameter in assessing our glaucoma patients.

ACKNOWLEDGEMENT

We are grateful to Courage Laboratory, Royal Eye Hospital Staff for their help, not least to Mrs. Penelope Wright for secretarial services.

REFERENCES

1. Aulhorn, E., & H. Harms. Early visual field defects in glaucoma. In: Glaucoma Tutzing Symposium, ed. W. Leydhecher. Karger, Basel, 151–186 (1967).
2. Carlow, T., J. Flynn & T. Shipley. Colour perimetry parameters. Doc. Ophthal. Proc. Series, Vol. 14: 427–429 (1976).
3. Drance, Sm. M., Early visual field defects in glaucoma. British Journal of Ophthalmology 56: 186 (1972).
4. Fishman, A. & A. Krill. Acquired colour defects in patients with open angle glaucoma and ocular hypertension. Colour vision deficiency II, International Symposium, Edinburgh. Mod. Prob. Ophthal. 13: 335–338 (1973).
5. Foulds, I. A. *et al.* Effects of raised I.O.P. in hue discrimination. Colour vision deficiency II, International Symposium, Edinburgh. Mod. Prob. Ophthal. 13: 328–334 (1973).
6. François, J. & G. Verriest. On acquired deficiency of colour vision. Vision Research I: 201 (1961).
7. Friedmann, A. I. Preliminary experiences with coloured filter in the Friedmann Visual Field Analyser Mark II. Journal Institute of Physics (1979 in print).
8. Greve, E. & W. M. Verduin. Two colour threshold in static perimetry. Colour vision deficiency II, International Symposium, Edinburgh. Mod. Prob. Ophthal. 13: 113–119 (1973).
9. Greve, E. Single and multiple stimulus static perimetry in glaucoma: The two phases of visual field examination. Thesis (1973).
10. Kitazawa, Y., O. Takahashi & Ohiwa. The mode of development and progression of visual field defects in glaucoma. A follow-up study. In: Third International Visual Field Symposium, Tokyo. Doc. Ophthal. Proc. Series, Vol. 19: 211–223 (1978).
11. Lakowski, *et al.* A study of colour vision in ocular hypertension. Canadian Journal of Ophthalmology 7: 86 (1972).
12. Lanthony, Ph. Perimétrie Colorée à stimuli multiples. L'Année Thérapeutique et Clinique en Ophthalmologie 25: 285–288 (1974).
13. Lichter & C. Standardi. Early glaucomatous visual field defects and their significance to clinical ophthalmology. In: Third International Visual Field Symposium, Tokyo. Doc. Ophthal. Proc. Series, Vol. 19: 111–118 (1978).
14. Verriest, G. Further studies on acquired deficiency of colour discrimination. Journal Opt. Soc. Amer. 53: 185 (1963).

Authors' address:
Courage Laboratory of Ophthalmology
Royal Eye, St. Thomas' Hospital
London SE1
Great Britain

AN ATTEMPT OF FLICKER PERIMETRY USING COLOURED LIGHT IN SIMPLE GLAUCOMA

IWAO IINUMA

(*Wakayama, Japan*)

ABSTRACT

An improved Goldmann perimeter was used, setting a rotating sector for flicker in the arm of the instrument, and a red or blue filter cap on the projector head. Each relative luminance of the red, blue or white light was controlled to be almost the same (1.00) and that of the background 0.0315 by the attached density filters and controllers. Isopter ranges of the visual fields originated from the same frequency and brightness of the flickering lights were usually the same in the same normal subjects and also in early glaucomas of satisfactory state notwithstanding any colour. In the case of testing advanced glaucoma with optic atrophy with red light, the isopter ranges were more depressed than the blue or white; however, in the case of testing early glaucomas of a progressive state with the blue, the results were sometimes more depressed than testing with the red or white.

INTRODUCTION

Mizukawa *et al.* (7), Nakabayashi and Takatsuki (8) studied disorders of the third visual neuron, including glaucoma, and reported that even if slight or no defect in the visual fields of the patients is detected by the original kinetic quantitative perimetry of Goldmann, more distinguishable defects are proven by the flicker perimetry.

Improving Yokoi's (12) and Yamasowa's (11) methods of flicker perimetry and colour lights, the nature of the defects in the glaucomatous field was studied in order to obtain more precise information in clinical situation.

METHODS AND MATERIALS

Thirty seven (27 female, 10 males) patients with a diagnosis of simple glaucoma without congenital dyschromatopsia seen in our clinic during the year 1979 were studied. Their ages ranged from 36 to 83 (average 66.5±12.1) years.

An improved Goldmann perimeter was used, setting a rotating sector as one half for flickering light source in the arm of the instrument (7, 8), and a red (dominant wavelength 626 nm; excitation purity 92%) or blue (485 nm; 64%) (Table 1) filter cap on the projector head. Each relative luminance of

Table 1. Colorimetric specification of the used filters.

Filter	C.I.E.			Dominant wavelength	Excitation purity
	x	y	Y		
Red	0.682	0.313	21.8%	626 nm	92%
Blue	0.207	0.290	9.3	485	64

Table 2. Combination of the density and colour filters for test objects.

Colour objects	Filters			Luminance*
	Colour	Density		
White		2	e	160.0 asb
Red	red	4	b	174.4
Blue	blue	4	e	148.8
Background				5.0

* In case of perfect fusion, the luminance of test objects corresponds to one half.

the red, blue or white colour was controlled to be almost the same (1.00) and that of the background was 0.0315 by the attached density filters and controllers (Table 2).

Each patient was tested with the pseudo-isochromatic plates of Ishihara and the kinetic quantitative perimetry of Goldmann. Following these, each patient was tested with critical fusion frequency (C.F.F.) test with red, blue or white light at the central fixation area and iso-frequency isopters from 10, or 15 times per second stepwise by 5, as 20, 25, . . . and so on, in the extra-central fields.

RESULTS

Depression of the C.F.F. at the central area was found in 73% in this study of glaucoma in comparison with normal subjects of the same age. Depression of isopters by the C.F.F. was shown in Table 3, in which stages of simple glaucoma were divided into 4 and phases of the colour C.F.F. into 3 groups:

Group I: Thirty eyes of 15 patients (40.5%) showed practically no difference among isopters from the three kinds of test object colours. The glaucoma cases in Group I were chiefly in early stage.

Group II: Thirty six eyes in 18 cases (48.7%) responded by showing the greatest contraction of the red isopters. The majority cases were classified as being in the advanced stage and with optic atrophy. Visual field defects in

Table 3. C.F.F. at the central area of glaucomatous fields.

	Eyes	Age	C.F.F./Sec.*	
		Mean ± S.D.	Min. – Max.	(Mean ± S.D.)
Glaucoma	74	66.5 ± 12.1	12 – 38	(W: 24.4 ± 6.8 R: 23.9 ± 6.2 B: 24.2 ± 6.5)
Control	30	68.7 ± 6.7	28 – 38	(31.5 ± 3.3)

* W, R, or B indicates respectively the white, red or blue test object. In case of the control, no difference is found among three colour objects.

this group using the Goldmann perimetry were moderately less depressed than by flicker perimetry, in comparison with Group I and III.

Group III: Eight eyes of 4 cases (2 females, 2 males) responded by showing the smallest blue isopters. They were classified as early stage but with progressive tendency.

DISCUSSION

An attempt to study the nature of glaucomatous field defects by using C.F.F. in colour (red, blue) or in white light of the same brightness and frequency was made. By use of the C.F.F. procedure which is based on the sensation of difference in brightness and its time, one may avoid the difficult judgement of the threshold point of colour saturation.

In Group I, the distinction between one isopter and another was decided by:

1. help provided by the probability of the next line, and
2. help provided by the standard deviation in the measurement.

In my experience there is about 3–10% standard deviation within about 30° area of the visual field.

It has already been reported (4) that colour sense in glaucoma patients is reduced in blue-yellow in early stage and in red-green in advanced cases. In my study, Group III patients would fit into the former classification (early) and Group II in the latter (advanced). The 4 patients of Group III had been examined over the span of several years for ophthalmological problems other than glaucoma and eventually developed glaucoma within the past 1 to 3 yeras. Clinically they have an early stage of simple glaucoma with progression of the disease.

In comparison with normal healthy individuals, C.F.F. values in glaucomatous eyes, at least except early stage, shows general depression at the central area and at peripheral isopters, especially in the Bjerrum area. Consequently, it is little wonder that both the red and blue sensations are more or less defective in glaucoma, even if the red may be super-depressed in optic atrophy in the advanced stage, presuming that the retina or choroid is the first to be affected in the eye of simple glaucoma patients.

Formerly, it has been said that perimetry by the red test object is useful for the early diagnosis of simple glaucoma according to Engelking (2), Suda *et al.* (10) and others. The results of this study show that the C.F.F. perimetry with blue object is also of value and is the procedure of choice as opinion of François *et al.* (3) and others (1, 6, 9).

REFERENCES

1. Andrezen, E. E. The threshold of colour vision in glaucoma. Vestn. Oftal. No. 6, 17–22 (1959) (in Russian).
2. Engelking, E. v. Graefes Arch. Ophthal. 116: 196 (1925), cit. S. Duke-Elder, System of Ophthalmology 11: 481 (1969).
3. François, J. Diagnostic et sémiologie du glaucome primaire. Ann. Oculist. (Paris) 197: 782–806 (1964).
4. Leydhecker, W. Glaukom. Ein Handbuch, 2. Aufl. Springer Verlag, Berlin (1973).
5. Kurata, K. A study on the discrimination of subjects with acquired anomalous colour vision. I: On the hue confusion of the glaucoma. Acta Soc. Ophthal. Jap. 69: 1998–2006 (1965) (in Japanese).
6. Makashova, E. V. Alterations in colour visual fields in glaucomatous patients. Oftal. Zh. 25: 47–49 (1970) (in Russian).
7. Mizukawa, T., M. Nakabayashi, R. Manabe, T. Otori & H. Kosaki. Studies on flicker fusion fields by an iso-frequency method. Med. J. Osaka Univ. 11: 155–164 (1960).
8. Nakabayashi, M. & R. Takatsuki. The diagnosis of disturbed neuron in the visual pathway using flicker perimetry and luminance perimetry. Acta Soc. Ophthal. Jap. 77: 1340–1349 (1973) (in Japanese).
9. Osiecka-Pilecka, H., H. Jaworowska & Wöjcik-Mazurowska. The examination of colour threshold of central vision in glaucoma. Klin. Oczna 36: 355–359 (1966) (in Polish).
10. Suda, K., T. Oyama & N. Miyata. Diagnostic value of red visual field in early glaucoma. Especially under low illumination. Acta Soc. Ophthal. Jap. 58: 642–647 (1954) (in Japanese).
11. Yamasowa, K. The specificity for spectral sensitivity in critical flicker fusion perimetry. Acta Soc. Ophthal. Jap. 77: 1325–1339 (1973) (in Japanese).
12. Yokoi, T. Color critical fusion frequency in the Bjerrum area. The basis condition for its measure. Acta Soc. Ophthal. Jap. 75: 2243–2248 (1971) (in Japanese).

Author's address:
Iwao Iinuma
Wakayama Rosai Hospital
Wakayama
Japan

SUBCLASSIFICATIONS OF RETINITIS PIGMENTOSA FROM TWO-COLOR SCOTOPIC STATIC PERIMETRY

ROBERT W. MASSOF & DANIEL FINKELSTEIN

(*Baltimore, Maryland, U.S.A.*)

ABSTRACT

On the basis of evaluations of rod sensitivity relative to cone sensitivity determined from perimetric dark-adapted absolute threshold measures to a short wavelength stimulus and a long wavelength stimulus, we have identified two forms of dominant retinitis pigmentosa (RP) and two forms of recessive and (or simplex) RP. Here we present examples of early and advanced cases from recessive and simplex pedigrees that illustrate the two forms of RP appear to represent different disease mechanisms, rather than different stages of disease progression.

Primary retinitis pigmentosa (RP) is an inherited retinal dystrophy characterized by nightblindness, field loss, intra-retinal bone-spicule-like pigmentation and other distinctive clinical signs. All the mendelian modes of inheritance are represented; therefore RP classifications based on genetic history have been exhausted. Evidence for subdivisions of the autosomal dominant and autosomal recessive RP groups has been adduced (1, 2). Here we present examples of static absolute threshold profiles in recessive and simplex RP patients that suggest that the previously described subgroupings represent different disease mechanisms rather than representing different stages of RP progression.

METHODS

Patients. Through the course of our study, data have been collected on 217 typical RP patients (25% dominant, 27% recessive, 43% simplex, 5% X-linked). To illustrate our arguments we present examples of data from 6 RP patients representing 1 recessive and 3 simplex pedigrees. The clinical findings are summarized in Table 1. Informed consent was obtained from each participant in the study.

Apparatus and procedures. The rationale and experimental methods are detailed in an earlier report (2); we present them here in summary form. Following 45 min of dark adaptation, absolute thresholds were measured at the fovea and at 2.5°, 5°, 10°, 15°, and from 20° through 80° in 10° steps along the horizontal and vertical meridians, employing the Tübinger perimeter. Thresholds were measured for both blue-green ($\lambda_{max} = 500\,nm$) and red

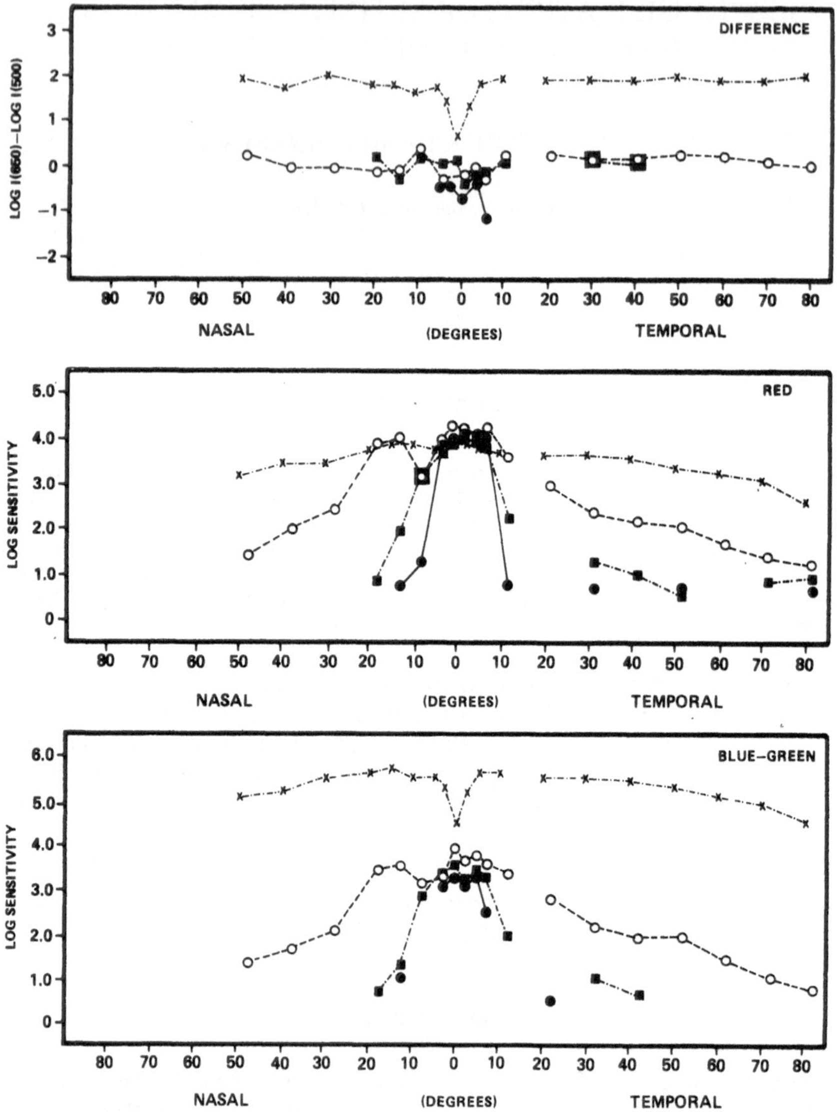

Fig. 1. Absolute sensitivity profiles measured with the blue-green stimulus (lower panel) and the red stimulus (middle panel) for 9-year-old patient A.1 (○——○), 12-year-old A.2 (■—·—·■) and 17-year-old A.3 (—●—). The differences between log threshold intensities (i.e. log of the ratio) for the red and blue-green stimuli are plotted in the upper panel. These data reflect dark-adapted spectral sensitivity. The rod determined value is close to 2.0 and the cone determined value is near, or less than zero. The means of the normal data, obtained in an earlier study (Massof and Finkelstein, 1979), are plotted for comparison (x—·—·x).

(λ_{max} = 650 nm) stimuli, subtending a visual angle of 2°, flashed for a duration of 500 msec. Absolute thresholds were defined as the mean of 3 to 5 repetitions of an ascending method of limits.

Of primary interest to the present study is the log of the ratio of the threshold luminance for the red stimulus to the threshold luminance for the blue-green stimulus. This ratio reflects dark-adapted spectral sensitivity. If only cones are present, the log threshold ratio will be close to, or less than zero; if rods mediate detection of both stimuli the log threshold ratio will be close to 2. An intermediate value represents a combination of rod and cone contributions to detection.

RESULTS

Fig. 1 illustrates static dark-adapted sensitivity profiles obtained along the horizontal meridian for patients A.1, A.2, A.3 (see Table 1). The lower panel of Fig. 1 illustrates data obtained with the short wavelength stimulus and the middle panel illustrates data obtained with the long wavelength stimulus. The top panel is a plot of sensitivity differences between the two stimuli, values that reflect dark-adapted spectral sensitivity. It can be seen in the lower and middle panels that there is an increasing loss of peripheral sensitivity with increasing age of the patient. In the top panel, it can be seen that cone spectral sensitivity values (≈ 0 log unit) are obtained all along the horizontal meridian, despite the differences between patients in degree of RP progression. Even though patient A.1 has normal fields, there is no evidence of rod function throughout the retina.

Figs. 2 and 3 illustrate sensitivity profiles on patients B.1, C.1, and D.1. For patient B.1 (Fig. 2) sensitivity losses are confined to a midperipheral ring (lower and middle panels). Despite 2 log unit sensitivity losses in the midperiphery, rod spectral sensitivity determined difference values of 2 log units are obtained (top panel) indicating concomitant rod and cone sensitivity losses.

Patients C.1 and D.1 (Fig. 3) have more advanced field loss than patient B.1, whose fields were nearly normal. As seen in the lower and middle panels of Fig. 3, sensitivities are nearly normal in the central 10° and in the far periphery. There is a ring scotoma in the midperiphery. The difference values in the top panel indicate rod spectral sensitivity, even at 10° temporal where there is a 2 log unit sensitivity loss for patient D.1.

DISCUSSION

The two different types of sensitivity profiles described here for recessive and simplex cases (i.e. one suggesting a diffuse loss of rod function, the other suggesting regionalized losses of rod and cone function) are also seen in dominant RP. The RP subtypes will be described in greater detail elsewhere. Here, we illustrate from comparisons of early and advanced cases that one type does not evolve into the other. Rather, they appear to represent different disease processes. Fig. 4 illustrates histograms of nightblindness onset for

Table 1. Summary of clinical findings

Patient	Sex	Age	Onset age nyctalopia	Mode of inheritance	Visual acuity	Goldmann visual fields
A.1	M	9	4	Recessive	20/40 20/30	Normal V/5 35° II/4
A.2	F	12	Early Childhood	Recessive	20/25 20/25	Normal V/5 35° II/4
A.3	F	17	4	Recessive	20/30 20/25	Normal V/4 20° II/4
B.1	F	13	No symptoms	Simplex	20/20 20/40	Normal with superior field defect V/4 and II/4
C.1	M	37	No symptoms	Simplex	20/30 20/40	Ring scotoma from 15° to 40° for V/4 and II/4 targets
D.1	F	46	44	Simplex	20/60 20/30	Ring scotoma from 15° to 50° V/4 and 10° II/4

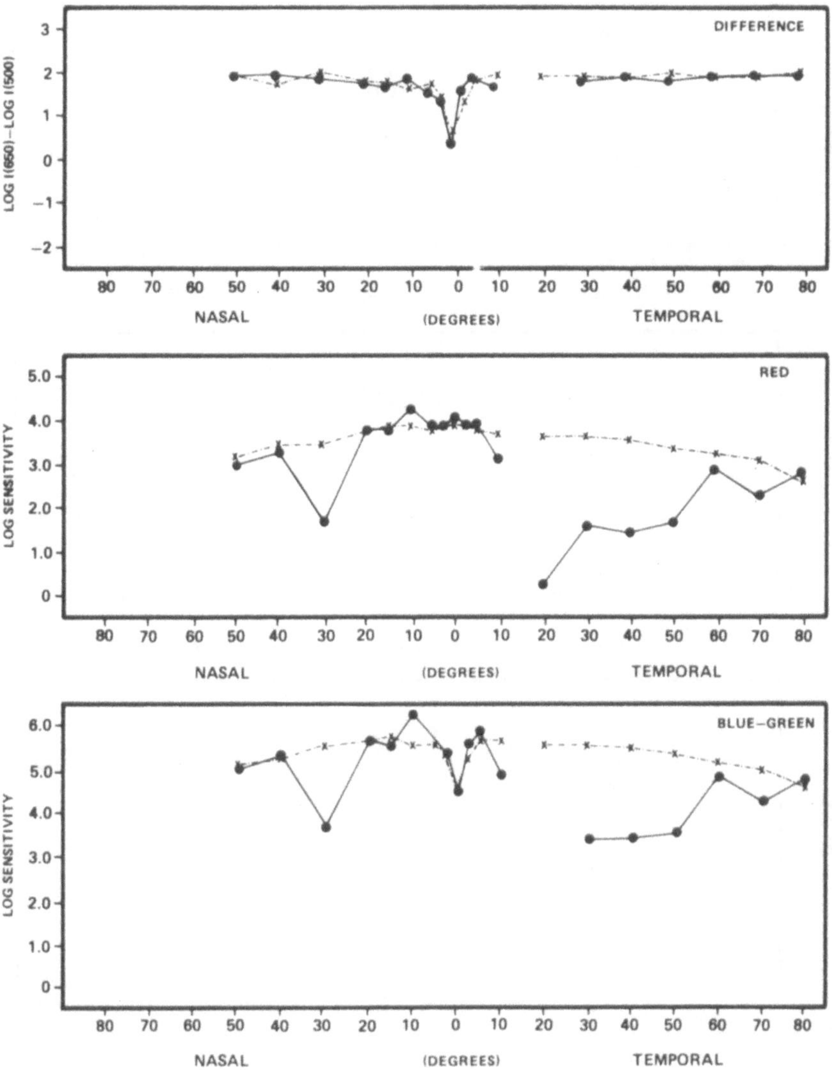

Fig. 2. Same as Fig. 1, but for patient B.1 (points), a 13-year-old simplex case who is asymptomatic.

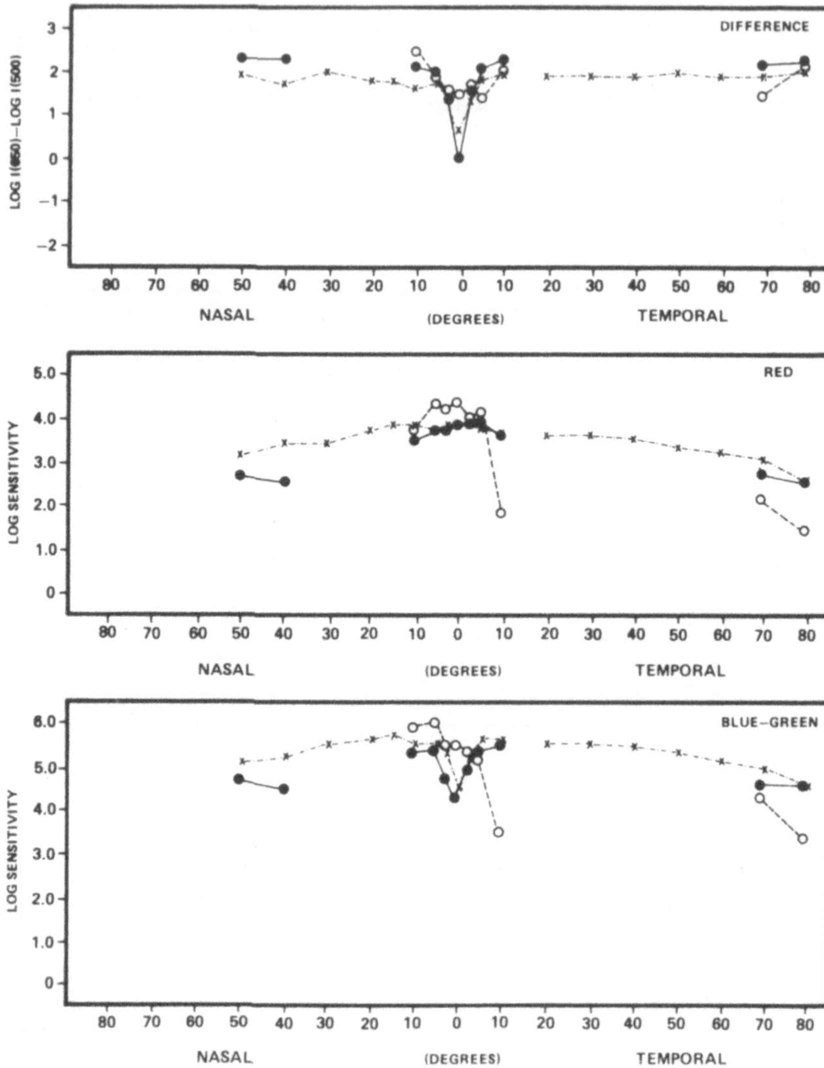

Fig. 3. Same as Fig. 1, but for patients C.1 (closed circles) and D.1 (open circles).

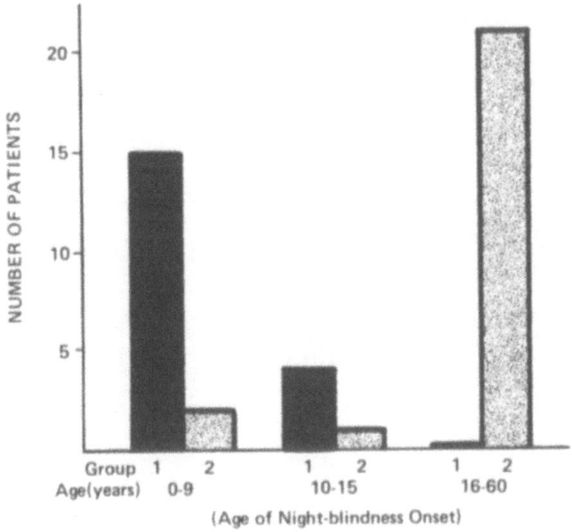

Fig. 4. Histograms representing the distributions of the age of nightblindness onset reported by the patients. The solid bars represent patients with threshold profiles similar to those in Fig. 1 (group 1) and the stippled bars represent patients with threshold profiles similar to those in Figs. 2 and 3 (group 2).

the two types of RP separated on the basis of sensitivity profiles. Those patients characterized by a diffuse loss of rod sensitivity (group 1) report nightblindness from infancy or childhood. Those patients characterized by a regionalized and combined loss of rod and cone sensitivity (group 2) report adulthood onset of nightblindness. We always see the same pattern within a pedigree.

REFERENCES

1. Marmor M. F. The electroretinogram in retinitis pigmentosa. Arch. Ophthalmol. 97: 1300–1304 (1979).
2. Massof, R. W. & D. Finkelstein. Rod sensitivity relative to cone sensitivity in retinitis pigmentosa. Invest. Ophthal. Visual Sci. 18: 263–272 (1979).

Supported by research grants from the National Institutes of Health (EY-01791) and the National Retinitis Pigmentosa Foundation.

Authors' addresses:

Robert W. Massof, Ph.D.
Wilmer Institute
Johns Hopkins University School of Medicine
601 N. Broadway
Baltimore, Maryland 21205

Daniel Finkelstein, M.D.
Wilmer Institute
Johns Hopkins University School of Medicine
601 N. Broadway
Baltimore, Maryland 21205

A REPORT ON COLOUR NORMALS ON THE FRIEDMANN MARK II ANALYSER

V. J. MARMION

(*Bristol, Great Britain*)

SUMMARY

The results indicate that the colour levels obtained from normal subjects with the Visual Field Analyser are comparable with a known standard. The Visual Field Analyser offers a simple scanning method for colour in the central twenty five degrees and in conjunction with the Visual Field Analyser Mark I offers a method for comparison of photopic and scotopic colour vision.

INTRODUCTION

The clinical practice of colour perimetry requires the adaptation of a normal perimeter with accepted colour filters within a specific range of blue, green and red. Further, the perimeter should be adaptable to cover both the photopic and scotopic levels of examination. Normal base line values of threshold measurement provide a guideline for the assessment of pathological changes. While the measurement is primarily of light appreciation and to a lesser extent of colour recognition, base line normals should be assessed in subjects with no colour vision deficiency. As colour appreciation is mainly within the central twenty five degrees, the visual field analyser Mark II should represent a useful clinical tool. The visual field analyser will present a flash stimulus on a neutral field at specific angles of incidence to the retina.

MATERIALS AND METHODS

The evaluation of colour normals was a three-phase process. Ten subjects (eighteen eyes) were examined. All were subjects with normal acuity and no demonstrable defect either on the D15 or Keely plates.

The first examination was performed on the Goldmann perimeter. Static perimetry in the 180°–360° axis was undertaken in a standard fashion, using a one millimetre test object. The following colours were examined: white, then green, red and blue in that order. Static profiles were obtained and summated and the means are shown in Figure 1 and the means and standard deviations in Table 1.

The second phase of the examination was with the visual field analyser,

Doc. Ophthal. Proc. Series, Vol. 26, ed. by E. L. Greve & G. Verriest

Table 1. Examinations on the Goldmann perimeter.

	25		20		15		10		5		0		5		10		20		25	
	M	SD	M	SD	M	SD	M	SD	M	SD	M	SD	M	SD	M	SD	M	SD	M	SD
W	27	20.2	20.1	11	13.3	4.86	9.8	2.81	7.2	2.2	3.5	0.5	7.5	2.04	11.8	2.9	21.4	6.4	23.0	5.7
G	129.4	81	86.6	39.3	53.0	19.7	41.5	20.1	28.8	11.3	11.4	3.3	28.9	7.3	49.1	13.0	119.4	9.77	132.0	71.6
R	714.8	372	522.5	231	394.3	185	280.6	144	173.7	75.4	51.4	22.8	175	38.7	343	129	664	378	749	358
B	637.5	226	479	167	328	112	238	63	193	67.6	143.8	55.2	194.5	69.2	275.6	86.1	500.6	202	662	274

Asb 1 mm Test Target 31.6 Asb luminosity of sphere.

Table 2. Examinations on the Friedmann analyser.

	25		20		15		10		5		0	5		10		20		25	
	M	SD	M	SD	M	SD	M	SD	M	SD	M	M	SD	M	SD	M	SD	M	SD
W	16.2	5.3	16.1	5.3	17.7	3.9	18.8	3.5	17.8	3.5	23.18	19.3	3.6	20	4.2	20	3.3	12.8	7.8
G	31.7	17.6	29.1	19	25.8	22	19.1	15	20.8	9.7	16.19	16.6	15.9	22.2	18.7	32.7	23.5	29.5	12.3
R	52.4	10.8	50.1	12.9	51.8	10.5	38.6	15.9	30.2	14.1	11.95	30.2	14.7	42.3	14.3	59.9	6.6	42.2	14.2
B	45.2	23.9	35.6	26	39.9	10.9	25.8	24.8	18.2	19.4	6.86	13.9	21.4	33.2	32.4	69.0	18.7	36.0	21.3

Filter settings % of 0

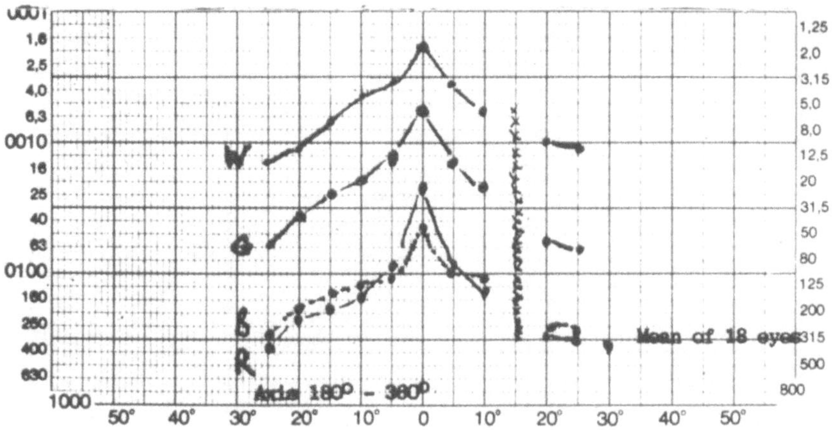

Fig. 1. Static colour profiles

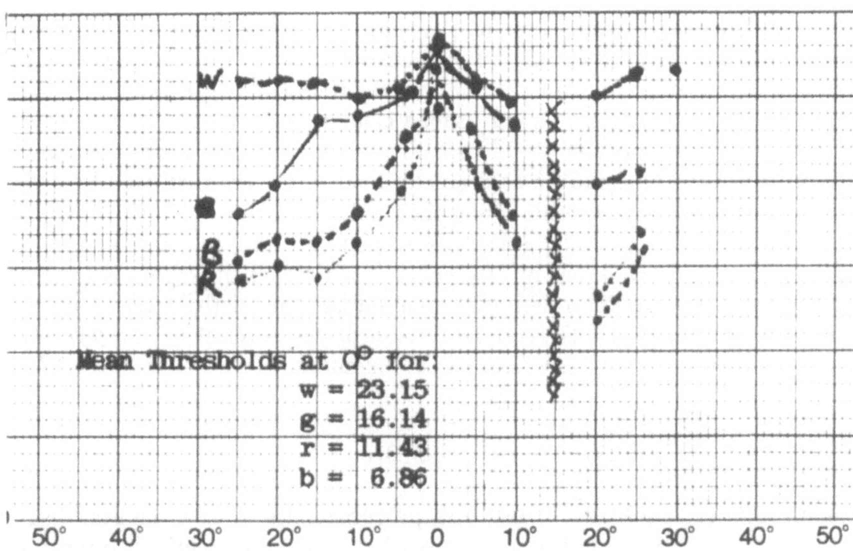

Fig. 2. Colour curves Friedmann analyser Mk 11

Mark II. This consisted of a routine scan with white, followed by green, red and blue. Examinations were conducted in a brightly illuminated room with a natural daylight fluorescent tube supplementing the normal background illumination of the Friedmann Analyser. All filter settings were taken from a supra-threshold level down to determine a threshold. The filter ratings for white and each colour in the 180°–360° axis, using those mainly below the horizontal meridian were then summated and transposed to provide a fraction of the macular threshold. The results were specifically recorded from areas which were close to 5, 10, 15, 20 and 25 degrees from fixation. The results are presented in Figure 2 and the means and standard deviations in Table 2.

The third phase of the examination was on dark adaptation. Five subjects

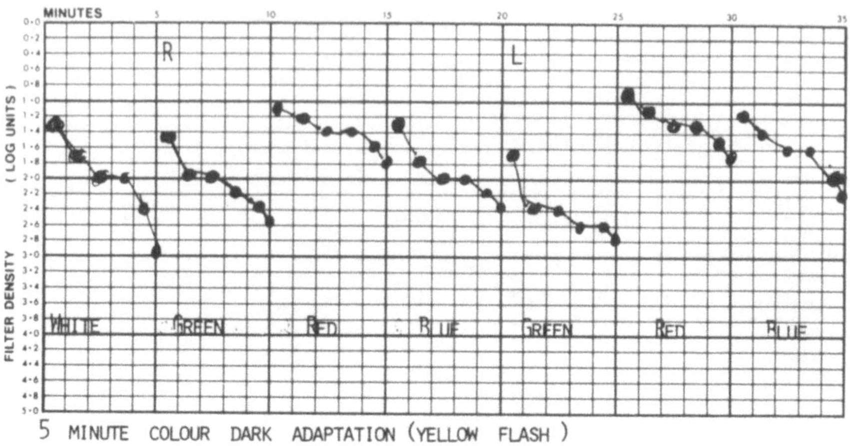

Fig. 3.

from the previous ten were examined, each eye individually on the Friedmann Mark I analyser, using the same filters, coupled with a 3 ND filter. The eyes were adapted to the standard natural daylight fluorescent light and then the eye to be examined was adapted using a camera flash covered by an Ilford 109 filter. Dark adaptation was then conducted in the standard manner, first to white and then repeated for each colour. Specifically the first five minutes, (cone adaptation), were examined and the results presented (Figure 3).

The results show a similar pattern of response in both methods of examination. In the relative levels of response to each colour the scatter is greater further away from fixation with each method and the relative levels of mean values are proportional. The results also show the reversal of the level of response to red and blue in the scotopic illumination.

DISCUSSION

Colour perimetry is a time consuming procedure. Its value in clinical diagnosis is well established (1). For comparability with other methods of examination the visual field analyser Mark II should provide in normals a comparable range of color threshold and meet some of the requirements as set out by Stiles (2). While an instrument should reveal a range and variation of a normal physiological parameter it is important to clarify that this is a subjective response and not an instrumental variation. It is in this context that a comparison with a known method is important. The different method of presentation of the stimulus and the different nature of the background, does not exclude a normal response. The results of the macular threshold with the Friedmann analyser suggest that there is a consistency with a previous experimental work of Wald (3). Any reduction of the scatter (standard deviation), would suggest a better form of examination.

The Friedmann analyser might offer the prospect of uncovering the presence of various cone clusters. Examination of the full field suggests that there are certain areas which have low threshold for colours in photopic conditions. This could be a modifying factor in the evaluation of various bitemporal field defects.

An interesting prospect arises from the difference between various colour factors obtained in light and dark adaptation. The visual field analyser presents within the one system of examination a simple method for examining colour cone function in light and dark.

REFERENCES

1. Hansen, E. Selective chromatic adaptation studies with special reference to a method combining Stiles two-colour threshold technique and static colour perimetry. Studentsamskipnaden i Oslo (1979).
2. Stiles, W. S. Colour vision: The approach through increment threshold sensitivity. Physics 45: 100–114 (1959).
3. Wald, G. The receptors of human color vision. Science 145: 1007–1016 (September 1964).

Author's address:
V. J. Marmion, F.R.C.S.
73 Pembroke Road
Clifton
Bristol, 8
Great Britain

THE SINE-BELL SCREENER

R. P. CRICK & J. C. P. CRICK

(*London, Great Britain*)

ABSTRACT

There is an urgent need and an important role throughout the world for a simple and very cheap instrument (approximately £5) which would be effective in detecting visual field loss and be relatively independent of refractive error. The Sine Bell Screening Perimeter has been devised with this object in view and particularly for visual field screening for glaucoma. The principle of the sine bell stimulus which has been employed in this simple multiple stimulus instrument has already been described elsewhere. It provides a rapid test with an easy method of scoring visual field performance and it allows control of fixation as well as being relatively independent of the patients' refractive error. The S.B. Screener brings a reasonably standardised visual field test within the reach of all those carrying out eye examinations and in particular encourages the early identification of glaucoma.

INTRODUCTION

While the general function of visual field recording is common to all perimeters they may have various levels of complexity and standardisation. An Octopus is essential for some purposes but for the worldwide detection of fairly gross glaucomatous field loss when otherwise no test would be made a very simple and inexpensive instrument may be appropriate if it is capable of giving reasonably reliable results. It is preferable for the test to be as independent of refractive error as possible so the principle of the sine-bell stimulus (1) has been incorporated. A numerical representation of the state of the visual field also aids classification. The sine-bell screener is a hand held device for use by general practitioners and all those involved in testing sight when the use of more complex equipment is precluded by lack of time or finance. It comprises a screen with windows and a sheet held closely behind the screen, the sheet bearing spot images; the spots being presented to the patient by sliding the sheet behind the screen so that the images can appear briefly at the windows. The windows and the images have ill-defined edges so that the stimuli have approximately a sine bell character.

The screen is in the form of an open ended envelope within which the sheet slides, the envelope having a different pattern of windows in its two sides, in this case a mirror image pattern. Thus the device is reversible and the number of available patterns doubled (Fig. 1).

Doc. Ophthal. Proc. Series, Vol. 26, ed. by E. L. Greve & G. Verriest

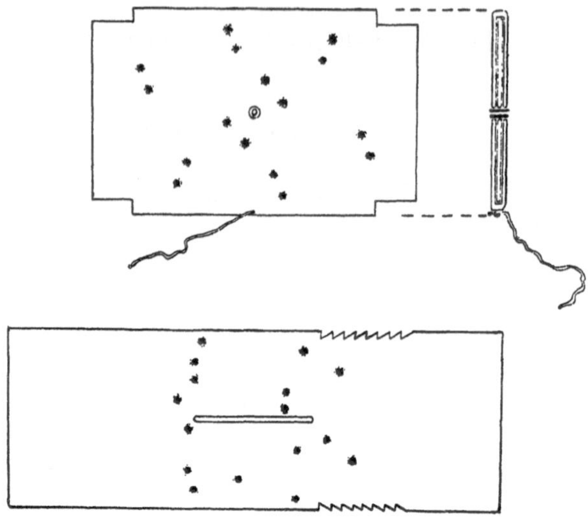

Fig. 1. Diagram of envelope and slide of sine-bell screener.

A convenient way of displaying a pattern briefly to the patient is to arrange for a series of notches or holes to be cut in or near the edge of the sheet which is pushed manually behind the screen to the extent of one notch at a time against a simple form of spring. In this way a reasonably constant time of display can be achieved. For fixation the screen has a central aperture and the sheet has an open or transparent slot through which the eye of the patient may be viewed through the screen and correct fixation assured.

It will be seen that there are 16 windows (Fig. 1) on each side of the envelope. The sheet has 16 printed images. The envelope has a central aperture through which a perforated rivet passes. This also locates the slot in the slide. The windows are apertures in photographic film printed with a graduated pattern of the required optical density.

In use the envelope is held away from the face of a patient at a distance which is determined by a distance cord fixed to the base of the envelope. The cord is 30 cm in length. The end of the cord is held against the cheek of the patient and when the cord is taut the device is at the required distance from the eye. The patient gazes at the white margin of the aperture in the envelope (Fig. 2). The practitioner looks through the aperture and ensures that the eye of the patient is fixed on the aperture. Then the practitioner places his finger in the first of a series of notches in the top edge of the sheet. The sheet is thereby pushed along to the extent of one notch. This has the effect of bringing into registration certain of the images with respective windows. Each image passes completely across the respective window and appears only briefly. The practitioner asks the patient which images were seen and makes a note. The process is repeated for each of the notches. The different notches bring into registration different images with different windows so as to give a variety of patterns of spots which are presented briefly to the patient's eye. A total of eight patterns is displayed. Then, the device is reversed and the pattern of windows and images on the reverse is the mirror image of the

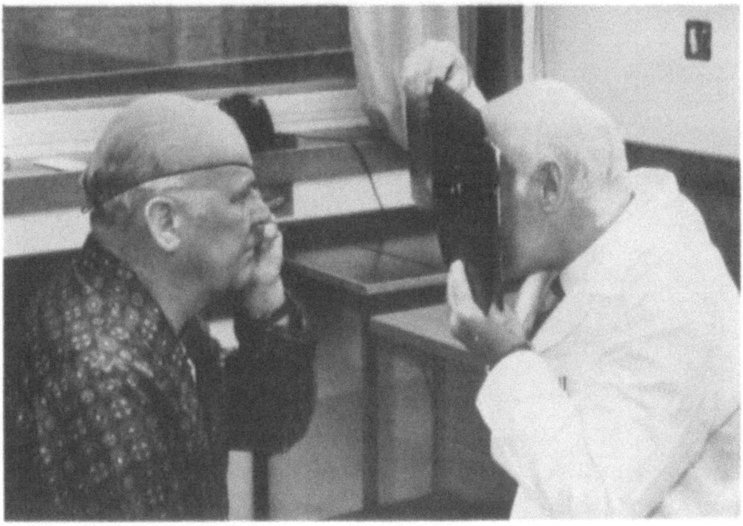

Fig. 2. Sine-bell screener (prototype) in use.

pattern on the front side. The process is repeated so that another eight patterns are displayed in turn to the patient. In this way a record can be made of the light sensitivity of different parts of the eye to the stimuli presented by the briefly appearing spots which are situated in the parts of the visual field shown experimentally to be most frequently impaired in glaucoma. Two, three or more spots, or single spots, may be displayed. It will be noted that no two images are on the same horizontal line.

The background presented by the basic shade of the envelope and sheet is grey. Although shown in Fig. 1 for the sake of illustration as dark spots, the windows and images give spots of lighter hue than the grey background. Grey is chosen instead of black in order to provide less variation of contrast between stimulus and background in lighting conditions which may be difficult to standardise accurately.

Referring now to Fig. 3 there is shown enlarged the nature of the density distribution of one of the windows (left). This is printed on photographic film across the window. The density of colouration (grey) diminishes from the outside to the centre of the window. The graduation of density is continuous and can be defined by a particular curve of density against distance.

The appearance of each spot to the eye depends not only upon the nature of the density distribution at the window but also on the nature of the image (right) which passes behind the window. It will be seen that in view of the graduated density pattern of the spots they have edges which are ill-defined. The curves of density distribution of the combination of the window and the image are such that when the window and the image are in registration the total density distribution is sinusoidal. This is represented by the curve in Fig. 3 which illustrates light intensity in the ordinate against distance across the spot in the abscissa. It is to be understood that the density distribution is

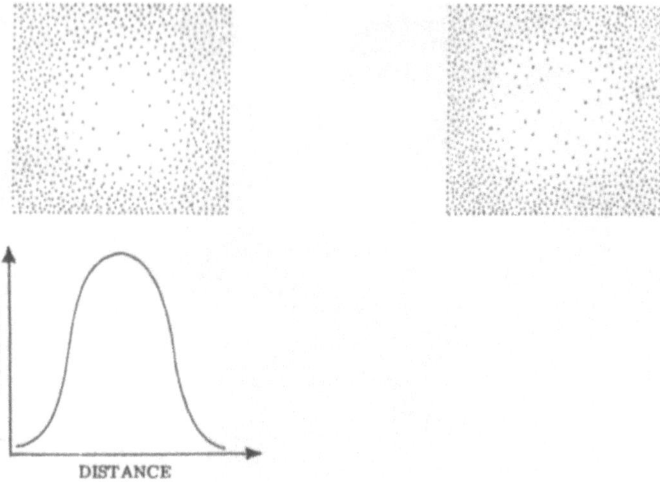

Fig. 3. Diagram showing indefinite edges to aperture and spots and the intensity of stimulus when they are momentarily superimposed.

symmetrical and is the same in all diameters of the essentially circular spot which appears to the observer. The most satisfactory size and brightness of the stimuli and the recommended ambient light are still under review.

In summary the features of the Sine Bell Screener are:

a) The Sine Bell character of the stimuli minimising the influence of 'form sense' and inaccurate refraction.
b) The use of multiple stimuli which shorten the test.
c) The simple slide mechanism for the presentation and change of stimulus patterns.
d) The mirror image double sided display allows a uniform distribution of stimuli and at the same time satisfies the requirement that there can only be one stimulus on the slide at each level. Additional slides can be made available to vary the stimulus patterns, intensity or quality.
e) The direct control of fixation by the observer and simple control of distance by the 'distance cord'.
f) The visual field assessment by simple scoring with or without note of the pattern of loss to this particular stimulus.
g) As the main medical objective of perimetry is to prevent loss of sight by detecting visual field defects which can be arrested by treatment, the distribution of stimuli in this test has been selected to be particularly applicable to glaucoma detection though other neurological conditions may be revealed. While a successful test does not exclude glaucomatous or other field loss the use of the simple sine-bell screener when a more expensive instrument is not available may help to remedy the frequent failure of recognition of established cases of glaucoma so that their treatment is not further delayed.

ACKNOWLEDGEMENTS

The assistance and encouragement of Mr Roger Barnes of Lederle Laboratories and Mrs Janice Krushner of Counsellor is gratefully acknowledged.

REFERENCE

Crick, J. C. P. & R. P. Crick. The application of signal processing theory to perimetry. 'Glaucoma Concepts' Ed. R. P. Crick, M.C.S. Consultants, Tunbridge Wells (1980).

Authors' address:
King's College Hospital
Denmark Hill
London SE5 9RS
Great Britain

THE SINE-BELL STIMULUS IN PERIMETRY

J. C. P. CRICK & R. P. CRICK

(London, Great Britain)

ABSTRACT

Signal processing theory may be used to describe the input to, and to some extent the response of the human visual apparatus. In perimetry it is desirable to separate the function of light sense from that of form sense. This requires the use of stimuli which contain the minimum of high spatial frequency components, which corresponds to a lack of an abrupt brightness step or sharp edge. A new design of standard stimulus is proposed which satisfies this requirement while remaining limited in extent, and is simply defined. The use of this sine-bell stimulus in perimetry would minimise the influence of visual acuity on the field and obviate the need to correct refraction error accurately. This would result in a quicker and more consistent test.

INTRODUCTION

Most people are aware that the quality of pictures transmitted to earth from space ships is enhanced by the techniques of image processing. This is made possible by treating the image as a 2-dimensional signal and applying the established methods of signal processing. The same theoretical approach may be made to the investigation of the visual field with the aim of making the test more specific and the results more consistent.

First we should like to elaborate on the concept of the visual signal. In this context, a 1-dimensional signal is the variation of one parameter as the single value function of another, the latter usually being time or distance. Familiar medical examples include palpation of the radial pulse where distension of the arteries is sensed in relation to time, and the electrocardiograph where a voltage between two points on the surface of the body is plotted on paper in relation to distance along the paper. In perimetry, we present the examinee with an area bearing a pattern of light and dark, typically being a relatively dark background with a small light area for fixation of gaze and one or more other light areas positioned within the normal field of view. As an area has two dimensions, this pattern may be analysed as a two-dimensional signal, being brightness in relation to distance in each of two directions at right angles. If this pattern is varied in time the signal takes on a third dimension, now being brightness in relation to two perpendicular distances and time. Thus the input to the patient's visual system may be regarded as a three dimensional signal.

Doc. Ophthal. Proc. Series, Vol. 26, ed. by E. L. Greve & G. Verriest

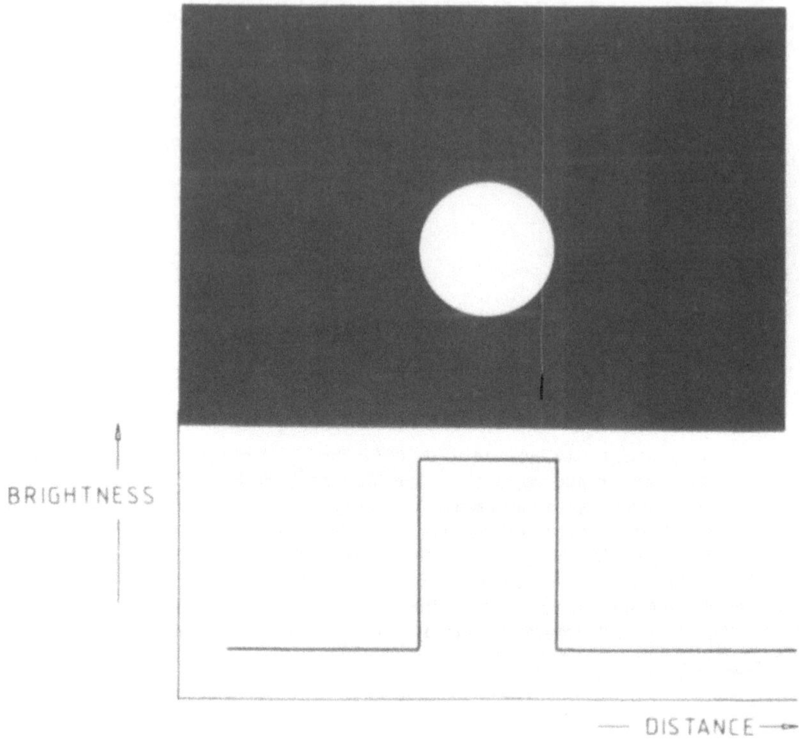

Fig. 1. Brightness plotted against distance across the diameter of a typical perimetric stimulus – a uniformly white disc with a relatively dark background – produces a 'square wave' pattern.

One of the cornerstones of the mathematical analysis of signals is the ability to represent them as the algebraic sum of a series of harmonically related sine wave components, the amplitudes of which may be derived by means of the Fourier transform. For example, if brightness is plotted against distance across a typical perimetric stimulus (Fig. 1), the resulting graph takes the form of a square wave. This same pattern may be synthesised by adding a series of sine waves as shown in Fig. 2, the first being the fundamental to which are added the third, fifth, seventh and further odd harmonics at progressively lower amplitudes. It may be seen that with just four components, a fairly good approximation to the square wave is achieved and this approximation is improved with the addition of further components. Plotting the amplitude (brightness contrast) of these components against their frequency (cycles per unit length) gives the frequency spectrum of this type of signal (Fig. 3).

In general, higher frequency components are present in any signals possessing sharp corners and loss of high frequencies (by filtering or damping for example) results in a more rounded looking pattern.

Signal processing theory is concerned not just in describing signals, but also in predicting the response of systems to them. In general, if the output of

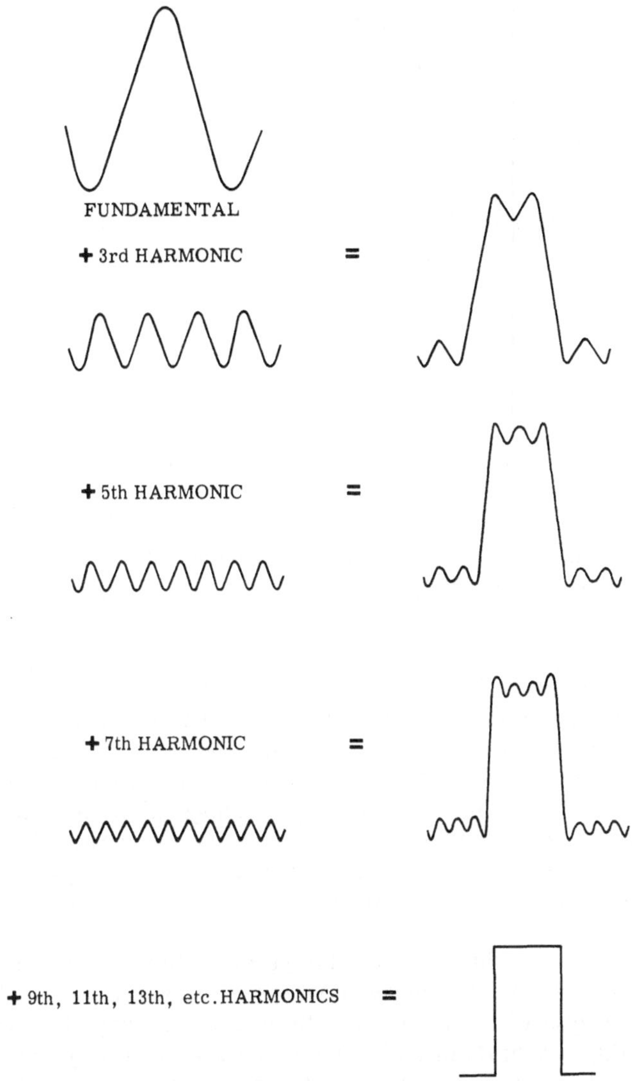

Fig. 2. The synthesis of a square wave by adding harmonic sine waves whose amplitudes may be determined by the Fourier transform.

a system bears some relation to the input, the relationship may be expressed as an equation. In one extremely important class of systems, this takes the form of a linear differential equation with constant coefficients. These are called linear systems and it should be understood that the name does not imply a simple straight-line relationship between the input and output. There are, however, two major properties of linear systems that make them particularly interesting. The first is superposition whereby the response to the sum of two signals is the same as the sum of the responses to each signal separately. The second, frequency preservation, means that the response to a continuous sinusoidal input is a sinusoidal output of the same frequency. As a conse-

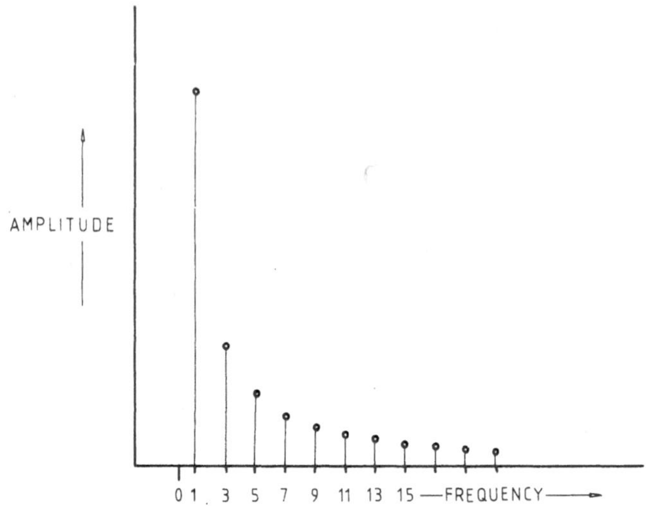

Fig. 3 Amplitude plotted against frequency for the sine wave components of a square wave to give its frequency spectrum.

quence of these properties, the behaviour of a linear system can be described using a Fourier series in the same way as a signal, the result being the frequency response, rather than the frequency spectrum. This is the form in which the performance of 'hi-fi' audio equipment is often presented and is similarly used in medicine in the 'pure tone audiogram'. In this test of hearing there is no measurable audio output, so the parameter measured is minimum intensity of input – a pure tone or sine wave – that is just heard. This threshold intensity, found for several different frequencies is plotted against the frequency.

The use of these techniques on audio systems with valuable results suggests that applying them to the human visual system may also prove helpful. For frequency analysis of the visual apparatus to yield meaningful results, it must be shown that it behaves in some circumstances as a linear system. This may be considered in two parts: the optical system and the receptor/neural processing system.

In assessing the performance of photographic and other lenses a useful parameter has been found to be the 'modulation transfer function' – MTF. This is obtained by using as the object, patterns of light and dark stripes such that a graph of brightness across them produces a sine wave pattern (Fig. 4). The contrast between the maximum and minimum brightness (i.e. the amplitude of the sine wave) of the image is then compared to that of the object. The transfer function for objects of different spatial frequencies may be plotted against the frequency (in lines per milimetre). The resulting frequency response of the optical system reveals its flare properties and resolution. The design and use of this test presupposes the 'linear' properties of the system, and the supposition is borne out by the usefulness and consistency of the results.

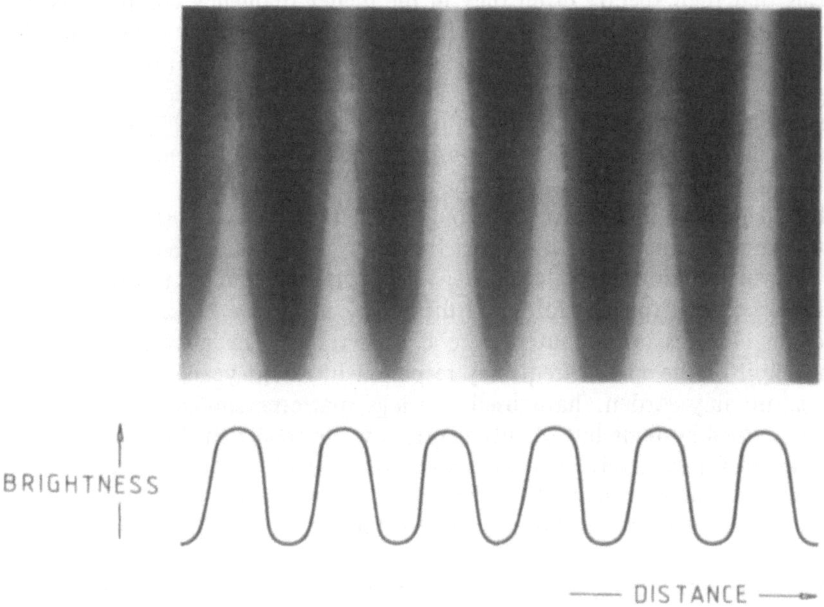

Fig. 4. Stripe pattern ('grating') with sine-wave plot of brightness against distance.

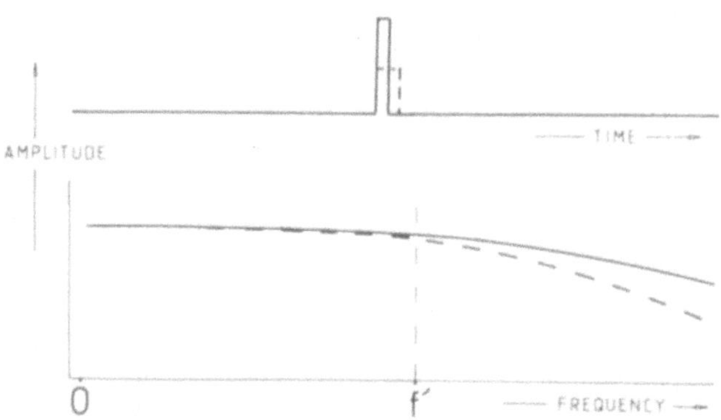

Fig. 5. Frequency spectra of two very brief pulses with the same product of amplitude x duration showing that the amplitudes of the lower frequency components of each are very nearly equal. To a linear system responding only to frequencies below f' these pulses will be equivalent inputs and result in similar outputs.

Characterising the response of the receptors and neural processors is more difficult because generally there is no objective output that bears a quantitative relation to the input and corresponds reliably with the subjective perception of the stimulus. One practically unambiguous 'output' is the yes/no response to threshold testing and for this reason it is by far the most widely used form of sensory measurement. Even with this limited response, however, there is some indication of linear system behaviour. Consider, for example, an input taking the form of a pulse of short duration. A frequency analysis of different such pulses which have the same product of amplitude and duration reveals that their spectra differ only in the higher frequency components. It would therefore be expected that a linear system whose frequency response was limited to those lower frequencies common to the different pulses, would respond to them all in a similar way (Fig. 5). That this has been found to be true, under certain conditions, for both very brief and very small visual stimuli is embodied in the laws of Bunsen-Roscoe and Ricco respectively, which have been employed extensively in the design of perimeters.

By analogy to audiometry, it would seem reasonable to assess the eye's performance by measuring its spatial frequency response. In the routine testing of visual acuity using the Snellen type, the object is of the maximum available contrast (black/white) and the ability to resolve lines, as parts of a letter, as close as one minute of arc apart is tested. This gives the absolute upper limit of the spatial frequency response. In recent years several investigators, notably Arden, have used 'gratings' patterns similar to those for testing optical systems but of sufficiently low contrast that threshold can be determined for relatively coarse gratings with up to 5° of arc between peaks. This allows contrast sensitivity to be plotted against spatial frequency to give a full spatial frequency response cruve for human vision (Fig. 6). Refractive errors have been found, not unexpectedly, to reduce sensitivity to high spatial frequencies while response to low frequencies is unaffected. In some other

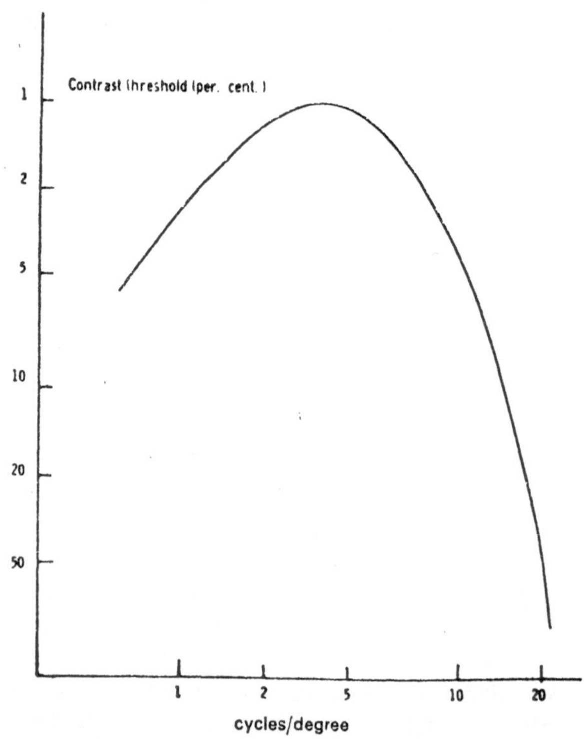

Fig. 6. Sensitivity (brightness contrast at threshold of perception) of normal subjects to gratings patterns plotted against the number of lines per degree (subtended at the eye) of the patterns to give a spatial frequency response graph for the human visual apparatus (modified from Arden, 1978).

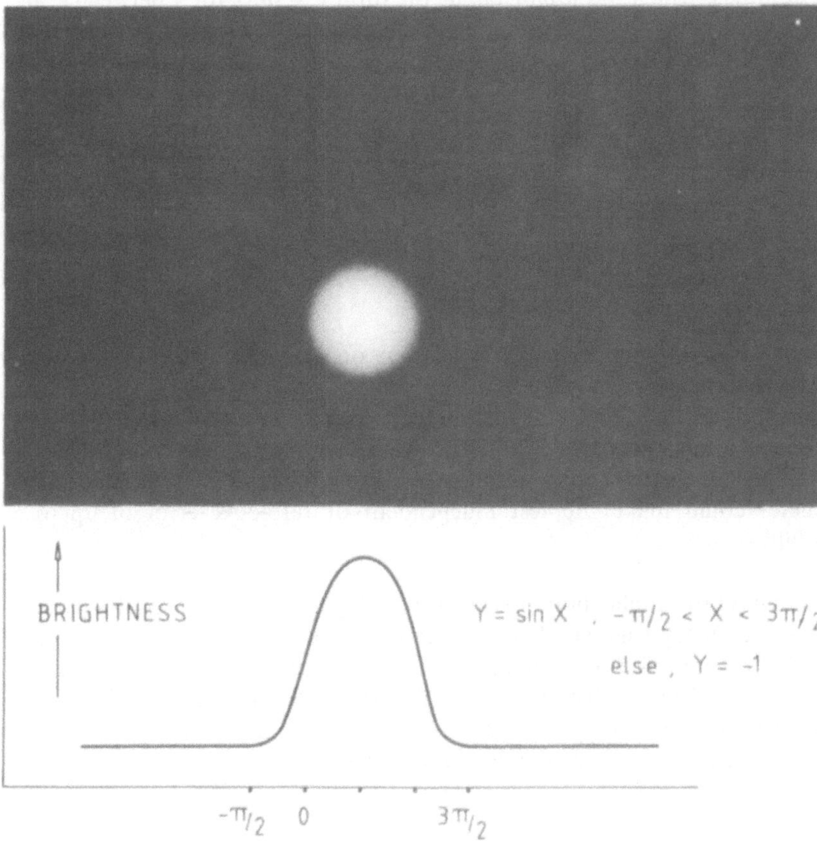

Fig. 7. **Sine-bell perimetric stimulus, and plot of brightness across a diameter (*cf.* Fig. 1).**

conditions the reverse seems to be true or there may be a depressed sensitivity over the whole frequency range.

Returning to the standard perimetric methods, refractive error may have a profound effect on the result, necessitating the time consuming assessment and correction of refraction prior to the test if meaningful and consistently comparable fields are required. If refractive error does not affect the response to lower spatial frequencies, why not devise a test employing a pattern containing only low frequencies? Or, put another way, why include in the stimulus, high spatial frequencies which mainly test form sense when the aim is to test the light sense in a part of the field? A pattern minimising high frequency content could easily be obtained by using light stimulus areas which have indistinct edges as opposed to the normal sharply defined disc stimuli. The design of stimulus with no high frequency components would have, as a plot of brightness across a diameter, a sin x/x function. This would not be practical as each stimulus would extend over the entire field. A design with limited extent and still having little energy in the high spatial frequencies is the sine bell stimulus, which has a plot taking the form $y = \sin x$ for x between $-\pi/2$ and $+3\,\pi/2$ (Fig. 7). A defining equation for brightness (B) in relation to distance (d) from the centre would be:

$$B = c + \frac{a-c}{2}\left(\cos\frac{\pi d}{r} + 1\right) \quad \text{for} \quad d \leqslant r$$

and $B = c$ for $d > r$

where a = brightness at the centre of the stimulus
c = brightness of the background
r = radius of the stimulus.

The sine bell stimulus, however, is just one of many possible similar designs which would in practice be equivalent provided abrupt edges are avoided.

The resolution of a static perimeter depends on the distance between adjacent stimulus positions. There is thus little to be gained from using stimuli of smaller diameter than this distance. The use of sine bell stimuli of large diameter could make the test independent of refractive error of up to 5 diopters.

In summary, the application of signal processing theory to the stimulus pattern used in perimetry suggests that redesign of the typically sharply-defined disc stimulus to minimise high spatial frequency components would reduce the influence of visual acuity on the resulting fields. Such a design, with a sine-bell brightness distribution, is described and will be assessed experimentally as a possible new standard stimulus for perimetry.

REFERENCE

1. Arden, G. B. Visual loss in patients with normal visual acuity. Trans. Ophthal. Soc. U.K. 98: 219–231 (1978).

Authors' address:
King's College Hospital
Denmark Hill
London SE5 9RS
Great Britain

CENTRAL FIELD SCREENER
A new tool for screening and quantitative campimetry

TOSHIFUMI OTORI, TAKASHI HOHKI & MASAHARU IKEDA

(Osaka, Japan)

ABSTRACT

A portable 'Central Field Screener' was designed for screening and quantitative campimetry. The new campimeter is the modification of Park Central Field Tangent Screen (Sola) and uses 46 static red diode targets and one target for fixation. These targets have the diameter of 3.0 mm, light up for 0.1–2.5 sec and flicker at the frequency of 5, 10, 15, 25, 30 and 35 Hz. Four symmetrical targets are exposed simultaneously at the distance of 50 cm and one or any number of these four targets can be extinguished at the examiner's will. A classical wand with a red diode target of 3.0 or 5.0 mm in diameter can be used at any time for on-the-spot confirmation of abnormal fields. Central Field Screener is also equipped with a daylight screen as in Autoplot Tangent Screen (Bausch & Lomb) and a portable quantitative light pointer with the neutral density filters of 1/4, 1/8, 1/16, 1/32, 1/64, 1/128 and 1/256. The diameter and the highest luminance of the projected target are 6.0 mm and approximately 70 asb respectively. This new campimeter has been found quite useful in detecting field changes of hemianopsia, hemianoptic scotoma, glaucoma fields, especially Bjerrum scotoma, central scotoma, enlarged blind spot and marked contraction.

INTRODUCTION

In recent years various types of screening campimeters and very expensive computerized automatic perimeters have been developed and used in the world. However, from our personal experience in clinical perimetry during the last 20 years it is deplorable that classical methods of campimetry are being forgotten. Based on our clinical experience with Goldmann perimeter and modified Autoplot Tangent Screen (Bausch & Lomb), we decided to develop a new portable screening and quantitative campimeter which simulated Park Central Field Tangent Screen (3). It is the purpose of this paper to describe the design and characteristic features of our new campimeter, 'Central Field Screener'.

MATERIALS AND METHODS

Fig. 1 is the whole view of our 'Central Field Screener'. This is as large as a medium-sized suitcase which can be opened and set up as in Fig. 1.

We employed one diode fixation target and 46 red diode targets whose

Doc. Ophthal. Proc. Series, Vol. 26, ed. by E. L. Greve & G. Verriest

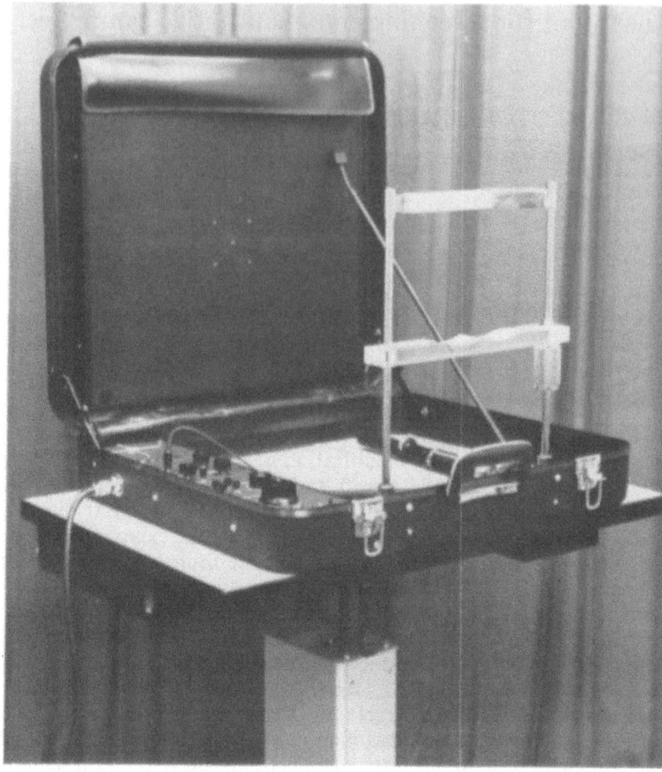

Fig. 1. The whole view of the 'Central Field Screener', opened and set up for the examination of the central field by multiple pattern method.

diameters were 3.0 mm. The front panel was holed to install 46 diode targets so that we could detect hemianopsia and early changes of glaucoma by multiple pattern method (1, 2).

Fig. 2 shows the location of 4 targets exposed simultaneously from positions 1 to 12 except for 2 targets in position 9. The two targets in position 9 are used for testing the blind spot.

In order to assure easy and quick determination of the field, 4 red diode targets light up simultaneously, one in each quadrant, by pressing the red button installed on the left control panel. The exposure time of the target is 0.1–2.5 sec and these targets flicker at the frequency of 5, 10, 15, 20, 25, 30 and 35 Hz. One or any numbers of these targets can be extinguished at the will of the examiner. This simultaneous exposure of four targets eliminates the difficulty of plotting the results by multiple pattern method.

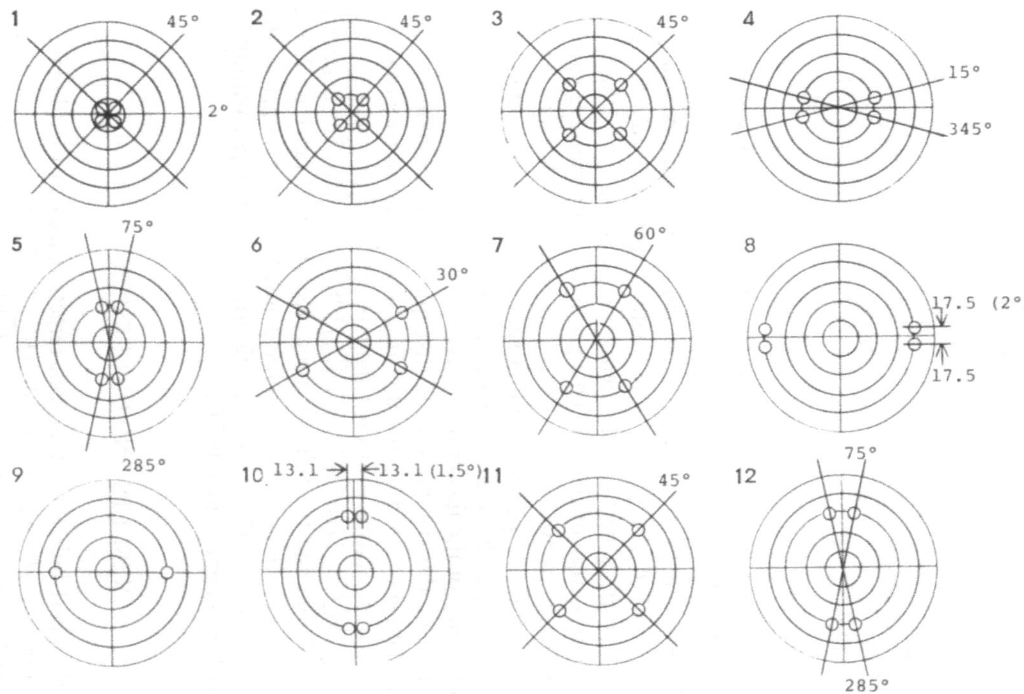

Fig. 2. Location of 4 targets exposed simultaneously from position 1 to 12.

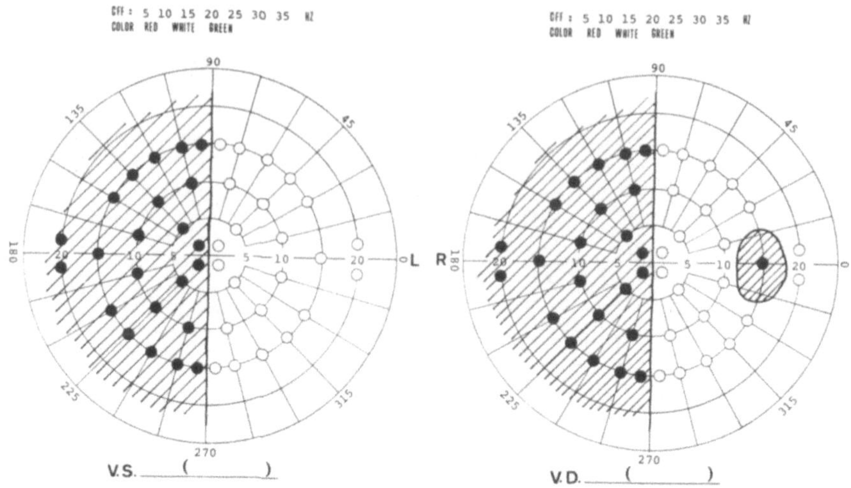

Fig. 3. Central field of a case of left homonymous hemianopsia in a 69-year-old female caused by infarction of the right occipital lobe.

We abandoned unexpectedness in the location and order of the exposure of targets. We simply asked the patient how many targets he could see and whether or not four targets were equally seen as in confrontation method.

On-the-spot confirmation of the field changes detected by multiple pattern method can be achieved by the use of a 3.0 or 5.0 mm red diode target on the wand. Classical absolute margin of the blind spot can be easily plotted with the red diode target on the wand. Flicker isopters are also obtained by changing the frequency of the flickering target.

Another feature of this campimeter is that quantitative campimetry can be done on the daylight screen by the use of a small quantitative projected light pointer. Our quantitative projected light point has 7 different neutral density filters of 1/4, 1/8, 1/16, 1/32, 1/64, 1/128 and 1/256. The diameter of the target is 6.0 mm and the target is projected at the distance of 75 cm from the screen to obtain the sharply defined margin of the target at the background luminosity of 10 asb. The luminosity of the target without a neutral density filger is approximately 70 asb.

RESULTS AND DISCUSSION

Black dots on the chart indicate the unseen targets in a case of left homonymous hemianopsia in a 69-year-old female (Fig. 3). The use of a red target on the wand and a quantitative projected light pointer reveals clear-cut hemianopsia, which corresponded well to the field determined with the Goldmann perimeter.

Our quantitative projected light pointer was found quite useful in detecting the subtle and earliest changes of hemianopsia in cases of chiasmal syndrome.

Fig. 4 shows a Bjerrum scotoma detected with a red diode target on the

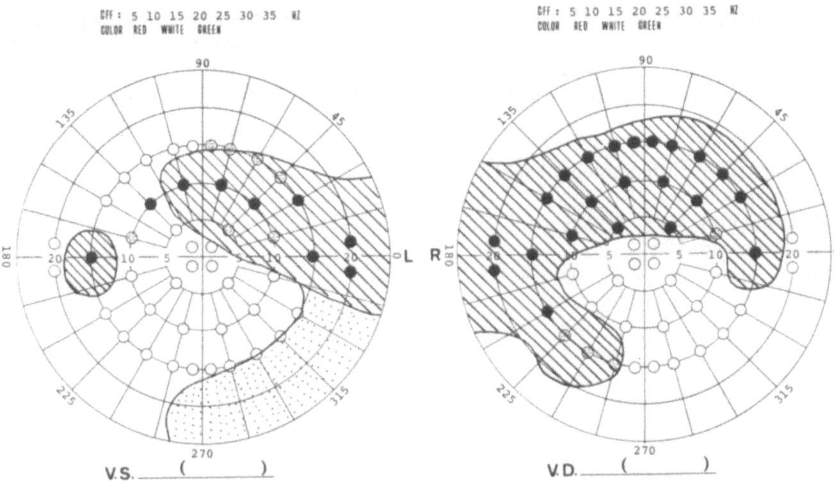

Fig. 4. Central field of a case of chronic simple glaucoma in a 53-year-old female.

wand in cases of chronic simple glaucoma. The abnormal findings with the screener are in good agreement with those of the Goldmann perimeter.

The present study revealed that this screener was quite useful in detecting the following field defects:

1) hemianopsia and hemianoptic scotoma
2) glaucoma field, especially Bjerrum scotoma
3) central scotoma
4) enlargement of the blind spot
5) marked contraction of the field.

CONCLUSION

It is concluded that our 'Central Field Screener' is quite useful as a screening and quantitative campimeter not only for in-patients but also from the viewpoint of space economy in modern examining rooms.

ACKNOWLEDGEMENT

Thanks are due to the technical assistances of Yasushi Obase, Kazuo Tohyama and Hiroshi Horiuchi.

REFERENCES

1. Friedman, A. I. Serial analysis of changes in visual field defects, employing a new instrument, to determine the activity of diseases involving the visual pathways. Ophthalmologica 152: 1–12 (1966).

2. Harrington, D. O. & M. Flocks. Visual field examination by new tachystoscopic multiple pattern method: A preliminary report. Am. J. Ophthalmol. 37: 719–723 (1954).
3. Sola International. The park central field tangent screen: Instruction manual.

Authors' address:
Department of Ophthalmology, Kinki University
School of Medicine
Toshifumi Otori, M.D., Sayama-cho, Minamikawachi-gun,
Osaka Prefecture 589
Japan

A NEW SCREENING METHOD FOR THE DETECTION OF GLAUCOMATOUS FIELD CHANGES
The flicker triple circle method

HIROSHI KOSAKI

(*Osaka, Japan*)

ABSTRACT

A report was made of a new screening method for detecting early glaucomatous field defects by the use of flicker campimeter. This method consisted of detection of depression of critical fusion frequency along the 10°, 15° and 20° lines. Studies of 45 eyes of incipient cases of chronic primary glaucoma and 32 eyes of normal subjects with this method revealed that the sensitivity of this method was as high as 78% in glaucoma cases. However, this method was so sensitive that false-positive results were obtained in 13% of the normal subjects.

INTRODUCTION

Since diagnosis of chronic primary glaucoma is not always easy to make with tonometric data, perimetry is very important to detect characteristic glaucomatous field defects. It is well known that glaucomatous nerve fiber bundle defect is sensitive to flicker campimetry of the Bjerrum area (1, 4).

It is the purpose of this paper to describe a new screening method for detecting early field changes of glaucoma using a modified Autoplot Tangent Screen.

MATERIALS AND METHOD

Using Bausch & Lomb Autoplot Tangent Screen and a flicker attachment designed by Dr. Nakabayashi (3) (Fig. 1), we examined the central field as follows (Fig. 2):

1) determination of the blind spot with a 6 mm target by kinetic method;
2) determination of the critical fusion frequency of the fixation point with a 15 mm flickering target;
3) detection of the depression of critical fusion frequency along the 10° line with the flickering target 10 Hz lower than that of fixation point. If there was no depression, the flickering target 2 Hz higher than that of the initial target was used for reappraisal;
4) detection of the depression of the critical fusion frequency along the 15° line with the flickering target 3 Hz lower than that of the 10° line;
5) detection of the depression of the critical fusion frequency along the 20° line with the flickering target 2 Hz lower than that of the 15° line.

Doc. Ophthal. Proc. Series, Vol. 26, ed. by E. L. Greve & G. Verriest

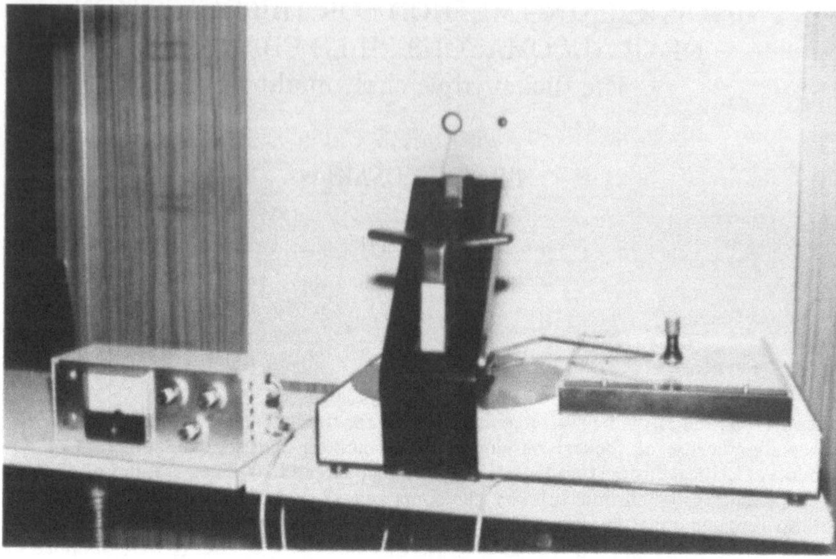

Fig. 1. Flicker campimeter Modified Autoplot Tangent screen by Dr. Nakabayashi.

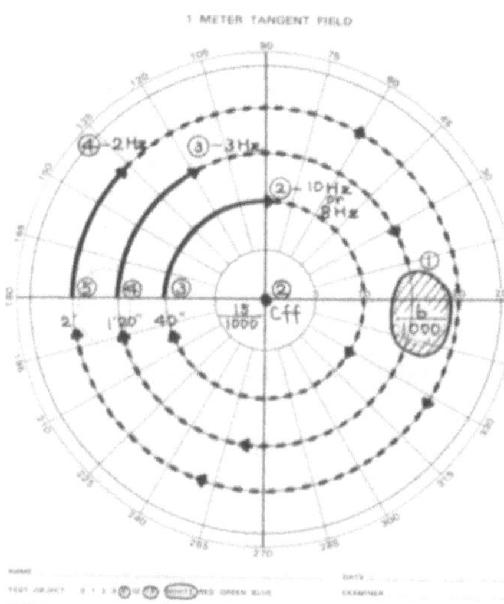

Fig. 2. The figure which explains our flicker triple circle method.

It took us 40 seconds for the test of the 10° line, 80 seconds for the test of the 15° line and 120 seconds for the test of the 20° line. Total time for screening was therefore about 5 minutes. All tests were performed by one technician to obtain uniform results. This method was performed on 45 eyes of incipient cases of chronic primary glaucoma and 32 eyes of normal subjects.

Glaucoma cases consisted of 28 eyes of open angle glaucoma and 17 eyes of closed angle glaucoma. The age of the patients ranged from 22 to 84 years with the average of 58.3 years. As reported previously, according to Kosaki's classification (2), I-1, I-2 and I-3 isopters were abnormal in IIa and not only all these isopters but also I-4 isopter was abnormal in IIb on the Goldmann perimeter. Field defects of 39 eyes were classified as IIa and those of 6 eyes were classified as IIb.

No abnormalities were detected in kinetic Goldmann perimetry of normal subjects. The age of normal subjects ranged from 17 to 75 years with the average of 41.3 years.

RESULTS

Case 1 was a 58-year-old female and she suffered from open angle glaucoma. Her intraocular pressure was controlled with 0.25% solution of β-blocker (Bupranolol) and her visual field was classified as IIb according to my classification (2). Arcuate scotoma in the superior Bjerrum area and superior nasal step were observed in her left eye (Fig. 3.1). As shown in Fig. 3.2, depression of the critical fusion frequency was suspected in the nasal area of the 20° line when the flickering target of 8 Hz was used and depression was suspected in the upper and nasal areas of the 15° line when the flickering target of 10 Hz was used and depression was noted in the nasal area of the 10° line when the flickering target of 13 Hz was used. In this case, the result of our screening method corresponded well to that of kinetic Goldmann perimetry.

Case 2 was a 67-year-old female and she suffered from closed angle glaucoma. Her intraocular pressure was controlled with 1% pilocarpine and her visual field was classified as IIa. Scotoma was found superior to the blind spot in her left eye (Fig. 4.1). As shown in Fig. 4.2, depression of the critical fusion frequency was noted both in the temporo-superior area and in the superior area of the 20° line when the flickering target of 8 Hz was used and depression was noted in the temporo-superior area of the 15° line when the flickering target of 10 Hz was used. The result of this case with our screening method corresponded well to that of kinetic Goldmann perimetry.

The results of our screening method in 45 eyes of incipient glaucoma cases was shown in Table 1. Depression of the critical fusion frequency was noted in 35 eyes (78%) and no depression was noted in 2 eyes (4%). Poor reproducibility or changeability of the results was observed in 8 suspected cases (18%).

The results of our screening method in 32 eyes of normal subjects were shown in Table 2. Depression was noted in 4 eyes (13%), abnormality was suspected in 11 eyes (34%) and no depression was observed in 17 eyes (53%).

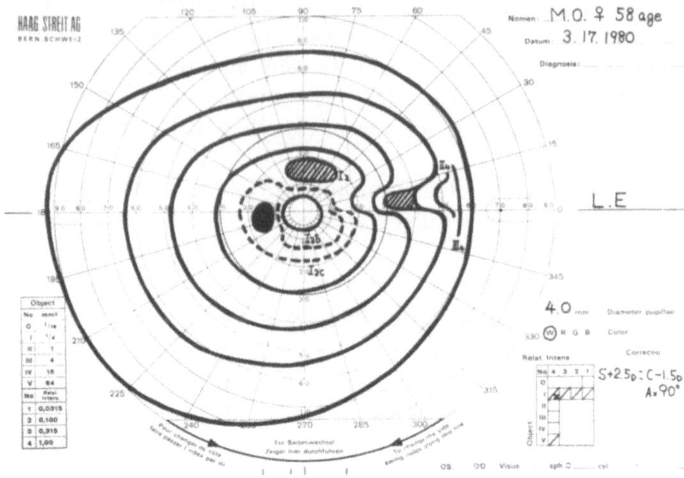

Fig. 3.1. Case 1. the result of kinetic Goldmann perimetry.

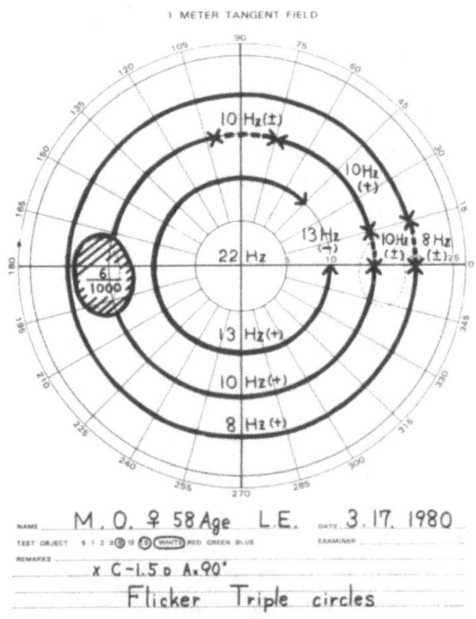

Fig. 3.2. Case 1. the result of flicker triple circle method.

Table 1. Results of our screening method in 45 eyes of glaucoma.

	No depression	Suspected	Depression
IIa	2	6	31
IIb		2	4
Total	2	8	35
%	(4%)	(18%)	(78%)

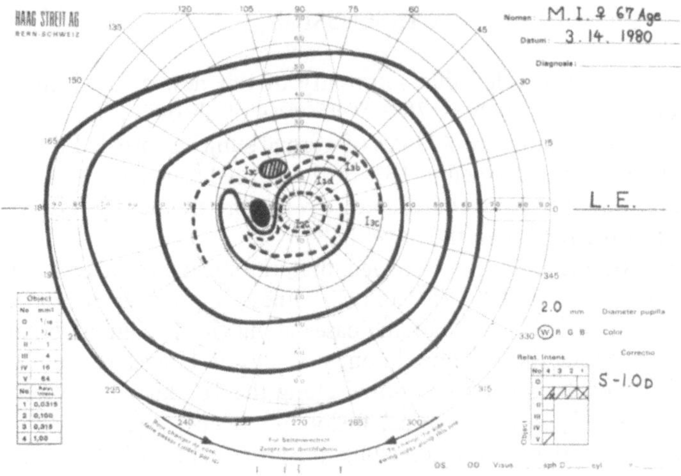

Fig. 4.1. Case 2. the result of kinetic Goldmann perimetry.

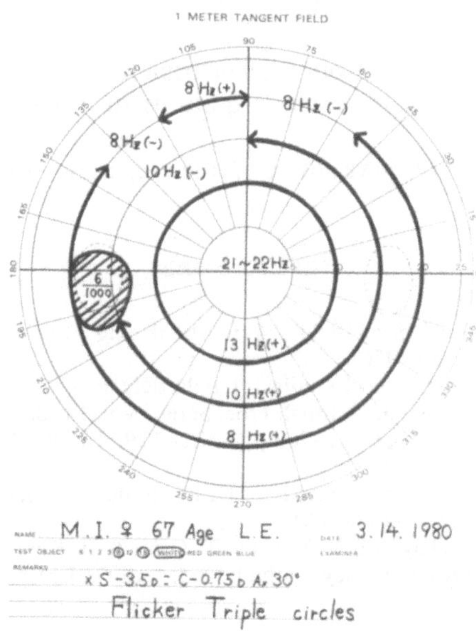

Fig. 4.2. Case 2. the result of flicker triple circle method.

Table 2. Results of our screening method in 32 eyes of normal subjects.

	No depression	Suspected	Depression
Eyes %	17 (53%)	11 (34%)	4 (13%)

DISCUSSION

The present study revealed that sensitivity of this new method, flicker triple circle method was as high as 78% of 45 eyes of chronic primary glaucoma. On the other hand, study of 32 eyes of normal subjects revealed that the false-positive results were obtained in 13% of the normal subjects.

It is interesting to note that depression is more frequently observed in the upper half of the field than the lower half.

Analyses of the data also revealed that the incidence of abnormal fields were not the same in 10°, 15° and 20° lines. Depression of critical fusion frequency was noted in 91% of the cases along the 15° line, 77% along the 20° line, 51% along the 10° line. In one case out of 43 eyes tested, depression of critical fusion frequency was noted along the 10° line. These results seem to suggest that the test of critical fusion frequency along the 15° and 20° lines may be sufficient for screening purposes, although the triple circle method is preferable.

CONCLUSION

It is therefore concluded that our 'flicker triple circle' method by the use of modified Autoplot Tangent Screen is quite useful for detecting early field changes of glaucoma.

Toshifumi Otori, M.D., gave advice on the preparation of this report.

REFERENCES

1. Harrington, D. O. The visual fields. A textbook and atlas of clinical perimetry. C. V. Mosby, St Louis (1976).
2. Kosaki, H. *et al.* Topographical studies of field defects in various stages of primary chronic glaucoma. Docum. Ophthal. Proc. Series, Vol. 14: Sec. International Visual Field symposium, Tübingen, 1976, pp. 121–129. Dr. W. Junk Publishers, The Hague (1978).
3. Matsuda, H. & M. Nakabayashi. Studies on a newly devised flicker campimeter. Jap. J. of Clin. Ophthal. 21: 673 (1967).
4. Mizukawa, T., M. Nakabayashi, R. Manabe, T. Otori & H. Kosaki. Studies on flicker fusion fields by an iso-frequency method. Med. J. of Osaka Univ. 11: 155 (1960).

Author's address:
Hiroshi Kosaki
1-51-10 Hannan-cho
Abenoku
Osaka 545
Japan

PROTOTYPE CAMPIMETER AS-2 AND ITS APPLICABILITY WITH BOTH EYES OPEN

AKIHIRO SUZUMURA

(Aichi, Japan)

ABSTRACT

In the present investigation the Suzumura spatial perimeter was modified and a new campimeter prototype was devised for use with both eyes open. The feature of the new device is its capacity for fixation with both eyes on a fixed point on a screen positioned only on the eyes of the subject tested, and the distance of the image formed is equivalent to that of the screen. Thus, the visual target is seen as if to actually appear on the screen. The results were as follows: (1) Central fixation is possible by the normal eye even if there is central scotoma, and error is small; (2) Fluctuation in ocular fixation is minimal; (3) Visual fatigue is marginal in central scotoma; and (4) Accommodation and pupillary athetosis are prevented from occurring at the time of measurement.

INTRODUCTION

The author (3) developed a campimetric method to measure binocular vision with both eyes open. Kato (2) clarified its clinical application. In the present study, the use of a clinically practical campimetric prototype is reported together with the test results.

MATERIALS AND METHODS

Figure 1 shows a view of the system developed by the author, and Fig. 2 presents the optical arrangement. The system uses a large beam splitter, and 60° visual field measurement is feasible. (The field can be enlarged to 120° with fixation point movement.) The light target is not a projected image but a spatial one positioned one meter (variable) in front of the light source by a light guide. Target conditions are the same as with the Goldmann perimeter. The target is moved manually and synchronized with the recorder. The screen is placed in the positioning area of the light object; light intensity is 31.5 asb (adjustable). Illumination is controlled from beneath the chin rest, and the fixation point is also projected simultaneously.

Subjects for basic Tests I and II were 5 persons of both sexes with normal vision, aged 24–25; in Test III, 5 children of ages 7 to 10 with normal vision were used. The diseased eye case had a visual field only in the paracentral area of the ruptured macula lutea.

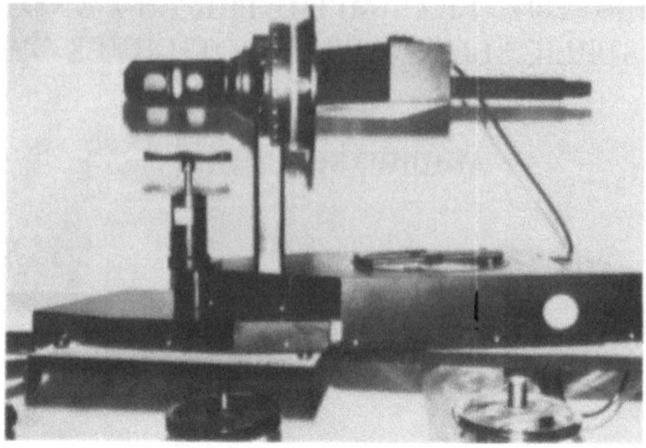

Fig. 1. External view of prototype campimeter AS-2.

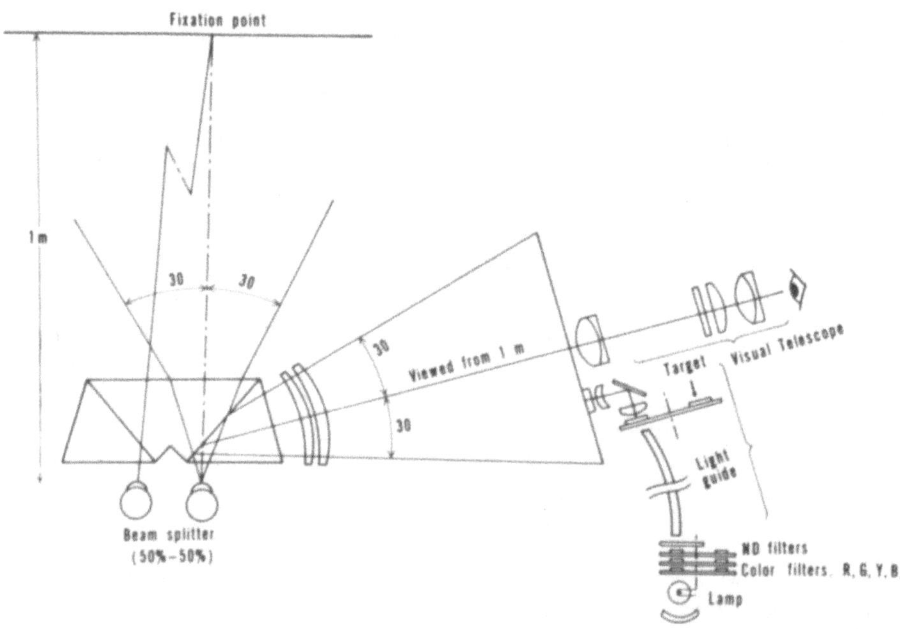

Fig. 2. Optical arrangement for AS-II campimeter with both eyes open.

RESULTS

Test I. Effects of fixation conditions on isopter

Measuring conditions: Fixed target fixation in the perimetric measurement with both eyes open (herewith BP) was with (1) binocular fixation; (2) measured eye fixation, and (3) non-measured eye fixation. In the case of (2) and (3), a diffusion glass was placed in front of the one eye beam splitter front surface, and only a clear field was presented. The Goldmann perimeter (hereafter GP) was used for the control measurements. The right eye was used for centrifugal and centripetal measurement in I-1 (light target).

Measurement results: Mean centrifugal values for the 5 subjects are shown in Fig. 3. BP (1) values were broadest and not so dispersed. BP (2) and (3) evidenced a narrower range. GP values were virtually the same as the BP (1) ones but showed great variation.

The difference in centrifugal and centripetal values is seen in Fig. 4. Other than for GP, extremely little difference was noted. From here on the visual field tended to show smaller values with a clear field and no fixation. The condition in which both eyes were left open resulted in stabler, more accurate values, with less fatigue.

Case of diseased eye. In the macula lutea breakdown case in which only the paracentral field remained, results were as shown in Fig. 5 for BP (1) and GP (2) measurement. In BP (1), fixation was correctly performed and an accurate field of vision obtained.

Test II. Effects of background space on isopter

Kato (2) reported stabilization in 'floating' accommodation and pupillary diameter oscillation in BP measurement. In this test, distance of the visual object was put at 1 m, and the fixation point distance was varied to 0.5, 1, 1.5 and 2 m for centrifugal and centripetal measurements. Table 1 shows the comparative results with the visual field area under centripetal measurement and with a 1-m fixation distance was taken as 1. Whenever there was little accommodation, the field was narrow and values very disparate. However, no statistically significant difference was observed.

Table 1. Visual field area changes in terms of fixation distance.

Subject	0.5 m	1 m	1.5 m	2 m	GP
H.I.	1.29	1	1.24	1.23	1.05
A.S.	1.12	1	0.89	0.92	0.99
M.W.	1.07	1	1.10	0.69	1.11
T.K.	0.88	1	1.00	0.94	1.04
N.T.	0.98	1	1.12	0.92	1.11
Mean	1.07	1	1.07	0.94	1.06
Deviation	± 0.138	1	± 0.119	± 0.171	± 0.045

Visual target I-1.
Background illumination: 31.5 asb.

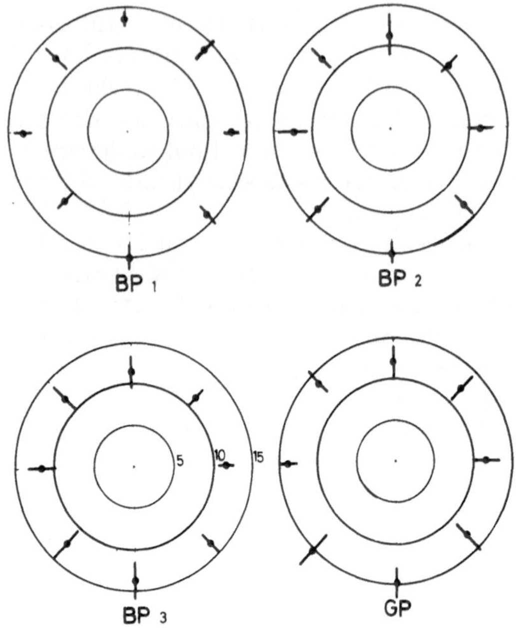

Fig. 3. Mean values from centripetal dynamic perimeter measurements, obtained from fixation by one or both eyes (right eye: mean from 5 subjects).

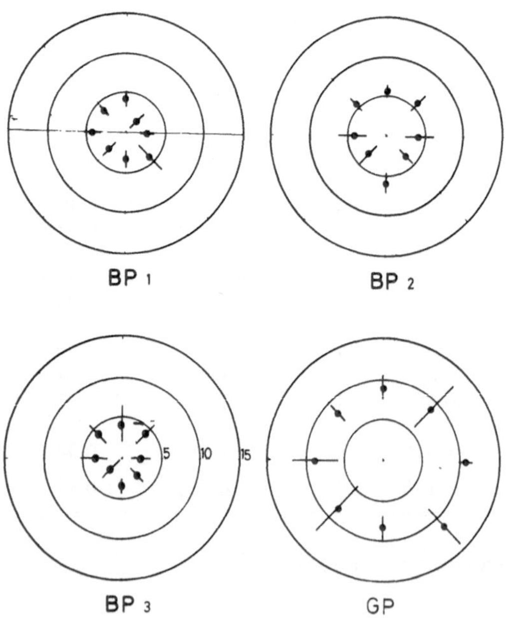

Fig. 4. Difference of fixation by both or one eye in terms of manifestation and disappearance regions.

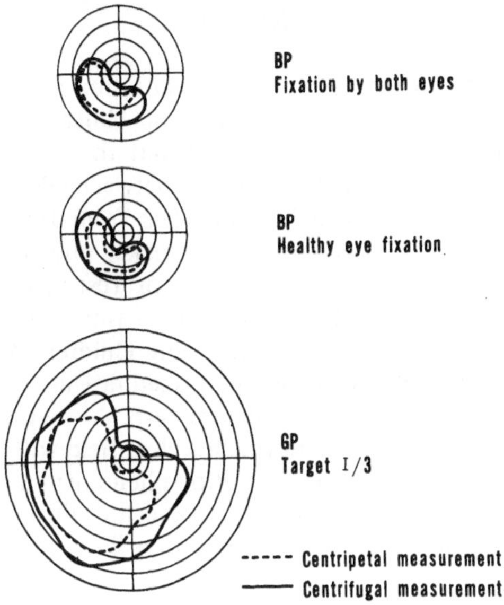

Fig. 5. Patient (K.S.) with breakdown of macula lutea.

Test III. Measurement of visual field in children

Results of children's tests with previous measurement methods have been inconsistent. Using children ranging in age from 8 to 10 years, the author investigated the stability of BP values and compared them with those from GP measurements. As shown by the comparative areas in Table 2, the BP and GP results were virtually the same with centripetal measurement; BP showed slightly broader values, and less divergence. However, GP values from centrifugal measurement were markedly greater. The BP-measured values approached those of adults, and they were obtained with virtually the same ease.

Table 2. Visual field area ratio in children.

Subject No.	GP		BP	
	Centrifugal	Centripetal	Centrifugal	Centripetal
1.	6.29	2.04	2.82	1.06
2	6.56	3.41	2.41	1.01
3	8.52	2.62	4.17	3.21
4	5.87	0.66	3.34	1.84
5	1.34	0.50	4.51	0.78
Mean	5.72	1.65	3.45	1.58
Deviation	±2.37	±1.16	±0.79	±0.89

1 = area of circle with 10° radius.

DISCUSSION

A system was devised to measure mono-ocular vision with both eyes open, namely, in the natural condition. Ashley (1) and Miller's systems, developed for the same purpose, have been employed, but they involve problems of astigmatism and imbalance of accommodation between eyes. The relationship between accommodation and visual field is clear from Test II. The value of the fixation measurement the present system makes possible in truly natural condition is clearly underscored by the results of Test I and the diseased eye findings. It was also obvious that consistent measurement is feasible even under difficult conditions, such as with young children. Moreover, results revealed less time for measurement and diminished fatigue.

As for measurement accuracy, the present tests showed a visual field narrowing tendency under conditions in which a clear field without fixation was presented to one eye, and a type of inhibition phenomenon was noted. However, this was not true with both eyes open, and thus the new system is considered in no way inferior to the method used thus far.

CONCLUSION

A new system was developed to measure mono-ocular visual field with both eyes in the naturally open condition. Measuring accuracy proved to be outstanding from tests, and measurement was also possible under difficult fixation conditions. An advantageous decrease in fatigue and increased ease of measurement were also quite evident. Another feature of the present system is that it makes possible measurement with the screen as the actual surface, and it is also thought to be an effective device for the ergoperimetry cited by G. Verriest.

REFERENCES

1. Ashley, J. C. Binocular instantly programmable automatic screener. Docum. Ophthal. Proc. Series, Vol. 14: Sec. International Visual Field Symposium, Tübingen. pp. 37–45. Dr. W. Junk Publishers, The Hague (1978).
2. Kato, K. A study of visual field under binocular condition. Folia Ophthal. Jap. 30: 128–140 (1979).
3. Suzumura, A. Variation of visual perception of spatial objects and development of perceptual aptitude. Acta Soc. Ophthal. Jap. 75: 1974–2006 (1971).

Author's address:
Akihiro Suzumura
Dept. of Opthalmology
Aichi Medical University
Nagakute-cho, Aichi-gun
Aichi Pref., 480-11
Japan

AN EVALUATION OF THE FRIEDMANN ANALYSER MARK II

V. J. MARMION

(*Bristol, Great Britain*)

ABSTRACT

The improved Visual Field Analyser Mark II represents a positive improvement with a better system of random sampling. There is a definable improvement in the method of multiple stimulus static perimetry in relation to the Visual Field Analyser Mark I.

INTRODUCTION

Techniques of examining the visual field have for the past thirty years been based on static or kinetic perimetry. Both required a logical programme sequence of examination, which naturally led to automation. Over the past decade the Friedmann Visual Field Analyser has introduced another concept, that of random sampling in a specified area of the central 25° (2). This technique has become firmly established and is attractive to the busy clinician and is, perhaps, simpler for the patient. The improved Visual Field Analyser Mark II offers cover of the blind spot, central 10°, nasal step and, in particular, the arcuate area. There is a better randomisation of the number of focii presented at any time and a degree of geometrical asymmetry is introduced in the patterns presented. The Visual Field Analyser Mark II therefore offers the possibility of covering a spectrum of defects with more accuracy.

MATERIAL AND METHODS

Ten patients of similar age and sex were examined. Five of these were glaucoma suspects with no expected visual field defect. Five were known glaucoma subjects with established field defects. All were examined on the Goldmann perimeter covering the central 30° along 15° meridiae in 2°5 steps using 2 different light thresholds with a 1 mm target. This examination was used as the baseline for the Visual Field Analyser examination which followed first the Mark I and then the Mark II. To compare the two instruments it was felt that neither an A, or a B run on the Visual Field Analyser Mark II provided a comparable number of positions for a valid comparison with Mark I. The whole of the upper and lower field filter settings for each instrument were recorded, summated and compared with the counts from within the corre-

Doc. Ophthal. Proc. Series, Vol. 26, ed. by E. L. Greve & G. Verriest

Table 1.

Glaucoma	Upper			Lower		
	Whole	10–20	*t*	Whole	10–20	*t*
Suspects						
VFA I	17.5 (2.91)	17.23 (3.04)	0.741	17.7 (3.29)	17.97 (2.29)	−0.547
VFA II	17.3 (1.8)	16.95 (2.16)	2.637S	17.48 (1.78)	16.95 (2.12)	3.090S
t	−0.755	−0.893		−1.416	−3.606S	
Patients						
VFA I	10.08 (5.84)	9.03 (5.95)	1.173	9.93 (6.73)	9.57 (6.83)	0.345
VFA II	10.01 (6.44)	9.35 (6.57)	1.233	9.66 (6.92)	8.54 (7.12)	1.776
t	−0.119	−0.340		−0.392	−0.982	

S = Significant.
SD shown in brackets to the right of mean.

sponding 10° to 20° area from fixation. A mean and standard deviation were obtained and a t-test applied to the results from within the instruments and between the two instruments. These are presented in the Table.

THE RESULTS

These show that in the recordings from the glaucoma suspect group, the variability (SD) is low, and the means are comparable. Statistical analysis, however, shows that there is a significant difference with the Visual Field Analyser Mark II in both the upper and lower fields between the arcuate area and the whole field and, in the case of the lower field, a significant difference between the arcuate area of each instrument. This could have been overlooked if a 0.4 log unit variability had been applied (3). In the glaucoma group, the degree of variability (SD) is greater although the means are similar. In the analysis between the whole and arcuate fields, although some results approach, they do not reach significance (95% level), and there is no significant difference between either instrument either for the whole or the arcuate area of the field.

DISCUSSION

The advent of a modification in the perimeter should offer both a quantitative and a qualitative progress. Qualitative improvement has been achieved with a range of controls, illuminated panels, continuous flow of filter selections and other features.

If this improvement is to be shown in clinical practice, it should be manifest in a quantitative and definable difference in the analysis of the field defects. As a control, a modified Armaly Drance technique was used (1). This was to provide a reference for the field defects and to reduce the elements of false positives or negatives. The Visual Field Analyser recordings are comparable yet, when analysed statistically, a significance appears in favour of the results obtained from the Visual Field Analyser Mark II indicating a discernable difference between the two instruments. It can therefore be anticipated that the Visual Field Analyser Mark II will fulfil the role ascribed to it in the detection and follow up phase more accurately than the Visual Field Analyser Mark I.

REFERENCES

1. Drance, S. M. A modification of the Armaly visual field screening technique for glaucoma. Canada J. Ophthal. 6: 283 (1971).
2. Friedmann, A. I. Serial analysis of changes in visual field defects, employing a new instrument to determine the activity of diseases involving the visual pathways. Ophthalmologica (Basle) 152: 1 (1966).
3. Greve, E. L. Visual field analyser and threshold. Brit. J. Ophthal. 55: 704 (1971).

Author's address:
V. J. Marmion, F.R.C.S., Ed.
73 Pembroke Road
Clifton
Bristol, 8
Great Britain

OPTIC NERVE FUNCTION IN THE TOXIC AMBLYOPIAS AND RELATED CONDITIONS

WALLACE S. FOULDS

(*Glasgow, Great Britain*)

There are of course many forms of toxic amblyopia and if we exclude ischaemic optic neuropathy and glaucoma, patients presenting with optic nerve dysfunction fall into four categories in order of frequency, namely the retrobulbar neuritis of multiple sclerosis, tobacco amblyopia, inherited optic atrophies and optic nerve compression.

Although this appears a disaparate group of conditions the differential diagnosis in this group can present difficulties. It is for this reason, and in order to assess the severity of the condition and its progress that cases falling within this group of disorders require careful visual assessment making use of all the powerful techniques we now have at our disposal.

The assessment of colour vision is an important measurable parameter and in cases of toxic amblyopia where error scores are often very high, automated equipment is a great help in the rapid computation of error scores and the plotting of results (11).

Much interest has been shown in recent years in such parameters as contrast sensitivity to grating patterns, for abnormalities in grating discrimination, not necessarily paralleling acuity may be seen in many optic nerve dysfunctions. To test grating resolution accurately is very time consuming and the simple grating test of Arden and Jacobsen (2) may be a useful addition to the armamentarium of clinical departments interested in optic nerve function. Electro-physiological tests are of course important and the ability to record visual evoked cortical potentials is mandatory as indeed is access to CAT scanning and sophisticated biochemistry in relation to the differential diagnosis of say compressive lesions from, for example, demyelination due to multiple sclerosis.

Returning to the toxic amblyopias and particularly tobacco amblyopia there is little new that can be said about the field defects in this condition, for it has been known for at least half a century that the defect in tobacco amblyopia is a bilateral centro-caecal depression and that the defect is more marked for a red or a green target than for a white target, a manifestation of the acquired red/green dyschromatopsia that these patients demonstrate. When one examines the centro-caecal depression by static perimetry, one frequently finds that the defect goes well beyond fixation and that often there are peaks and troughs within the centro-caecal area (Fig. 1a).

As is well known, when smoking is stopped vision gradually recovers over a

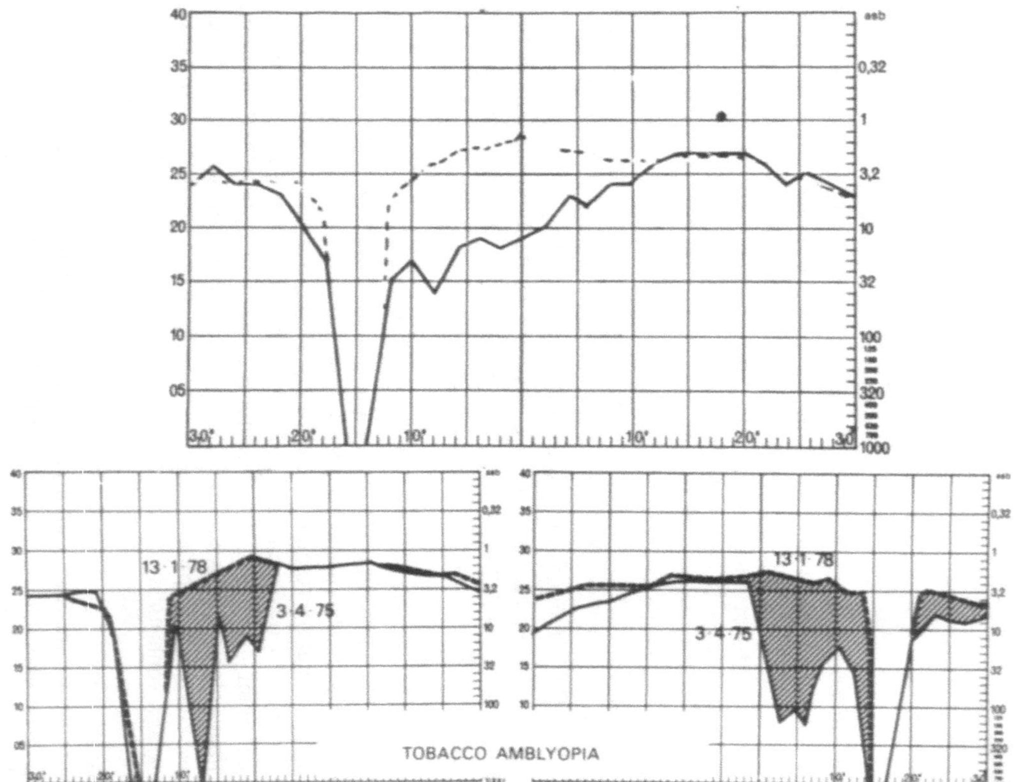

Fig. 1. Static perimetry in tobacco amblyopia. The depression of centro-caecal field often crosses the mid-line (a). During treatment the juxtapapillary defect recovers more rapidly than the central (b).

period of three to nine months, and during recovery there is a tendency for the juxtapapillary defect to recover more rapidly than the central defect, so that a peak is often seen between the blind spot and fixation (Fig. 1b).

As is well known the accompanying red/green defect also improves with cessation of smoking, although a residual and often permanent defect of colour vision is common (4).

The contrast sensitivity to gratings is interesting in tobacco amblyopia. In the untreated condition, contrast thresholds are high for grating patterns of all spatial frequencies (Fig. 2a), but recovery is first heralded by a decrease in the threshold for low frequency gratings (Fig. 2b). Even when visual acuity has completely recovered however contrast threshold for high frequency gratings often remains elevated and this with the common residual colour defect indicates that not all the damage in this form of toxic amblyopia is reversible (Fig. 2c).

Obviously many other measurable parameters can be demonstrated as being abnormal in tobacco amblyopia. Thus, dark adaptation curves from the centro-caecal retina are manifestly abnormal as compared to those derived from the temporal retina. In general however, such measurements do not add to our diagnostic accuracy and are not routinely carried out by us in such patients.

Out main interest in tobacco amblyopia has been biochemical and our current thoughts are that the condition is a defect of sulphur metabolism which results in the abnormal detoxication of cyanide derived from tobacco smoke, resulting in the production of a detoxication product 2-immino-4-thiazolidine carboxylic acid, which may interfere with myelination via its effect on choline synthesis. The evidence for abnormal sulphur metabolism in tobacco amblyopia includes lower than expected thiocyanate levels, which are usually high in tobacco smokers; low levels of red cell glutathione, a rich source of sulphydryl groups and low levels of sulphamino acids, especially cystine, in the plasma. Correction of the relative sulphur deficiency by, for example, giving the sulphamino acid cystine, rapidly normalises the biochemical picture and leads to recovery of vision even when smoking is continued (6, 7, 8).

The predilection which this type of optic nerve damage has for the centrocaecal area of the field is not understood nor are the reasons why differing field defects are seen in other types of toxic optic neuropathy. Thus, quinine amblyopia is characterised by loss of peripheral field while in ethambutol optic neuropathy the defect may be a bi-temporal one indicating chiasmal damage (3).

Ethambutol toxicity shares with many optic neuropathies the features of good recovery of function in the presence of sometimes severe optic atrophy as seen ophthalmoscopically and illustrates the difficulty in assessing potential function from the appearance of the disc.

It is interesting that ethambutol has been shown to reduce plasma zinc levels (10) and it is now thought that zinc deficiency may be an important causal mechanism underlying the neuropathy. We ourselves have confirmed zinc deficiency in a number of toxic amblyopias, but have not so far had the opportunity to try zinc supplementation as a therapy in these cases. Another

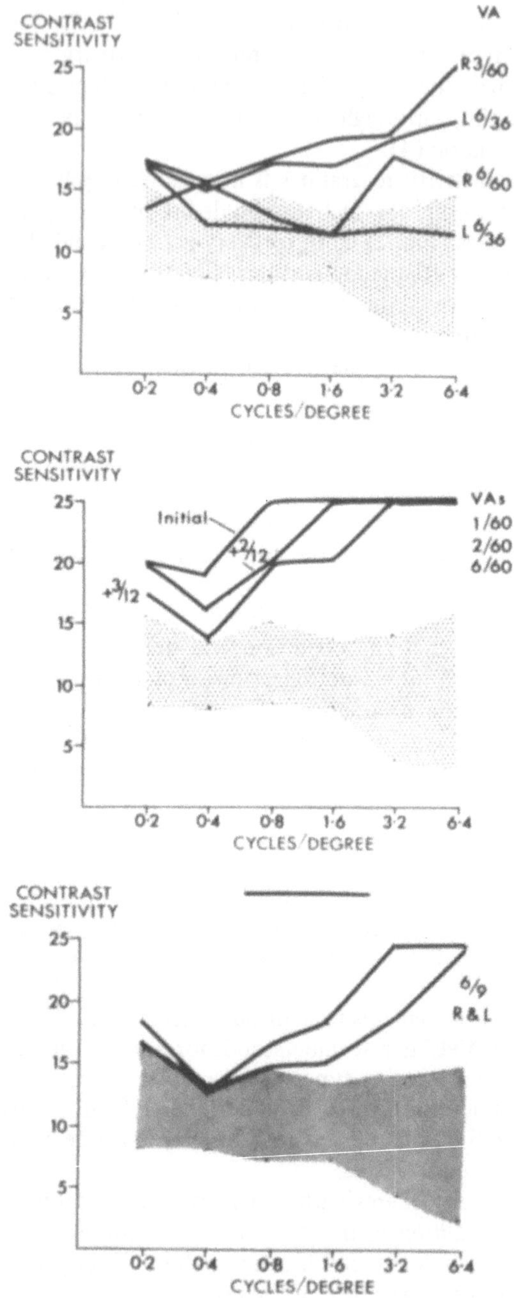

Fig. 2. Contrast threshold to gratings in tobacco amblyopia. Before treatment thresholds are elvated for all spatial frequencies (a). During treatment recovery is heralded by a decrease in threshold for gratings of low frequency (b). Contrast threshold for high frequencies may remain poor after good visual recovery (c).

factor of importance in ethambutol toxicity is that many of the patients we have seen have demonstrated abnormal renal function probably causing higher than expected ethambutol levels in the plasma on standard dosage.

Returning to tobacco amblyopia and its biochemistry, before we became aware of the sulphamino acid deficiency in these cases, it was known that many of them showed deficiency of Vitamin B12 and responded to treatment with Hydroxocobalamin (5, 9). This is of course explicable in view of the known role that B12 has in the interconvertibility of the sulphamino acids, a role which it shares with folic acid and with piridoxine. We have seen a few folate deficient patients present with field defects identical to those seen in tobacco amblyopia, and these patients have recovered vision when treated with folic acid. The reported response of nutritional amblyopia in the U.S.A. to treatment with piridoxine might have a similar basis. On one occasion a patient who had had a bowel resection and was protein deficient, presented with a similar field loss and recovered vision on protein supplementation.

The biochemistry of tobacco amblyopia leads us straight to the inherited optic atrophies for Leber's hereditary optic atrophy shares some of the same biochemical peculiarities that are shown by patients with tobacco amblyopia. Thus, patients with Leber's atrophy have low red cell glutathione levels and low levels of plasma cystine, while those patients with Leber's atrophy who smoke have lower than expected levels of thiocyanate in the plasma and urine. In addition some patients with Leber's hereditary optic atrophy recover vision when treated with cystine and hydroxocobalamin. Nine out of 22 cases treated within a month of onset of the visual loss recovered near normal vison and recovery of vision occurred even in the presence of marked optic atrophy.

It seems unlikely that the visual recovery in nine out of 22 cases of Leber's hereditary optic atrophy could occur by chance, but it is disappointing that 13 of the cases did not improve, suggesting that some other factor has still to be identified.

As is well known the onset of the optic nerve defect in Leber's hereditary optic atrophy is abrupt and both eyes are usually affected within a few days of each other. At the onset the discs are swollen and hyperaemic but as a rule they do not leak fluorescein on angiography in contrast to the retro-bulbar neuritis of M.S. where leakage from the discs may be seen even in those patients presenting with retro-bulbar neuritis in the absence of papillitis. The field defect in Leber's atrophy is traditionally described as central, absolute and steep-edged and indeed this is often the case. However many other varieties of field defect may be seen including generalised depression and not infrequently depression in the centro-caecal area similar to that seen in tobacco amblyopia (Fig. 3). A red/green colour defect is characteristic and often easily recorded even when the acuity is very poor. Once again contrast sensitivity to gratings of low spatial frequency may be retained while that for high frequency is lost.

It is of interest that patients with Leber's atrophy treated with dietary cystine, persistently show low cystine levels in the plasma, suggesting either an inability to absorb cystine adequately or possibly a failure of renal tubular reabsorption, an aspect which is currently being studied.

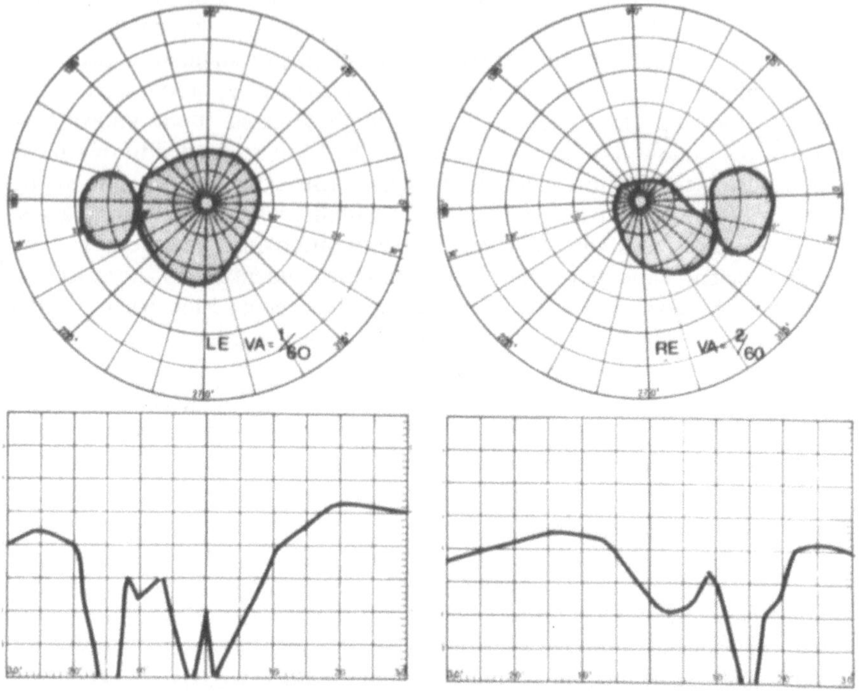

Fig. 3. Static perimetry in Leber's hereditary optic atrophy. The field defect in this case resembles that seen in tobacco amblyopia.

It is important to differentiate Leber's hereditary optic atrophy from the other inherited atrophies for the prognosis varies greatly in the different types of hereditary atrophy and of course the inheritance must be known if adequate genetic counselling is to be given.

Apart from Leber's hereditary optic atrophy the only inherited optic atrophy seen with any frequency is dominantly inherited optic atrophy and occasionally Wolfram's syndrome (12) where the optic atrophy is combined with diabetes mellites, diabetes insipidus and deafness.

The inheritance of Leber's hereditary optic atrophy has of course some of the hall-marks of a sex linked recessive inheritance although males never transmit the disease either directly or indirectly. To make the diagnosis there must be at least one maternally related relative. In dominant optic atrophy the inheritance is autosomal dominant and both males and females transmit this disorder. In our experience the onset of dominant optic atrophy is commonly in the first decade of life while in Leber's hereditary optic atrophy the second decade is the commonest time of onset.

The acuity in dominant optic atrophy is commonly of the order of 6/36 while in Leber's hereditary optic atrophy it tends to be much poorer in the region of 1/60 to 3/60. In dominant atrophy there is often an irregular enlargement of the blind spot with some depression of the centro-caecal static profile. Unlike Leber's hereditary optic atrophy dominant atrophy is often characterised by a yellow/blue colour defect in contrast to the red/green

Table 1. Differential diagnosis of inherited optic atrophies.

	LHOA.	DOA.	'DIDMOAD'
HEREDITY	ATYPICAL RECESSIVE	AUTOSOMAL DOMINANT	AUTOSOMAL RECESSIVE
OPTIC DISC	ATROPHIC	MODERATELY ATROPHIC	SEVERELY ATROPHIC
COLOUR VISION	RED/GREEN DEFECT	BLUE/YELLOW DEFECT	RED/GREEN → ACHROMATOPSIA
FIELD DEFECT	CENTRAL OR CENTRO-CAECAL	PARACAECAL	PERIPHERAL CONSTRICTION

defect associated with Leber's atrophy. So far we have found no characteristic biochemical abnormality in patients with dominant atrophy.

In relation to Wolfram's syndrome we have followed three cases of this rare condition for more than 10 years. The condition is a distressing one which is inexorably progressive and may lead, as in one of our cases to complete blindness. The clinical picture in our cases has been a progressive loss of peripheral field and an acquired dyschromatopsia which initially has been red/green and subsequently anarchic going on to complete achromatopsia.

Clinically, one can differentiate these three inherited optic atrophies on the basis of their different inheritance, the degree of optic atrophy, the colour defect and the nature of the field defect (Table 1).

In considering the differential diagnosis of these conditions not only must toxic and nutritional causes be considered but also M.S. and chiasmal and optic nerve compression.

Although the retro-bulbar neuritis of M.S. usually presents with a unilateral central scotoma the presentation may be bilateral and the field defect very variable. A proportion of M.S. patients present with chiasmal or retrochiasmal lesions with corresponding field defects which are as a rule of a temporary nature (8).

In M.S. visual recovery may be very rapid or very slow and of course multiple attacks of retro-bulbar neuritis are not uncommon. Uhthoff's phenomenon, i.e. worsening of acuity and of field on exercise is common in M.S. and in our experience does not occur in tobacco amblyopia or in the inherited optic atrophies. The effect can be well demonstrated in M.S. by the ingestion of a small amount of iced water which may be rapidly followed by improvement in vision and in field. The mechanism underlying the phenomenon is still not understood.

Arden claims (1) that in retro-bulbar neuritis the contrast threshold for gratings is elevated in a bi-phasic fashion and that this test is a very sensitive indicator of sub-clinical damage in the unaffected eye. We have confirmed

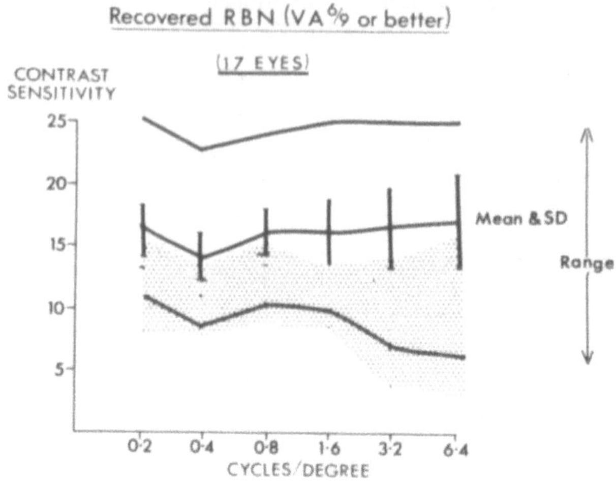

Fig. 4. Contrast threshold to grating pattern in healed retro-bulbar neuritis. Mean threshold is elevated for all spatial frequencies, but there is considerable overlap with normal values.

that in healed retro-bulbar neuritis the mean threshold for contrast sensitivity to gratings is raised for gratings of all frequencies tested, but the overlap with the normal range is considerable (Fig. 4). Our experience has been that the latency of the V.E.R. is a better guide to sub-clinical damage in apparently unaffected eyes.

The other important differential diagnosis in this group of conditions is of course optic nerve or chiasmal pressure. Chiasmal pressure may sometimes present with what may appear to be a centro-caecal defect and often the field defect unexpectedly crosses the mid-line. The case histories of two Doctors illustrate fairly well the difficulties sometimes encountered in the case of pituitary tumours.

The first was an Ophthalmologist in training who complained that his co-student was unable to improve his acuity beyond 6/9 in the left eye. His fields showed a depression in the para-caecal and peri-caecal area, a Farnsworth Munsell 100 Hue test showed an elevated error score and a red/green defect and there was a loss of contrast sensitivity to higher frequencies. The possibility of multiple sclerosis was considered, but more detailed investigation of the fields confirmed the bi-temporal nature of the loss and a pituitary tumour confirmed by radiology and EMI scan was removed with complete recovery of all functions.

The other Doctor complained that colour vision was defective in the left eye. The acuity was 6/5 in the right eye and 6/6 in the left. The discs were deeply cupped and kinetic fields showed arcuate defects. The left eye showed a significant red/green dyschromatopsia. Oblique static perimetry showed depression in the Bjerrum area and in addition an upper temporal depression. Static retinal sensitivity values showed lower values temporal to the mid-line in each upper field. EMI scan confirmed a pituitary tumour and again its removal was followed by excellent recovery of visual parameters.

One of the features of nearly all of the conditions mentioned is the great capacity the optic nerve has to recover function, even after developing clinical optic atrophy and sometimes after very extended periods of visual loss. When one looks at some of the cases of Leber's atrophy who have recovered vision steadily over a period of two to three years one wonders what process is occurring during this time, but is thankful for the innate resilience of the tissues which is rather out of keeping with our general views on the behaviour of the central nervous system.

ACKNOWLEDGEMENTS

The majority of patients described in this paper were seen in the Optic Nerve Clinic of the Tennent Institute of Ophthalmology by Dr. J. M. Bronte-Stewart, to whom I am greatly indebted. The colour vision assessments, visual field studies and so on were carried out by Miss E. McClure, Senior Optician in the Tennent Institute. I am grateful to the many Ophthalmic Surgeons in the West of Scotland who referred cases for investigation and I should like to thank Mrs. A. Currie for the preparation of figures and Miss O. M. Rankin for secretarial assistance.

REFERENCES

1. Arden, G. Visual loss in patients with normal visual acuity. Trans. Ophthal. Soc. U.K. 98: 219–231 (1978).
2. Arden, G. & J. J. Jacobsen. A simple grating test for contrast sensitivity. Invest. Ophthalmol. 17: 23–32 (1978).
3. Bronte-Stewart, J., A. R. Pettigrew & W. S. Foulds. Toxic optic neuropathy and its experimental production. Trans. Ophthal. Soc. U.K. 96: 355–358 (1976).
4. Chisholm, I. A. Vitamin B12 and cyanide relationships in tobacco amblyopia and related diseases. Thesis for degree of M.D., University of Glasgow (1969).
5. Chisholm, I. A., J. Bronte-Stewart & W. S. Foulds. Hydroxocobalamin versus cyanocobalamin in the treatment of tobacco amblyopia. Lancet II: 450 (1967).
6. Foulds, W. S., I. A. Chisholm & A. R. Pettigrew. The toxic optic neuropathies. Brit. J. Ophthalmol. 58: 386–390 (1974).
7. Foulds, W. S. & A. R. Pettigrew. Tobacco alcohol amblyopia. In: Controversy in Ophthalmology (R. J. Brockhurst, S. A. Boruchoff, B. T. Hutchinson & F. Lessell, eds.), Saunders, Philadelphia (1977), p. 851.
8. Foulds, W. S., J. Bronte-Stewart & E. McClure. The diagnosis and prognosis of demyelination in the optic nerve. Proc. Con. Ophthalmologicum, Kyoto (Koicha Schimizu, ed.), Int. Cong. Series No. 450, XXIII: Exerpta Medica, Amsterdam/ Oxford (1978).
9. Heaton, J. M., A. J. A. McCormick & A. G. Freeman. Tobacco amblyopia, a clinical manifestation of Vitamin B12 deficiency? Lancet II: 286 (1958).
10. Saraux, H., B. Bechetoille, B. Non & B. Curtois. The diminution in the level of serum zinc during some toxic optic neuropathy cases. Ann. Oculist 208: 29 (1975).
11. Taylor, W. O. G. & G. B. Donaldson. Recent developments in Farnsworth's colour vision tests. Trans. Ophthal. Soc. U.K. 96: 262–264 (1967).
12. Wolfram, D. J. Diabetes mellitus and simple optic atrophy among siblings. Report of 4 cases. Mayo Clin. Proc. 13: 715 (1938).

Author's address:
Wallace S. Foulds
Tennent Institute of Ophthalmology
University of Glasgow
Glasgow
Great Britain

FUNDUS CONTROLLED PERIMETRY IN OPTIC NEUROPATHY

YOJI OGITA, TAKAYUKI SOTANI, KAZUTAKA KANI & JO IMACHI

(*Nishinomiya, Japan*)

ABSTRACT

Fundus controlled perimetry was carried out observing the fundus by means of an infrared television funduscopy in cases of optic neuropathy, such as Leber's disease, infantile dominant optic atrophy, multiple sclerosis and optic atrophy of unknown origin, in which six cases were treated with craniotomy. Isopters were drawn on the fundus picture by means of static perimetry. The isopters showed very complicated shape compared with those obtained by conventional perimeters. High sensitive areas appeared at the fovea and/or at the retina along the superior and inferior temporal retinal vessels about 5 or 15 degrees apart from the disc in the recovery period of the disease. There was a correlation between the foveal sensitivity and the visual acuity.

INTRODUCTION

In order to measure central visual fields, projection perimeter, campimeter, multiple stimulus static perimeter or scotometric plates are commonly used. In these perimeters, patient's fixation is not exactly monitored, so that it would be very difficult to take an accurate measurement of central scotomata by conventional methods. We have developed fundus controlled perimetry (1, 3), which enables us to monitor patient's fundus as well as test object, so this method is useful in evaluation of some ocular disease especially with central scotoma. In this paper, the visual field was measured by fundus controlled perimeter in seven cases of optic nerve disease, such as Leber's disease, infantile dominant optic atrophy, multiple sclerosis and optic atrophy of unknown origin, in which six cases were brain surgically treated.

METHODS

Central visual fields were measured using a fundus controlled perimeter (Fig. 1) under the following conditions: background 10 asb (5.6 trolands), white; test object, 7′ in diameter, white, 200 msec in duration, 1000 asb (560 trolands) in maximal brightness with attenuation in 0.1 log unit steps. Detailed descriptions of the fundus controlled perimeter were previously reported (2).

Static perimetry was carried out observing the patient's fundus on the

Doc. Ophthal. Proc. Series, Vol. 26, ed. by E. L. Greve & G. Verriest

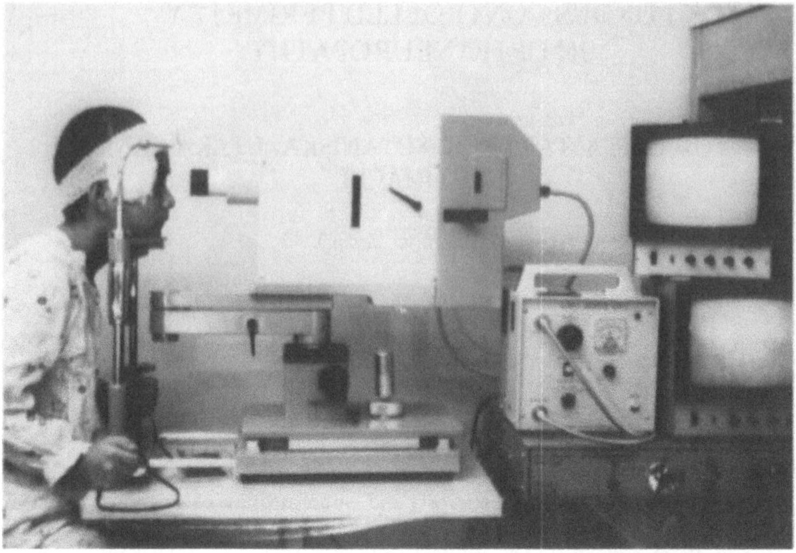

Fig. 1. Fundus controlled perimeter.

television screen. The test object was exposed briefly (200 msec) and, if it was not recognized, it was slightly moved and exposed again. This procedure was repeated until the object was recognized. The border points between 'seeing' and 'not seeing' were connected and the isopter was drawn. This method is tentatively called 'static isoptometry' (3).

RESULTS

Case 1. Leber's disease

A 30-year-old male had noted firstly a central scotoma in the right eye in May 1977, and four months later in the left. He was referred to our clinic on October 19, 1977. The visual acuity was 0.04 in the right, and 0.07 in the left. Two cousins on the mother's side had optic atrophy and underwent the brain surgical treatment. Right frontal craniotomy was performed on November 16, 1977. The arachnoid membrane around the optic nerves and the chiasm was thick, turbid and adherent to the surrounding brain tissues. This membrane was removed in order to improve the circulation of cerebrospinal fluid around the chiasm.

Fundus perimetry five months after the surgery revealed a large central scotoma extending from the disc to the macular area (Fig. 2 left). Three months later the area of the central scotoma slightly diminished and light sensitive areas were found along the superior temporal retinal vessels (Fig. 2, right).

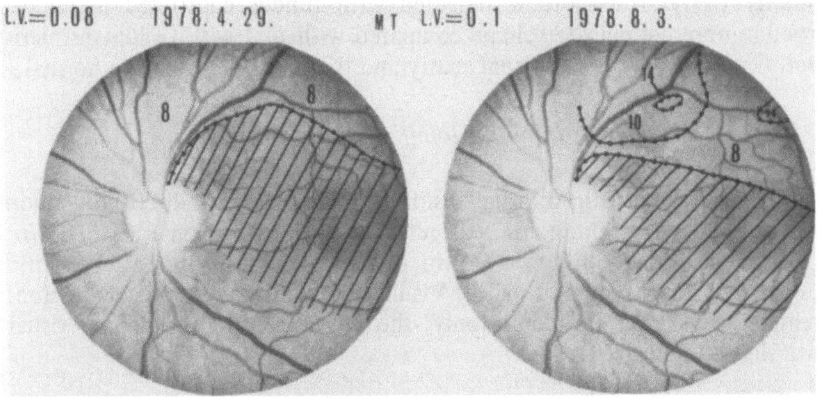

Fig. 2. Visual field by fundus controlled perimetry in case 1, left eye. The shaded part of the retina shows an area where the sensitivity was under 0 log unit (1000 asb). The number indicates the retinal sensitivity by 10 times the value of log unit. Isopters were obtained by means of static isoptometry.

Case 2. Multiple sclerosis

A 19-year-old female noted loss of vision in both eyes in September 1977. Since that time her visual acuity had fluctuated between 0.02 and 1.5 in both eyes. She came to our clinic because of a new loss of vision in the right eye on August 18, 1979. Her eye movements by electro-oculogram showed stair case pattern. Hypesthesia was noted in both upper extremities. Fig. 3 shows her visual fields measured with Goldmann perimeter (right) and fundus controlled

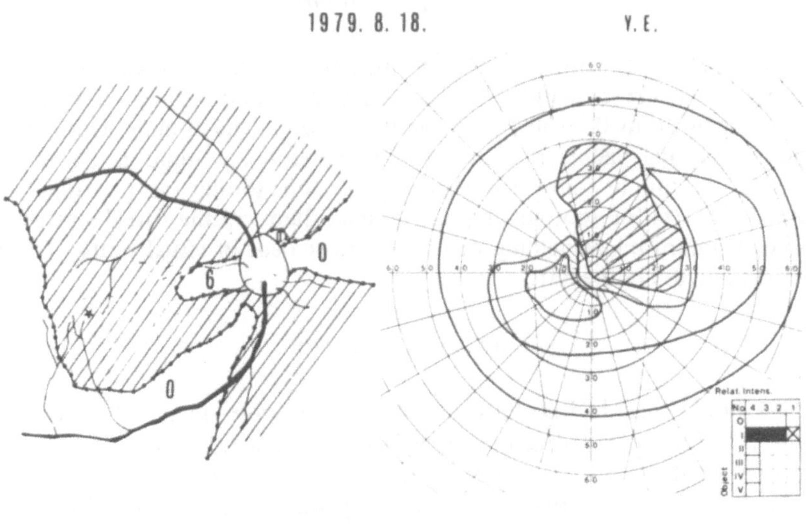

Fig. 3. Visual field of case 2, right eye obtained by fundus controlled perimeter (left) and Goldmann perimeter (right). Visual field by Goldmann perimeter is drawn upside down as against fundus picture.

perimeter (left). The scotoma detected with fundus controlled perimeter showed a more complicated shape compared with that with Goldmann perimeter. On September 5, the visual acuity and the visual field became normal.

Case 3. Infantile dominant optic atrophy

An 8-year-old boy noticed visual insufficiency which was discovered upon entering elementary school. He was referred to our clinic on June 6, 1976. His corrected visual acuity was 0.2 in the right and 0.3p in the left. Optic discs showed slight temporal pallor. Visual fields showed general depression. Seventeen days after the craniotomy, the retinal sensitivity and the visual acuity slightly improved.

Case 4. Optic atrophy

An 11-year-old girl lost her vision in the right eye in January 1978 and in the left in December. Her vision did not improve in spite of steroid therapy. She was admitted to our hospital on July 14, 1979. Her visual acuity was 0.08 in the right and 0.15 in the left. Within a large central scotoma with 1000 asb object, the sensitivity remained only at the fovea. The craniotomy was performed on September 12, 1979. The scotoma diminished, and in the left eye it was divided into two parts by the 0.2 log unit sensitive area. On December 20, her vision became 0.1 in the right and 1.0 in the left. The foveal sensitivity remarkably improved.

Case 5. Optic atrophy

A 16-year-old male with visual loss in his both eyes since February 1979 was referred to our clinic on July 7, 1979. His visual acuity showed diurnal variation ranging from 0.2p in the morning to 0.07 in the evening. Optic discs showed temporal pallor. A faint foveal sensitivity was found in the central scotoma with fundus controlled perimetry. The craniotomy was performed on July 23. The central scotoma gradually diminished and the foveal sensitivity markedly improved coinciding with an improvement of visual acutiy, 0.9 in the right and 0.8 in the left.

Case 6. Optic atrophy

A 50-year-old male had begun to notice visual disorder in the left eye since January 1978. The visual acuity progressively declined. On January 7, 1980, his visual acuity was 1.2 in the right and hand movement in the left. Steroid treatment was not effective. The craniotomy was performed on February 4. Three days after the operation, he felt brighter and fundus controlled perimetry revealed a high sensitive area along the superior temporal retinal vessels just above the fovea. One and a half months later, a very small sensitive area appeared adjacent to the fovea and his visual acuity became 0.2.

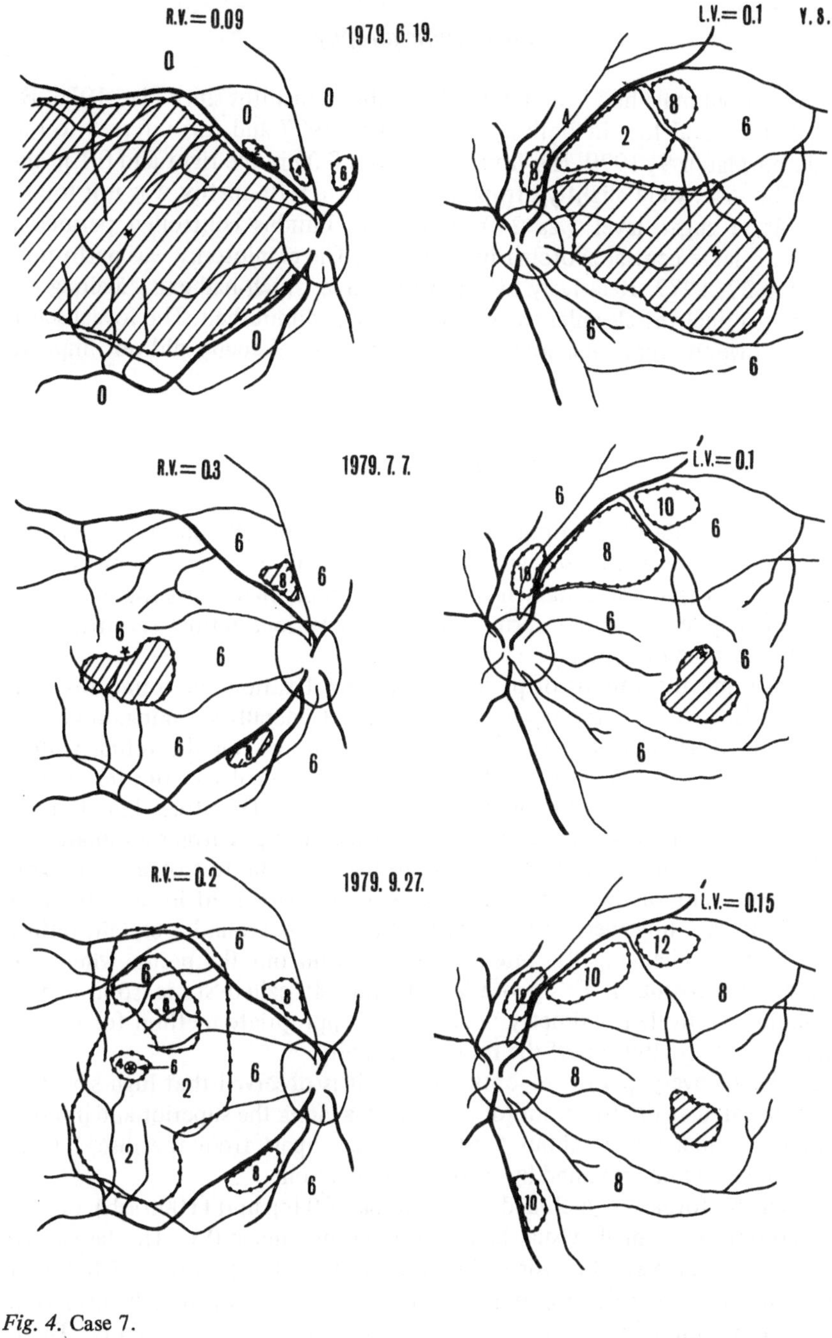

Fig. 4. Case 7.

Case 7. Optic atrophy

A 46-year-old male had been treated for diabetes mellitus since May 1976. He noted the visual loss in both eyes in January 1977 and was referred to our clinic on March 9, 1979. His visual acuity was 0.09 in the right and 0.1 in the left. The discs were slightly atrophic. A diabetic retinopathy was not found. The blood sugar level was 240–400 mg/dl. Fundus controlled perimetry showed a large central scotoma in both eyes. The craniotomy was performed on June 27, 1979. Relatively high sensitive area which had existed along the superior retinal vessels enlarged and the scotoma diminished. The foveal sensitivity, however, remained lower level and the visual acuity did not improve (Fig. 4).

DISCUSSION

Central scotomata of the optic nerve diseases were exactly detected using the fundus controlled perimeter with high reproducibility. A large, homogenous, round shaped scotoma obtained with Goldmann perimeter was found to have an extremely complicated form consisting of various retinal sensitivity by fundus controlled perimetry.

Monitoring the fundus of patients with poor fixation, we found that the eye very frequently made saccadic movements. Generally speaking, in kinetic perimetry, it is necessary that the test object moves on the retina with a constant velocity. However, if the retina moves irregularly, the test object does not move on the retina with constant velocity. Therefore, kinetic perimetry would not be an adequate method for measuring central scotomata.

In static perimetry, it was difficult to maintain the test object on a certain fixed point of the retina throughout the measurement in poor fixation patient. It was, however, easy to scatter the objects around a certain retinal locus without changing the intensity and to find out the points where the object was recognized. This procedure, tentatively called 'static isoptometry' in fundus controlled perimetry would be an appropriate method for detecting the exact distribution of the retinal sensitivity.

In the recovery period of optic disease, it is observed that high sensitive areas appeared at the fovea and/or at the retina along the superior and inferior temporal retinal vessels about 5 to 15 degrees apart from the disc, but its significance will be remained by further investigation.

When the fovea was included in a scotoma of 0 log unit (1000 asb), even if the scotoma was small, visual acuity was always under 0.1. The larger the central scotoma was, the worse the visual acuity. In cases in which foveal sensitivity was over 0.2 log unit, the visual acuity was generally over 0.2. Fig. 5 shows the relation between foveal sensitivity and visual acuity. There would be statistically significant correlation, when a coefficient of ranking correlation is calculated as $rs = 0.89$, $p < 0.01$. Making a comparison between the sensitivity of the fovea and the surrounding retina, visual acuity was good when the fovea was more sensitive than the surrounding retina.

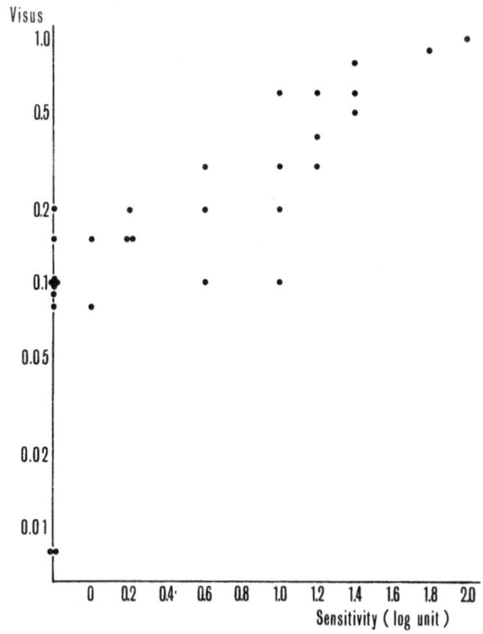

Fig. 5. Correlation between foveal sensitivity (abscissa) and visual acuity (ordinate).

REFERENCES

1. Kani, K., N. Eno, K. Abe & T. Ono. Perimetry under television ophthalmoscopy. Docum. Ophthal. Proc. Series 14: 231–236 (1977).
2. Kani, K. & Y. Ogita. Fundus controlled perimetry. The relation between the position of a lesion in the fundus and in the visual field. Docum. Ophthal. Proc. Series 19: 341–350 (1979).
3. Kani, K. & Y. Ogita. Fundus controlled perimetry. Folia Ophthal. jap. 30: 141–147 (1979).
4. Shimo-oku, M., N. Okamoto, I. Okuzawa & J. Imachi. The surgical treatment of retrobulbar neuritis. Special reference to pathological studies in one case. Docum. Ophthal. Proc. Series 17: 175–184 (1978).

Authors' address:
Department of Ophthalmology
Hyogo College of Medicine
Mukogawacho 1-1, Nishinomiya
Hyogo-ken 663
Japan

THE PERICOECAL AREA IN OPTIC SUB-ATROPHY

E. GANDOLFO, G. CALABRIA & M. ZINGIRIAN

(Genoa, Italy)

ABSTRACT

Static exploration with 'close single stimuli' that we devised for the pericoecal area examination was used for a perimetric evaluation of patients with optic sub-atrophy. The graphic (e.g. densitometric) representation of the results yields a fairly good display of the perimetric damage of this region. In turn the numerical representation of the whole defect in this area (pericoecal formula) offers a very useful indication for the quantitative follow-up of these cases.

INTRODUCTION

The study of the visual field pericoecal area holds great interest because of the presence of the blind spot and threshold gradient irregularities which are due to angioscotomata and other factors not well known (1–5). As we have demonstrated in detail by means of an original method of static perimetry (5), both coecal scotoma and the above mentioned sensitivity drops show a great variability even in normal subjects (1–5). An examination of those patients suffering from optic sub-atrophy by our method was considered useful in evaluating the sensitivity behaviour in the pericoecal area with reference to various optic nerve diseases.

MATERIALS AND METHODS

We tested a group of patients with optic sub-atrophy due to different optic nerve diseases by means of our original method (5) of pericoecal static perimetry (105 points evenly distributed in the pericoecal area, as shown in Fig. 1). For our research we utilized a modified static equipment of the Goldmann perimeter. We examined 20 subjects. Of them:

- 5 were affected by toxic neuropathy (due to alcohol-tobacco or occupational intoxication);
- 5 were affected by optic nerve damage of a demyelinating type (multiple sclerosis);
- 5 were affected by vascular optic sub-atrophy (as a result of either an acute anterior optic neuropathy or a chronic angio-sclerotic optic neuropathy);

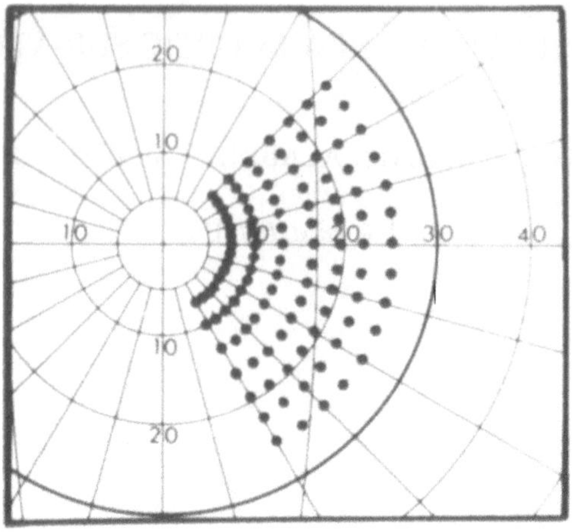

Fig. 1. Stimuli distribution in pericoecal area.

- 5 were affected by optic sub-atrophy of an inflammatory origin (as a result of a papillitis or optic neuritis).

Our patients' ages ranged from 12 to 74. Only those patients expected to co-operate during such a long and complex test were chosen. The test was carried out after correction of refractive errors and presbyopia when present. We used the object surfaces I and II of the Goldmann series. The results were plotted on a special scheme utilizing a grey scale or a conventional colour scale (Fig. 2). This type of representation was perfected with the co-operation

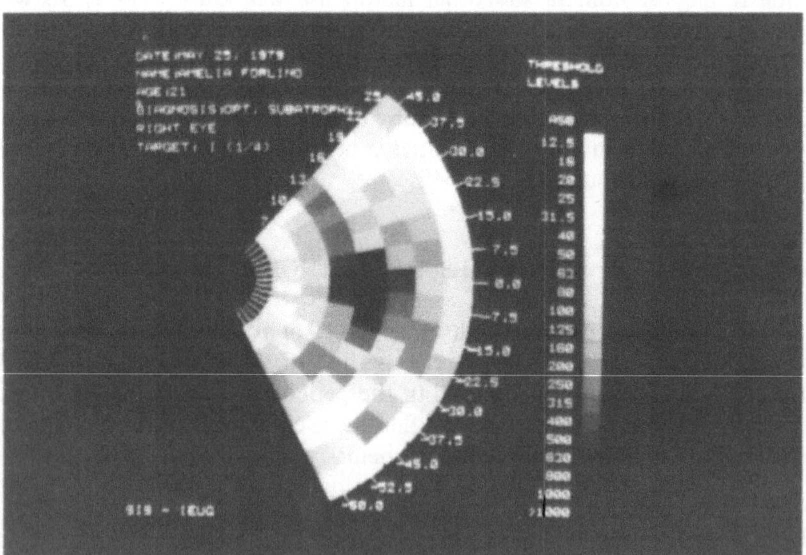

Fig. 2. Densitometric computed representation of the pericoecal sensitivity utilizing a grey scale.

of the Bioengineers of the Genoa University Institute of Electrotecnics (5). We also calculated the overall mean sensitivity value for every patient in order to obtain an immediate impression of the functional status of the pericoecal visual field (pericoecal formula).

RESULTS

In general, a great variability is evident according to the severity of the functional damage. Some subjects (group 1) maintain an almost normal pericoecal sensitivity, whereas others (group 2) show a severe sensitivity fall within the examined area.

Group 1 includes for the most part young patients affected by optic subatrophy of a toxic, inflammatory or demyelinating origin. These subjects consistently lack a central scotoma during standard kinetic perimetry and only show moderate threshold elevation during static examination of the central visual field (Fig. 3).

Group 2 includes older patients affected by vascular optic neuropathy or those subjects suffering from relapsed optic nerve involvement caused by multiple sclerosis. These subjects often have an easily detectable central scotoma or altitudinal visual field defects (Fig. 4).

Nevertheless, a certain threshold flattening in the pericoecal area is detectable also in patients with minimal visual field damage.

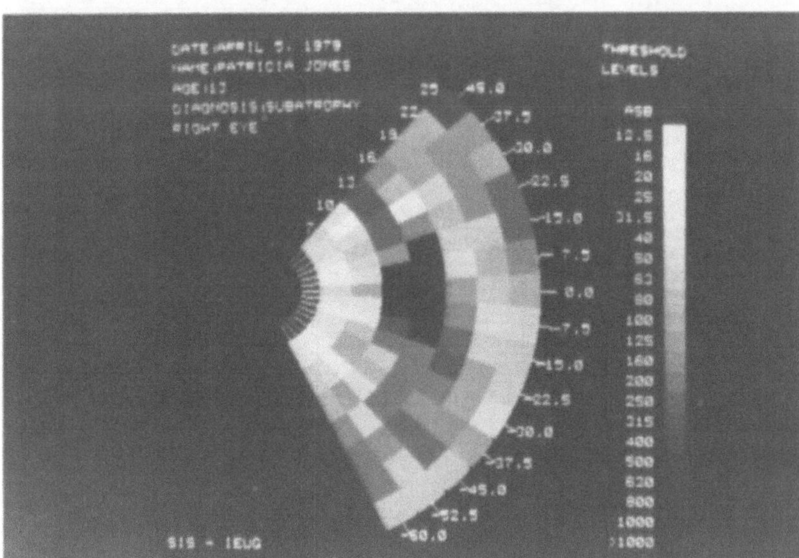

Fig. 3. Pericoecal area showing moderate threshold elevation only.

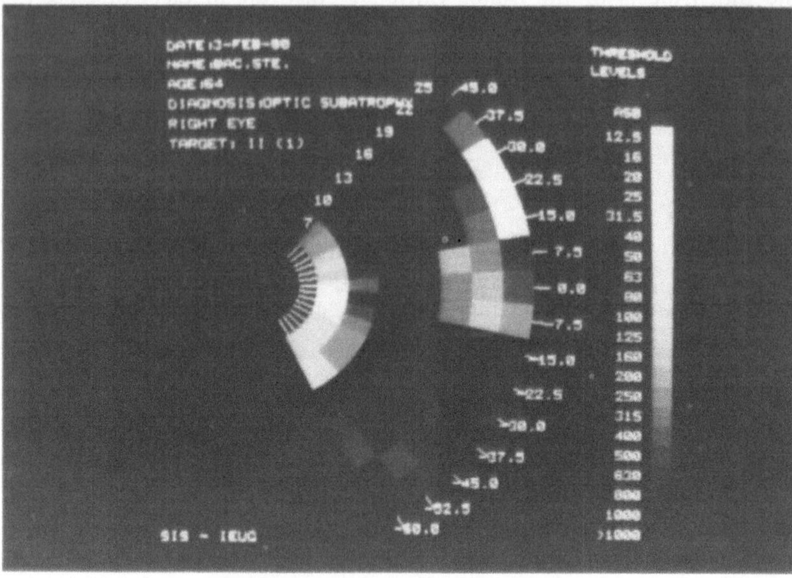

Fig. 4. Pericoecal area showing severe damage of the sensitivity.

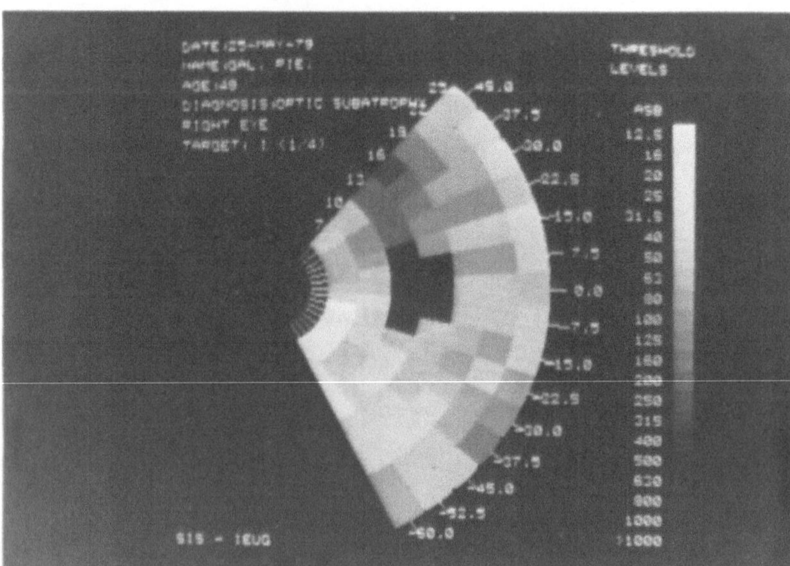

Fig. 5. Pericoecal area showing evident threshold flattening and modest gradient irregularity.

A deepening of the sensitivity drops due to angioscotomata does not take place, but rather an increase in the threshold level occurs in the usually more sensitive zones. It follows that we can observe a less evident threshold irregularity in comparison with normal subjects (Fig. 5).

Such a situation is more evident in seriously compromised cases in which the presence of angioscotoma or other sensitivity drops is not at all detectable. All details disappear in a general wide threshold elevation (Fig. 6).

It can also be noted that there is often a great difference between threshold levels above and below the blind spot. Such sensitivity behaviour is peculiar to the cases in which optic sub-atrophy follows from an acute anterior ischaemic optic neuropathy. This is explained by the frequent presence of altitudinal hemianoptic visual field defects (Fig. 7).

It should also be noted that our pericoecal static method confirmed the presence of optic nerve damage in some cases in which ophthalmoscopy had shown optic sub-atrophy but routine visual field examinations were negative. The comparison between the mean sensitivity value of the affected eye and the non-affected contro-lateral eye allowed us to obtain this result.

CONCLUSION

Our static pericoecal perimetry shows precision and usefulness in evaluating the functional status of patients suffering from optic sub-atrophy. This method is not a routine examination to be carried out in all subjects, but it may

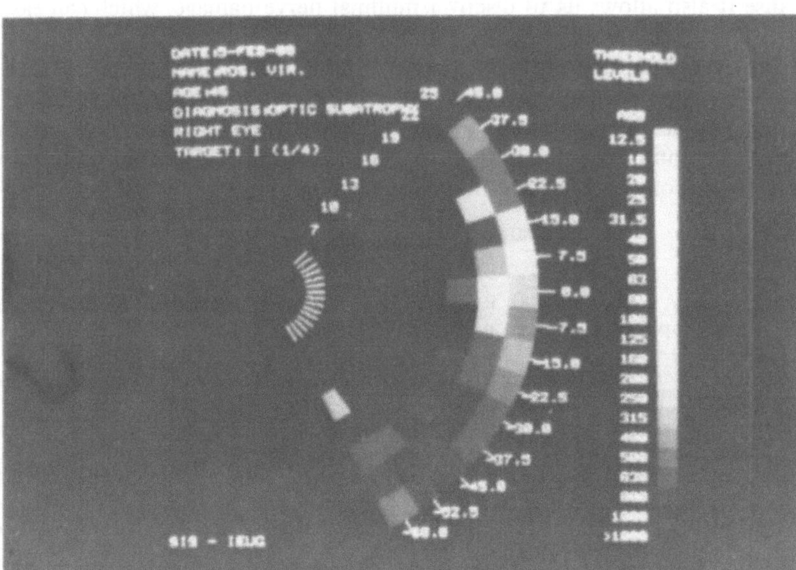

Fig. 6. Pericoecal area showing the absence of detection of sensibility drops due to angioscotomata.

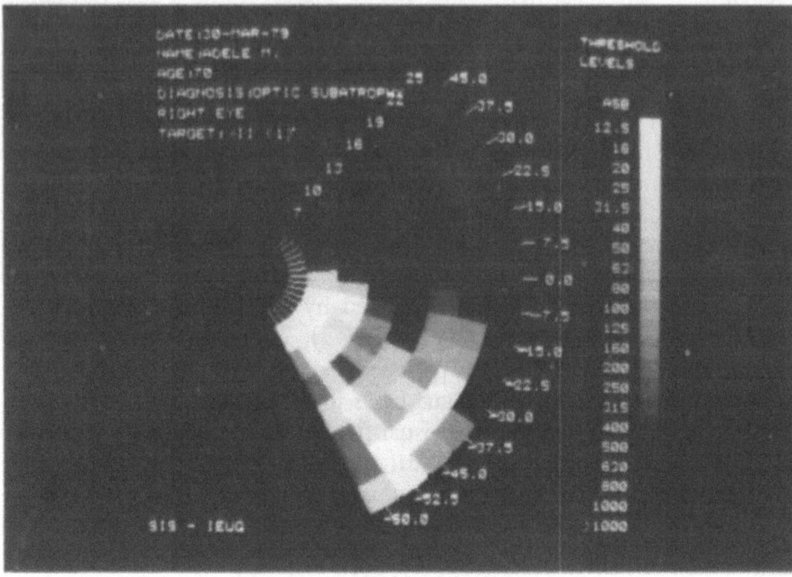

Fig. 7. Pericoecal area showing great difference between threshold levels above and below the blind spot.

substantially increase our knowledge about optic nerve diseases especially in hospitalized patients. Our test is useful in cases of diagnostic uncertainty because it also allows us to discover minimal nerve damage, which can easily escape detection during standard examinations.

The overall mean sensitivity value within the examined area provides a reliable index in evaluating every variation during the patients' follow-up.

The graphically computed method of representation with grey or conventional colour scales allows us to obtain images easily interpreted and immediately comparable with successive examinations.

REFERENCES

1. Benjumeda, A., S. Rodriguez Rubio & J. D. Campos. Perimetria estatica circular seriada. Topografia normal de la mancha ciega. Arch. Soc. Esp. Oftal. 34: 635–644 (1974).
2. Dubois Poulsen, A. Le champ visuel. Topographie normale et pathologique de ses sensibilités. Paris, Masson, pp. 257–277, 301–308 (1952).
3. Greve, E. L. Single and multiple stimulus static perimetry in glaucoma: the two phases of perimetry. Doc. Ophth. 36: 147–155 (1971).
4. Israel, A. Perimetric study of the blind spot with static perimetry. Mod. Probl. Ophth. 6: 62–70 (1969).
5. Zingirian, M., G. Calabria & E. Gandolfo. The pericoecal area: a static method for investigation. In press (1980).

Authors' address:
University Eye Clinic
Viale Benedetto XV, n°5
16132 Genoa
Italy

KINETIC PERIMETRY (IN THE PLATEAU REGION OF THE FIELD) AS A SENSITIVE INDICATOR OF VISUAL FATIGUE OR SATURATION-LIKE DEFECTS IN RETROBULBAR ANOMALIES

CONSTANCE R. FITZGERALD, JAY M. ENOCH & LEONARD A. TEMME

(Gainsville, Florida, U.S.A.)

ABSTRACT

A series of patients with radiation damage has been studied. Retinal vascular changes shown by fluorescein angiography were accompanied by local alterations in the sustained- and transient-like functions. When no retinal manifestations were found, and in all cases where the optic nerve was involved, visual fatigue or saturation-like effects were noted which were revealed as reductions in sensitivity in time. These could be surprisingly subtle. Because of amplification effects, small reductions in sensitivity in time are readily revealed in the plateau region of the central kinetic field. In every instance these effects, once discovered, could be verified using flashing repeat static tests. Comparable results were obtained in all patients tested.

Patients with malignancies in and about the visual pathways have been treated with radiation therapy at this institution and have allowed us the opportunity to determine radiation effects on the optic nerve posterior to the lamina cribrosa. In localizing these effects, changes observed include a time-dependent reduction in sensitivity, nerve fiber bundle defects, and chiasmal defects. A patient showing these changes will be presented as an example of the group as a whole. Patients who have received radiation are unique because of the duration required for the development of the time-dependent reduction in sensitivity (17). An initial isopter may even show relatively normal function. Often, only with repeated testing will the time-dependent lesion be shown. The nerve fiber bundle defects which are observed are not associated with glaucomatous cupping of the optic disc. The finding of these nerve fiber defects emphasizes the point that such defects need not be pathopneumonic of glaucoma (13, 14). It also emphasizes the point that current automated testing which will adequately show such nerve fiber bundle defects is not presently organized to assess the presence of time-dependent reductions in sensitivity which would help to make the distinction between this group of radiation patients and others with retro-laminar pathology from a glaucomatous patient with a nerve fiber bundle defect.

The time-dependent changes in sensitivity are seen in the plateau portion of the island of vision. Middle isopters are, therefore, most affected. The effects we observe are compatible with changes of the myelin as is seen in patients with retrobulbar optic neuritis associated with multiple sclerosis (8, 10, 11, 12, 26). Investigators studying the effect of radiation on the nervous system of both experimental animals and patients receiving radiation

Doc. Ophthal. Proc. Series, Vol. 26, ed. by E. L. Greve & G. Verriest

in and about the nervous system note that myelin dissolution related to ischemia may be seen secondary to small vessel occlusion characteristic of radiation therapy throughout the body (1, 18, 19, 21, 23).

Although the effect of radiation on the retina is appreciated (4, 5, 6, 7, 20, 22, 24, 25), this delineation of changes in a particular section of the optic nerve is, to our knowledge, the first to be spelled out. In some cases, tests of intraretinal neural connections (sustained-like and transient-like functions) have been normal unless concomitant radiation retinopathy has been observed (10). In those patients in whom radiation retinopathy is observed, changes in the sustained-like and/or transient-like functions may also be found.

METHODS

Kinetic testing

The patient closes his eyes for a period of 4–5 minutes which sharply reduces the light level and eliminates form vision. This serves to enhance sensitivity and provides a common baseline for measurement. The period with the eyes closed is repeated before each isopter is measured. Retesting is performed to confirm the findings.

In all patients a light adaptive response occurs shortly after opening the eyes. This causes a modest drop in sensitivity during the first minute of testing. Sensitivity then stabilizes. As in all measures of threshold there are fluctuations in response.

If the 'island of vision' is slowly 'sinking', an orderly fall-off or reduction in sensitivity is measured rather than simple fluctuant behavior about a mean. This test works only if other sources of variance are minimized. That is, image quality and pupil size cannot be fluctuating (e.g., the patient is provided with a maximum plus, minimum minus sphere refraction for the test distance to sharpen the image and to stabilize accomodation), lamp output is uniform and stable, background luminance is on the linear portion of the Weber function, since the effects described are also dependent on background field level.* Fixation is monitored. In summary, fluctuant behavior from other physical and physiological causes is minimized, so that the characteristic visual response determined in time may be evaluated (8, 10, 16).

The alteration measured in these patients is a generally reproducible time-dependent response. In Fig. 1, where the slope is steep (towards the periphery and in the very center of the field), small changes in sensitivity will not greatly alter the measured kinetic isopter. Where the plateau is flat small changes in sensitivity become amplified. Therefore if that which is described is occurring, there should be a clear shrinkage of mid-field isopters, in time, after a period of eye closure. Different strategies for revealing these alterations in mid-plateau isopters are shown in Fig. 2.

In specific pathologies or in different parts of the field, sensitivity may

* The 31.5 asb or 10 cd/m^2 setting of the Goldmann Haag-Streit perimeter is on the lower bound of this response state.

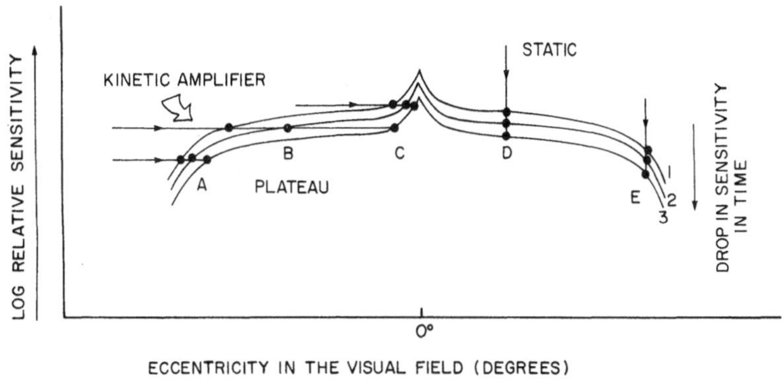

Fig. 1. Assume a cut is made through the 'island of vision'. The central area of peak sensitivity is surrounded by a relatively flat or plateau zone of the visual field. Sensitivity again falls towards the other bounds of the field. In the normal, it is generally found that the 'island' is relatively stable in time, while in post-lamina cribrosa lesions it seems to 'sink' in time, slowly in radiation damage cases, often faster in other conditions.

In kinetic perimetry the flatness of the plateau portion of the field amplifies small changes in sensitivity, leading to predictable contractions of field (see Fig. 2).

reach a level which can be sustained or the process of loss of sensitivity may continue so long as an effect can be measured.

Static techniques

Flashing Repeat Static Test (FRST). As in the case of the kinetic test, the eye is *sharply focused on the cupola* with a maximum plus, minimum minus sphere correction – only here the image quality was optimized at the point at which the test was conducted rather than the fixation point. The patient adapted to the cupola light level, a 'pre-test' sampling of the static threshold was determined in order to determine where to start the process after the five minute eye closure (2, 8, 9, 10, 13, 14, 26).

The test target was flashed (pulsed) for two reasons (a) in order to distinguish a reduction in sensitivity due to the visual saturation or fatigue-like effect considered here from local adaptation defects (8, 26), (b) to force patient re-evaluation of threshold with each audible opening of the shutter. Flash duration is longer than the critical duration and shorter than saccadic eye movement latency (ca. 200 msec once or twice per second). A small size target is used when possible. Testing is from not seeing to just seeing so that the luminance of the test target does not alter light adaptation level. Lowering background cupola level often prevents reduction in sensitivity in time and raising the level generally enhances it (8, 11, 15, 26).

When the patient opens his eyes after the five minute closure, he is instructed to look at fixation but attend the test point. Wandering fixation is a cause of variance. Normally just after eye closure there is a modest drop in sensitivity due to light adaptation; if there is an initial increase in sensitivity it usually means the patient did not remember where to expect the stimulus to appear. After an initial minute of light adaptation, in the normal eye the

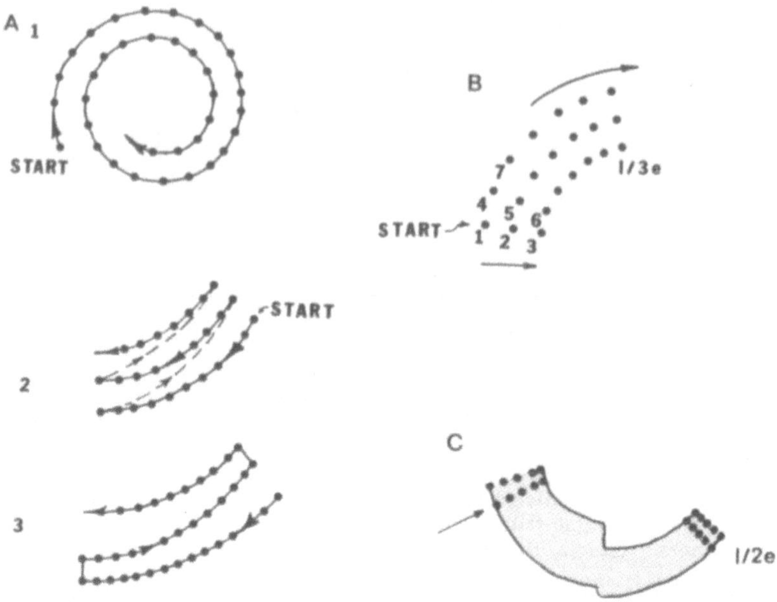

Fig. 2. When conducting kinetic perimetry in this group of patients, various techniques were used to show the time-dependent reductions in sensitivity:

A1. A continuous isopter may be determined. A determination is made in a given meridian, then the meridian is altered in an orderly clockwise or counter-clockwise manner circling of the fixation point. This results in a helical contraction of field. A2. On some occasions an arc of an isopter can be tested again and again. A3. A variant of A2 is to go back and forth sequentially, in the same arc or portion of the visual field.

B. The same technique as that used in A was used, but three or four sequential determinations are made in each meridian before altering meridian (see patient reported below). This was useful when considering the relative rates of fall-off in sensitivity in different meridians.

C. In a given arc showing a reduction in kinetic field sensitivity in time there is often a tendency for the field to contract with repeated kinetic 'passes' and then to firm-up or harden. A modest number of repeated passes were made in a given meridian until the response showed signs of 'firming-up'. Then the neighbouring meridian was tested. A halftone pattern may be used to characterize the zone of time-varying response.

static (flashing) threshold usually steadies and the *mean* response varies little over the five minute period of repeated re-evaluation of the threshold.

An inherent characteristic of threshold determinations is that they fluctuate. The interest here is not in the fluctuations *per se*, but rather *mean sensitivity reductions* during the five minute period of repeated threshold evaluation in patients with radiation damage. Changes may be small after radiation, i.e., reductions in sensitivity of only a few tenths of a log unit are noted. In other involvements of the post-lamina cribrosa visual pathway a more profound fall-off in sensitivity has often been found (references, this laboratory).

Techniques for obtaining sustained-like and transient-like functions are described elsewhere (10, 13, 14). These tests sample spatial interactions between the flashing test target (same as used in the FRST) and special background fields. The sustained-like function is altered in the presence of pathology affecting both the inner and outer plexiform layers while the transient-like function is affected by anomalies affecting the inner plexiform layer. Each function apparently may be affected independently.

RESULTS

A 26-year-old male patient was treated with radiation therapy for carcinoma of the nasopharynx. A 6500 rad tumour dose using opposed lateral and anterior fields from a Cobalt 60 source was used. The patient has been without visual complaints following radiation therapy. His first ophthalmology examination by us was conducted six years after his treatment. At that examination, visual acuity was 20/20 in each eye, applanation pressures were 16 and 14 mm Hg. Pupils were 3 mm in each eye with normal reactions. Normal motility, full confrontation fields and normal biomicroscopy were recorded. On ophthalmoscopic examination, vessels showed normal caliber with small microaneurysms surrounding the perifoveal avascular zone in each eye. Discs showed no glaucomatous cupping. Fluorescein angiography was performed and showed perifoveal microaneurysms with leakage. In addition, the capillaries of each disc appeared somewhat larger than usual.

Central visual fields of patient J.W. are presented (Figs. 3A and 3B). All points tested, with repeated sampling on individual isopters, showed a shrinkage of the field on both sides of the vertical meridian. A bitemporal difference in the two fields suggesting chiasmal involvement was also noted. To affirm that this did not represent an artifact of the testing approach, after periods of rest with eyes closed, the patient was tested at selected individual points on both sides of the vertical meridian in the left eye and near the horizontal meridian (Fig. 4). By testing these individual paired points near transitions and sampling back and forth, the real nature of the anomaly was shown. This anomaly included an alteration of the vertical meridian as well as a step on the horizontal meridian. This patient, therefore, showed changes characteristic of a chiasmal defect, as well as a nerve fiber bundle defect. A similar nerve fiber defect was also shown in the right eye (Figs. 3A, 5). Fig. 5 is a blow-up of the isopter on Fig. 3A and shows points where supplemental testing was conducted. At all points sampled, the flashing repeat static test (FRST) was abnormal. Sample data from both eyes are shown (Fig. 6). Points where both the sustained- and transient-like functions are normal in the right eye are especially notable because certain points involve the field area where a nerve fiber bundle defect is present. At other points, there was a reduction of the transient-like function. For example compare OD points 11 and 4. The transient-like function was normal at point 11 but essentially extinguished at point 4 (Fig. 7). This patient showed psychophysical changes compatible with retinal and optic nerve radiation damage.

It is of interest that a patient with Cushing's disease tested in a comparable way showed similar abnormality in the FRST and characteristic chiasmal defects. Those data are not included, because of manuscript length considerations.

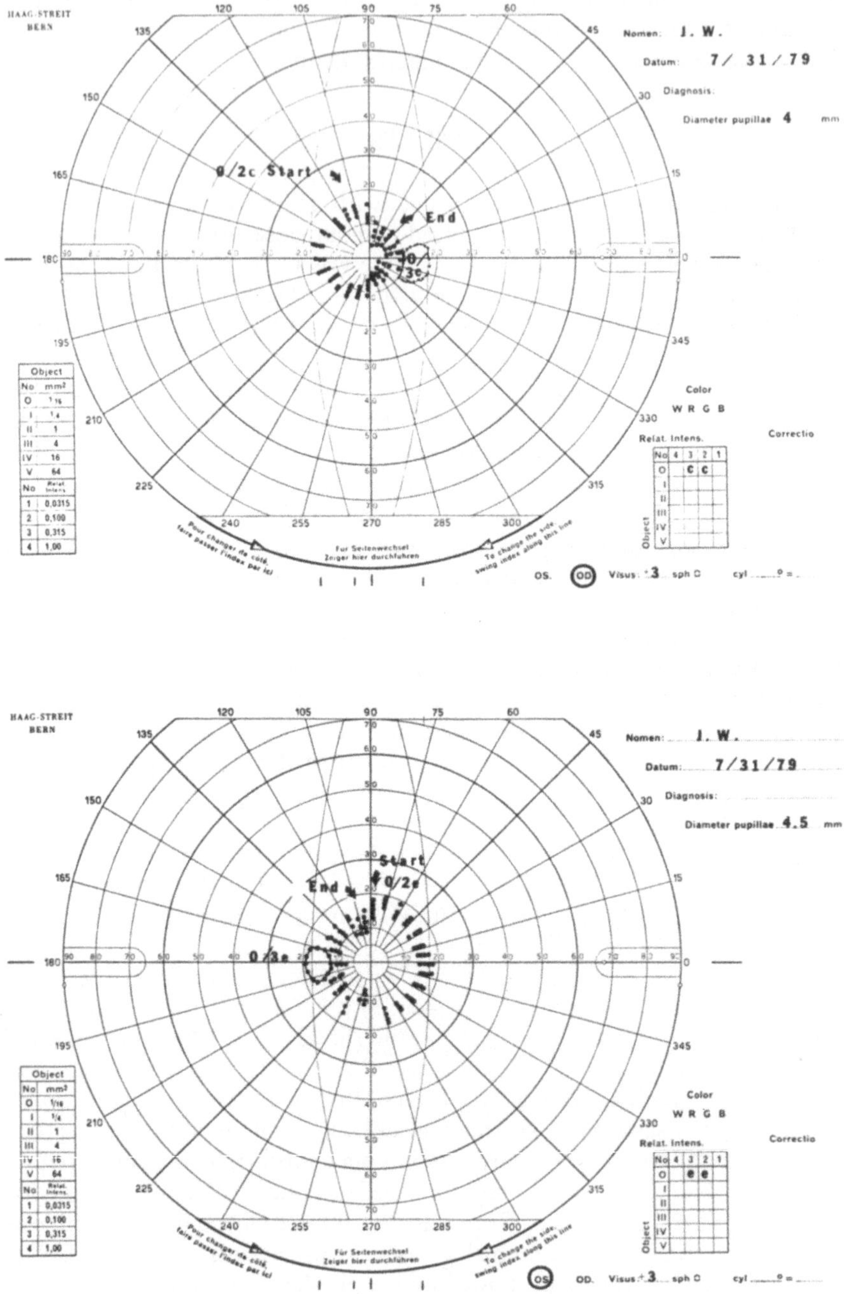

Fig. 3. Patient J.W.: Kinetic fields using technique shown in Fig. 2B. A: O.D.; B: O.S.

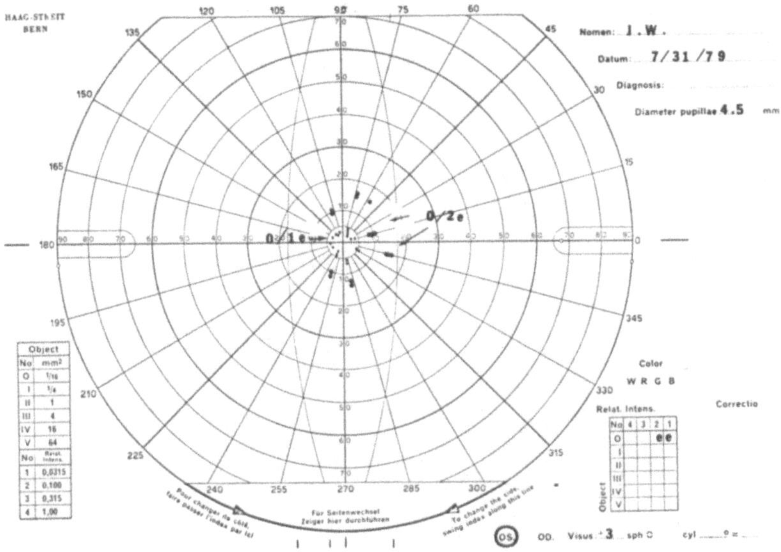

Fig. 4. Patient J.W.: Repetition of key points after eye closure to establish further t differences revealed in Fig. 3B in the vertical meridian and the nerve fiber bundle defe (nasal step) on the horizontal meridian.

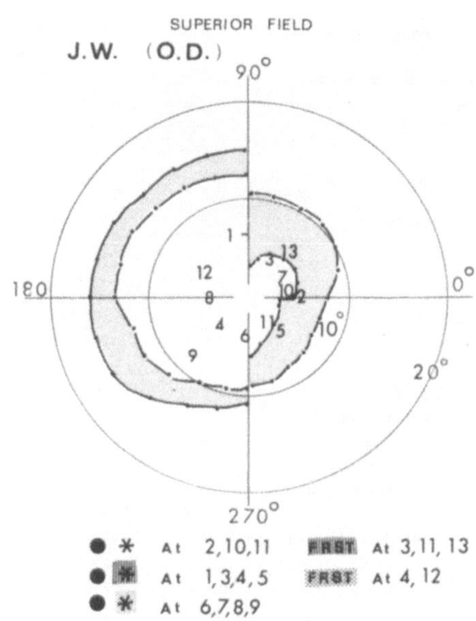

Fig. 5. Magnified representation of the bounds of the isopter shown in Fig. 3A. Overlaid are numbers indicating points where added tests were conducted. The flashing repeat static test (FRST) was abnormal at all points tested, more so at 3, 11 and 13 than at 4 and 12. The sustained- (disc shaped symbol) and transient-like (asterisk shaped symbol) functions were normal at points 2, 10 and 11. At test points 1, 3, 4 and 5 the transient-like function was essentially eliminated and at points 6–9 it was meaningfully reduced.

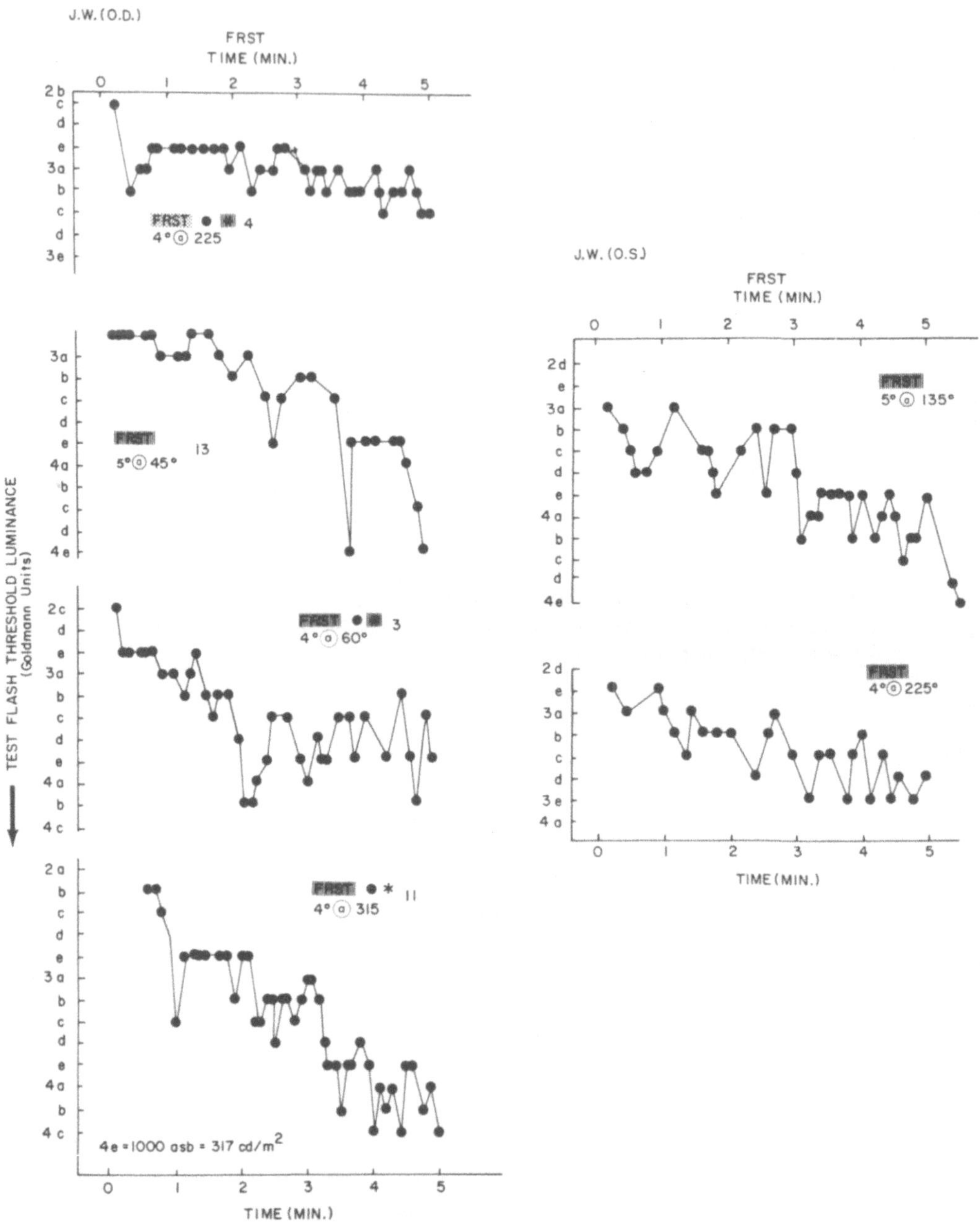

Fig. 6. Patient J.W.: Flashing repeat static test (FRST) data obtained at selected points in both eyes. Sensitivity increases upward on the ordinates. Goldmann units are used, with each step corresponding to 0.1 log unit. At point 4 (Fig. 5) the FRST is only modestly affected, at all other points O.D. (number 13, 3, 11) and O.S. (at 5° eccentricity on the 135° half-meridian, and 4° eccentricity on the 225° half meridian) the FRST was more severely affected. The abscissa is a measure of time in minutes after the eyes were opened following a 5 minute eye closure. Thresholds were determined from non-seeing to just-seeing. A Goldmann 0 target was used.

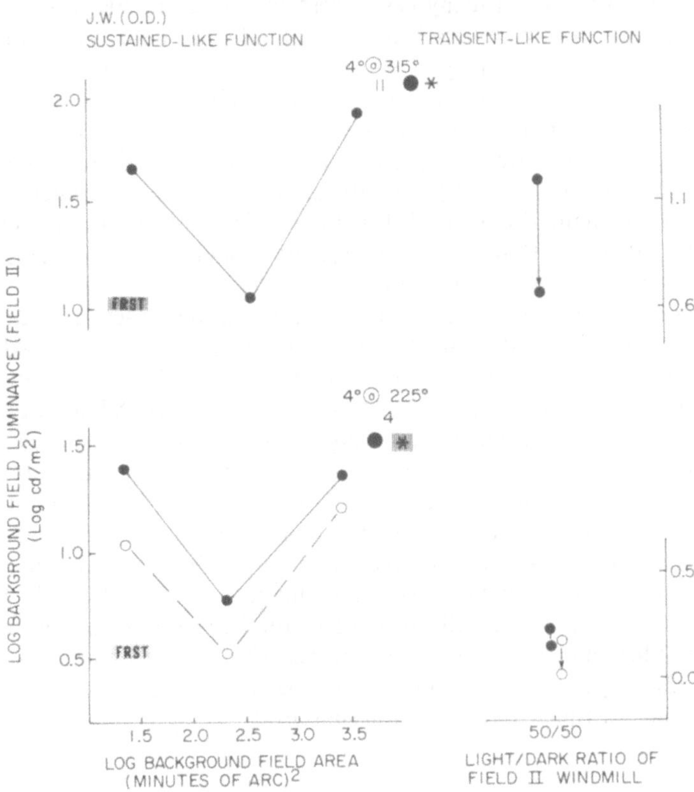

Fig. 7. Patient J.W., right eye: Sustained- and transient-like functions at two test points are shown. At 4° eccentricity on the 315° half-meridian (point 11, Figs. 5, 6) both functions were normal. It is obvious that at 4° eccentricity on the 225° half-meridian (point 4, Figs. 5, 6) the transient-like function is abnormal (i.e., its magnitude approaches zero). This point corresponds to an area where microvascular changes are visible on the fluorescein angiogram.

The ordinate is a measure of luminance of the background field needed to just bring the flashing test target to threshold (both tests). In the case of the transient-like function, the upper point corresponds to the non-rotating windmill background condition, and the arrow points to the measurement made when the windmill was rotated. For the sustained-like function the abscissa is a measure of background field diameter. The windmill target had four vanes covering 50% of the background field.

DISCUSSION

It has been our assumption that small vessels serving the post-lamina cribrosa optic nerve or optic pathways become occluded with resulting ischemia leading to damage to the myelin and subsequent optic atrophy in patients who have received radiation therapy in and about the visual pathways. In these evaluations we measure response of still surviving cells. The time-dependent reduction in sensitivity seen in radiation patients is similar to that seen in many cases of retrobulbar optic neuritis as may be seen in multiple sclerosis

(8, 10, 11, 12, 14, 26). In many cases these changes in the FRST are accompanied by alterations characteristic of nerve fiber bundle defects and chiasmal type lesions. Such changes may be present with or without alterations in the sustained-like and transient-like function depending on whether or not small vessel changes are present in the retina.

In the patient presented, retinal effects manifested as alterations of the transient-like function (Fig. 5). In others, the sustained-like function was affected, or a combination of both functions (17). It is not clear as yet why one or the other function is more susceptible in individual cases. This is an issue which must be pursued in future studies.

Patients with glaucoma tested carefully for time-dependent reduction in sensitivity show none although they do have changes in the sustained- and transient-like function in the region of nerve fiber bundle defects (16). A patient such as the one presented shows the presence of radiation damage both to the optic nerve posterior to the lamina cribrosa and changes that are based in the neural retina itself as demonstrated here by the alteration in transient-like function (10). Although additional patients are being studied using this technique, our limited sample represented by the case presented suggests that the time-dependent reduction in sensitivity, especially combined with nerve fiber bundle defects and chiasmal defects, places the lesion in the axon of the ganglion cell posterior to the lamina cribrosa. This means that nerve fiber bundle defects are not necessarily pathopneumonic of glaucoma. It also suggests that automated perimetric routines should include a way of testing for time-based reductions in sensitivity.

REFERENCES

1. Buys, N. S. & T. C. Kerns, Jr. Irradiation damage to the chiasm. Amer. J. Ophthal. 44: 483–486 (1957).
2. Campos, E. C., J. M. Enoch, C. R. Fitzgerald & M. D. Benedetto. Simple available psychological techniques provide early diagnosis in optic neuritis. Documenta Ophthal. (Submitted).
3. Caveness, W. F., L. Roizin, J. R. M. Innes & A. Carsten. Delayed effects of X-irradiation on the central nervous system of the monkey. In: Response of the nervous system to ionizing radiation. Ed. by Thomas J. Haley and Ray S. Snider. Boston, Little, Brown & Company (1964).
4. Chan, R. C. & L. J. Shukovsky. Effects of irradiation on the eye. Radiology 120: 673–675 (1976).
5. Chee, P. Radiation retinopathy. Amer. J. Ophthal. 66: 860–865 (1968).
6. Cibis, P. A., W. K. Noell & B. Eichel. Ocular effects produced by high-intensity X-radiation. Arch. Ophthal. 53: 651–663 (1955).
7. Cibis, P. A. & D. V. L. Brown. Retinal changes following ionizing radiation. Amer. J. Ophthal. 40: 84–88 (1955).
8. Enoch, J. M. & R. Sunga. Development of quantitative perimetric tests. Documenta Ophthal. 26: 215–229 (1969).
9. Enoch, J. M., R. Berger & R. Birns. A static perimetric technique believed to test receptive field properties: Extension and verification of the analysis. Documenta Ophthal. 29: 127–154 (1970).
10. Enoch, J. M. Quantitative layer-by-layer perimetry. Invest. Ophthal. 17: 199–257 (1978).

11. Enoch, J. M., E. C. Campos & H. E. Bedell. Visual resolution in a patient exhibiting a visual fatigue or saturation-like effect: Probable multiple sclerosis. A.M.A. Arch. Ophthal. 97: 176–178 (1979).
12. Enoch, J. M., E. C. Campos, M. Greer & J. Trobe. Measurement of visual resolution at high luminance levels in patients with possible demyelinating disease. International Ophthal. 1: 99–104 (1979).
13. Enoch, J. M. & E. C. Campos. New quantitative perimetric tests designed to evaluate receptive field-like properties in diseases of the retina and optic nerve. In: Electrophysiology and psychophysics: Their use in ophthalmic diagnosis. Ed. by S. Sokol. International Ophthalmology Clinics. Boston, Little, Brown, Inc. (1980).
14. Enoch, J. M., C. R. Fitzgerald & E. C. Campos. Quantitative layer-by-layer perimetry: An extended analysis. New York, Grune & Stratton, Inc. (1980).
15. Enoch, J. M., C. R. Fitzgerald, E. C. Campos & L. A. Temme. Different functional changes recorded in open angle glaucoma and anterior ischemic optic neuropathy. Documenta Ophthal. (Submitted, 1980).
16. Fankhauser, F. & J. M. Enoch. The effects of blur on perimetric thresholds. A.M.A. Arch. Ophthal. 86: 240–251 (1962).
17. Fitzgerald, C. R., J. M. Enoch & L. A. Temme. Psycho-physical assessment after radiation therapy in and about the optic nerve and anterior visual pathway. A.M.A. Arch. Ophthal. (Submitted).
18. Godwin-Austen, R. B., D. A. Howell & B. Worthington. Observations on radiation myelopathy. Brain 98: 557–568 (1975).
19. Harris, J. R. & M. B. Levene. Visual complications following irradiation for pituitary adenomas and craniopharyngiomas. Radiology 120: 167–171 (1976).
20. Hayreh, S. S. Post-radiation retinopathy: A fluorescence fundus angiographic study. Brit. J. Ophthal. 54: 705–714 (1970).
21. Llena, J. F., G. Céspedes, A. Hirano, H. M. Zimmerman, E. H. Feiring & D. Fine. Vascular alterations in delayed radiation necrosis of the brain. Arch. Pathol. Lab. Med. 100: 531–534 (1976).
22. MacFaul, P. A. & M. A. Bedford. Ocular complications after therapeutic irradiation. Brit. J. Ophthal. 54: 237–247 (1970).
23. Mastaglia, F. L., W. I. McDonald, J. V. Watson & K. Yogendran. Effects of X-radiation on the spinal cord: An experimental study of the morphological changes in central nerve fibres. Brain 99: 101–122 (1976).
24. Perrers-Taylor, M., D. Brinkley & T. Reynolds. Choroido-retinal damage as a complication of radiotherapy. Acta Radiol. 3: 431–440 (1965).
25. Shukovsky, L. J. & G. H. Fletcher. Retinal and optic nerve complications in a high dose irradiation technique of ethmoid sinus and nasal cavity. Radiology 104: 629–634 (1972).
26. Sunga, R. & J. M. Enoch. Further perimetric analysis of patients with lesions of the visual pathways. Amer. J. Ophthal. 70: 403–422 (1970).

This research has been supported in part by National Eye Institute Grants EY-01418 and EY-02303 (to JME) and in part by a NEI Post-Doctoral Fellowship No. EY-05047 (to LAT), NIH, Bethesda, Maryland.

Authors' addresses:
Department of Ophthalmology
and
Center for Sensory Studies
University of Florida, College of Medicine
Box J-284, JHMHC
Gainesville, Florida, 32610, U.S.A.

STATIC AND ACUITY PROFILE PERIMETRY IN OPTIC NEURITIS

CHRIS A. JOHNSON & JOHN L. KELTNER

(Davis, Calif., U.S.A.)

ABSTRACT

Luminance thresholds for detection (static profile perimetry) and resolution (acuity profile perimetry) were determined across the central visual field of 12 patients with optic neuritis. Loss and recovery of detection and resolution properties were generally equivalent with respect to their magnitude and time course. In one particularly interesting case of prolonged recovery, detection properties began to improve slightly before any enhancement of resolution properties were noted. Beyond this initial state of recovery, both functions again showed parallel improvements with time. These data are consistent with previous results for other types of optic nerve dysfunction. In contrast, many other visual disorders (e.g. cataracts, amblyopia, retinal diseases) typically display a large dissociation between detection and resolution properties, with resolution exhibiting greater loss (and in some instances, greater recovery) than detection. Our findings suggest that the combination of static and acuity profile perimetry may become a valuable differential diagnostic technique for optic nerve disease. A preliminary working hypothesis is proposed to account for the present results.

INTRODUCTION

Acuity profile perimetry is a method of clinically evaluating resolution properties on a point-by-point basis across the central visual field. This technique was developed for the Tübinger perimeter by Aulhorn and colleagues (1, 2) and has subsequently been examined by other investigators (3, 4, 7). In combination, static and acuity profile perimetry can provide valuable information about the relationship between detection and resolution characteristics at various locations in the visual field.

We have recently performed static and acuity profile perimetry in the central visual field (30° radius) of normal observers (4), patients with cataracts, amblyopia, retinal disease or optic nerve dysfunction, and individuals suspected of malingering (5, 6). These preliminary findings indicate that for visual disorders other than optic nerve disease, resolution sensitivity is more affected than detection sensitivity. Also, the loss and recovery of detection and resolution properties can sometimes be relatively independent. In contrast, most patients with optic nerve dysfunction exhibit approximately equivalent amounts of loss and recovery for detection and resolution sensitivity. These results suggest that static and acuity profile perimetry may be useful as differential diagnostic tests for optic nerve disease.

Doc. Ophthal. Proc. Series, Vol. 26, ed. by E. L. Greve & G. Verriest

This paper specifically describes our findings in patients with optic neuritis (6 with idiopathic optic neuritis and 6 with optic neuritis associated with multiple sclerosis). This disease follows a systematic course of loss and recovery of visual function, and thus represents an appropriate type of optic nerve dysfunction to study alterations in detection and resolution properties. A particularly interesting example of a patient (optic neuritis associated with multiple sclerosis) with prolonged recovery of detection and resolution properties is presented.

METHODS

Thorough descriptions of the principles and techniques of static and acuity profile perimetry have been provided in previous publications (2, 4, 5). The procedure basically consists of luminance thresholds for detection (static perimetry) and resolution (acuity profile perimetry) using the circle and square target pairs on the Tübinger perimeter. At each visual field location, detection sensitivity is measured for circular targets by an ascending method of limits according to the standard procedures of static perimetry. Resolution sensitivity is determined by presenting a random sequence of circle and square stimuli belonging to a specific target pair. The minimum threshold for reliably distinguishing between the circle and square targets is defined by varying the stimulus luminance according to a staircase procedure. Sensitivity profiles for static and acuity perimetry are generated by performing these determinations at successive visual field locations.

For each pair, the basis for distinguishing between the circle and square targets is defined by the distance between the outer edges of the circle and the corners of the square. This distance equals 0.15 times the diameter of the circle, and represents the minimum angle of resolution. For example, a 10′ diameter circle will have a 1.5′ minimum angle of resolution for the circle-square target pair, thereby corresponding to a Snellen visual acuity of 20/30 (see Johnson *et. al.* (4) for a further description). Previous studies have shown that the circle-square target pairs produce results similar to those obtained with other types of acuity targets (2, 5).

Twelve patients with unilateral optic neuritis were evaluated. Six of the patients (ages 28 to 68) had optic neuritis associated with multiple sclerosis and six patients (ages 18 to 66) exhibited an idiopathic optic neuritis. Static and acuity profile perimetry was performed with three stimulus pairs, consisting of the 10′ (20/30 acuity), 26′ (20/80 acuity) and 66′ (20/200 acuity) diameter targets.

RESULTS

Fig. 1 presents static and acuity sensitivity profiles for the 10′ (20/30 acuity), 26′ (20/80 acuity) and 66′ (20/200 acuity) diameter targets in the right eye of a normal observer. The results were obtained for the horizontal meridian, although profiles along other meridians exhibit similar results. Note that the static profile is only modestly affected by target size, becoming somewhat

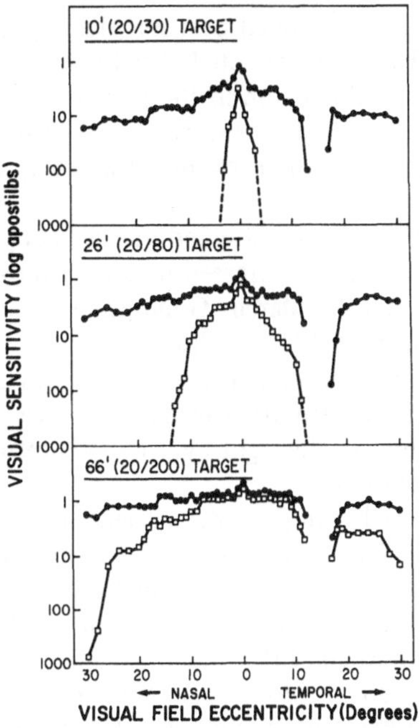

Fig. 1. Static (filled circles) and acuity (open squares) profiles obtained for the 10′ (20/30 acuity), 26′ (20/80 acuity) and 66′ (20/200 acuity) targets in the right eye of a normal observer.

flatter with larger stimuli. On the other hand, the acuity profile is very steep for small targets and broadens out considerably for larger stimuli. The relationships for static and acuity profile sensitivity in normal eyes may be used as a basis for comparison with the results in optic neuritis.

Twelve patients with unilateral optic neuritis were evaluated with static and acuity profile perimetry. No differences were found between the patients with idiopathic optic neuritis and patients with optic neuritis associated with multiple sclerosis. In general, the recovery of detection and resolution properties was approximately equal in each of these patients. In one or two instances, recovery of detection sensitivity slightly preceded resolution sensitivity for the smallest targets. Some of the patients recovered so rapidly that it was not possible for us to document many intermediate stages of improvement. A particularly interesting example in which we were able to obtain data for various stages of recovery is presented below.

A 30 year old female patient was seen on June 24, 1977, with a 10–12 day history of film over her right eye and pain with motion of the eye. Examination at that time revealed a best corrected visual acuity of 20/15 OU with color desaturation in the right eye. Visual fields, fundus exam, pupillary response, skull x-rays and laboratory evaluation were essentially normal and no other neurologic symptoms were present.

The patient did well without recurrence of symptoms until December 13, 1977, when she was seen with a one week history of rightsided headaches behind her right eye with pain on right gaze. Two to three days following the onset of pain, a film again developed over her right eye. She denied all other neurologic symptoms. Her best corrected visual acuity was 20/50 OD, 20/15 OS, with definite loss of color vision in the right eye. Visual fields showed a dense inferior altitudinal defect in the right eye. There was a 2+ Marcus Gunn pupil in the right eye. Fundus exam showed very mild temporal pallor of the right optic disc.

On December 20, 1977, best corrected visual acutiy was 20/20 −2 OD, 20/15 OS. Color vision was still decreased in the right eye. Visual fields were unchanged and there was a 2+ Marcus Gunn pupil in the right eye with mild temporal pallor noted in the right optic disc.

On January 3, 1978, best corrected visual acuity was 20/20 OD, 20/15 OS. Color vision showed mild desaturation in the right eye. Pupil exam revealed a trace Marcus Gunn pupil in the right eye. Fundus exam showed mild temporal pallor as noted previously.

The last recorded visual acuity in the patient on January 18, 1978, was 20/15 −1 OD and 20/15 OS. A visual evoked potential on that date showed a prolonged latency in the right eye with normal values in the left eye, despite the recovery of visual acuity in the right eye. Skull and optic foramen films and sinus x-rays were normal. CBC, sed rate, Serology and ANA were all normal. Two-hour postprandial blood sugar was normal. The patient was felt to probably have multiple sclerosis with two attacks of retrobulbar neuritis, one mild attack in June, 1977, with a more severe attack but with almost complete recovery in December, 1977.

Fig. 2 presents static and acuity sensitivity profiles for the 10′ (20/30 acuity) diameter target for this young female patient with optic neuritis in the right eye. Testing was performed along the vertical (90°–270°) meridian over a period of approximately five weeks. Similar evaluations for the left eye were normal throughout the five week period, and are not presented for the sake of brevity.

On her initial visit (Fig. 2a), the static profile for the right eye revealed a dense inferior paracentral scotoma between fixation and 20° eccentricity, whereas no acuity profile was able to be plotted. Fig. 2b, c and d display the static and acuity profiles for the 10′ (20/30 acuity) target on successive visits. Note that there is a progressive improvement up to nearly normal levels, and that both static and acuity profiles appear to recover at approximately the same rate. However, the steep profile of the acuity data for the 10′ (20/30 acuity) target is only able to provide information about the recovery of visual function within the central 3° radius of the visual field. A larger target (66′ diameter, 20/200 acuity) was therefore used to evaluate the relationship between detection and resolution sensitivity for paracentral regions of the visual field.

Static and acuity profiles for the 66′ (20/200 acuity) target are presented in Fig. 3a–e for five successive testing sessions. The recovery of detection and resolution properties near fixation again appear to be approximately equivalent. However, beyond 10° eccentricity in the inferior visual field, the results suggest that detection properties (static profile) began to improve slightly before resolution properties (acuity profile) began to recover. Beyond this initial recovery lead by detection properties, the rate of improvement

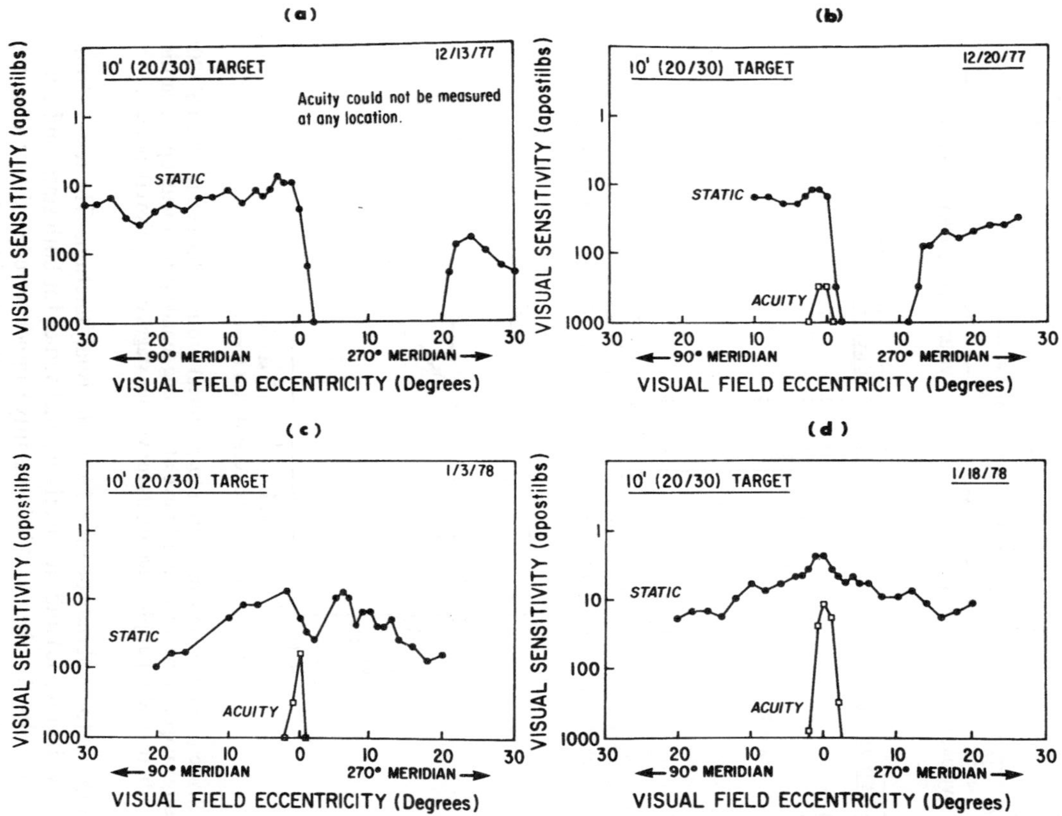

Fig. 2. Static (filled circles) and acuity (open squares) profiles obtained for the 10′ (20/30 acuity) target in the affected right eye of a young female patient with optic neuritis. (a), (b), (c) and (d) display the results for various stages of the recovery process.

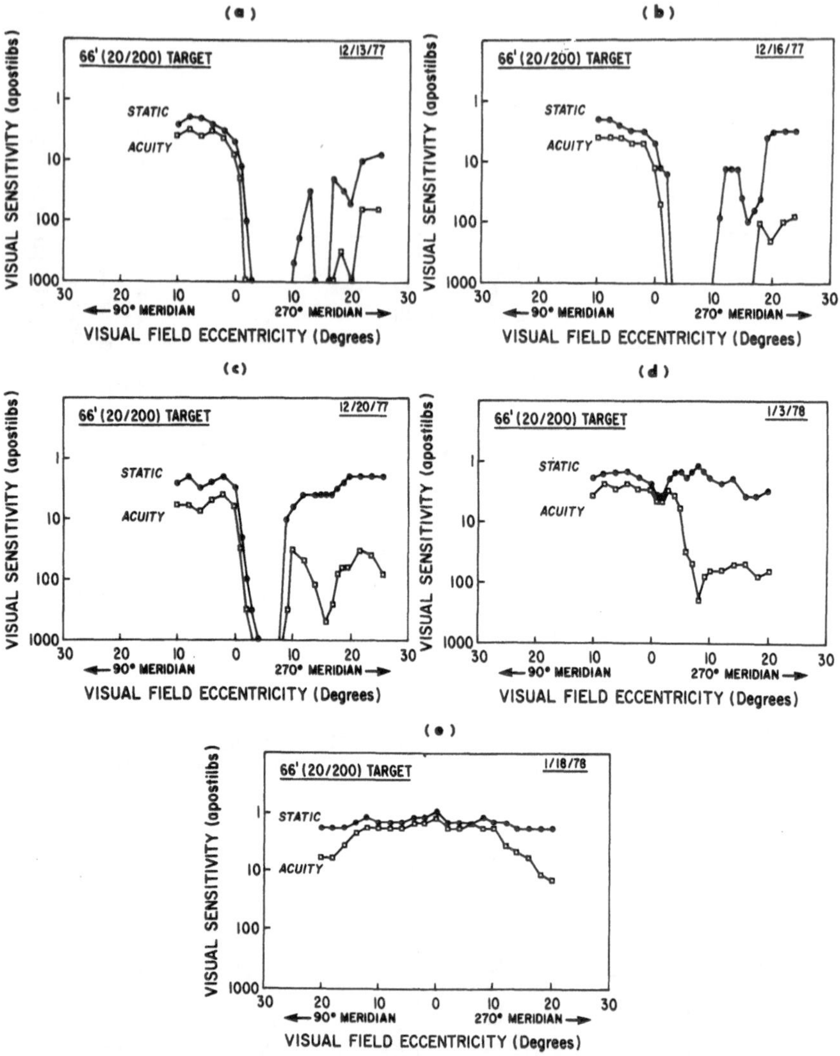

Fig. 3. Static (filled circles) and acuity (open squres) profiles obtained for the 66′ (20/200 acuity) target in the affected right eye of a young female patient with optic neuritis. (a), (b), (c), (d) and (e) display the results for various stages of the recovery process.

again appears to be about the same for both visual functions. The results from the final visit (Fig. 3e) indicate nearly normal values for both static and acuity profiles. Results for the 26′ (20/80 acuity) target were consistent with the findings for the other targets and are not shown for the sake of brevity.

DISCUSSION

Our present findings indicate that the loss and recovery of detection and resolution properties in optic neuritis are similar to that of other optic nerve disorders, since both visual functions seem to be affected by an equivalent amount (5). Some of the patients with optic neuritis exhibited a rapid recovery that did not allow us to sequentially evaluate the relationship between detection and resolution sensitivity at various stages of improvement. In the one example for which this type of documentation was possible, most of the results showed a parallel rate of improvement for detection and resolution properties. In one portion of the inferior paracentral visual field, it appeared that detection sensitivity began to recover slightly before improvements in resolution sensitivity. Beyond this initial stage, the recovery process was essentially parallel for both functions. In general, optic nerve disorders affect both detection and resolution properties equally (5).

In contrast to the findings for optic nerve disease, previous studies have shown that most patients with cataracts, amblyopia or retinal disorders exhibit a much greater deficit for resolution sensitivity than for detection sensitivity (5, 6). Also, the recovery of detection and resolution properties in retinal disorders can sometimes be relatively independent and show a substantial dissociation between detection and resolution sensitivity.

The results of static and acuity profile perimetry in various patient populations may be interpreted in terms of signal processing and signal transmission characteristics of the visual system. Since the optic nerve is responsible for conveying information from the retina to higher centers, disorders of this portion of the visual pathways will primarily alter signal transmission. Thus, both detection and resolution information will be affected by approximately equivalent amounts. On the other hand disorders such as amblyopia and retinal disease will exert a major influence on signal processing, which will produce greater deficits for resolution properties than for detection properties. Degraded retinal images (produced by cataracts or other opacities of the ocular media) will also affect resolution properties to a greater extent than detection properties.

The above analysis in terms of signal transmission vs. signal processing losses of the visual pathways provides a parsimonious interpretation of our clinical findings for static and acuity profile perimetry. In addition, it suggests that this technique may be a useful differential diagnostic tool, particularly with regard to optic nerve disorders.

REFERENCES

1. Aulhorn, E. Über die Beziehung zwischen Lichtsinn und Sehschärfe. Graefes Arch. Ophthal. 167: 4–74 (1964).
2. Aulhorn, E. & H. Harms. Visual perimetry. In: D. Jameson & L. Hurvich, eds, Handbook of sensory physiology, Vol. VII/4. New York, Springer-Verlag (1972).
3. Forstot, S. L., G. G. Weinstein & K. B. Feicock. Studies with the Tübingen perimeter of Harms and Aulhorn. Ann. Ophthalmol. 2: 843–854 (1970).
4. Johnson, C. A., J. L. Keltner & F. G. Balestrery. Effects of target size and eccentricity on visual detection and resolution. Vision Research 18: 1217–1222 (1978).
5. Johnson, C. A., J. L. Keltner & F. G. Balestrery. Acuity profile perimetry: Description of technique and preliminary clinical trials. Arch. Ophthalmol. 97: 684–689 (1979).

6. Keltner, J. L., C. A. Johnson & I. J. Cowley. Acuity profile perimetry in a unique case of bilateral central serous retinopathy. Ann. Ophthalmol. 12: 726–731 (1980).
7. Sloan, L. L. The Tübinger perimeter of Harms and Aulhorn. Arch. Ophthalmol. 86: 612–622 (1970).

Supported in part by National Eye Institute Academic Investigator Award No. EY-00095 (to CAJ).

Authors' addresses:
Chris A. Johnson, Ph.D.
Dept. of Ophthalmology

and

John L Keltner, M.D.
Depts. of Ophthalmology,
Neurology and
Neurological Surgery
University of California, Davis
Davis, CA 95616
U.S.A.

VISUAL FIELD LOSS AND PUPILLARY DYSFUNCTION

H. STANLEY THOMPSON

(Iowa City, Iowa, U.S.A.)

The relative afferent pupillary defect (RAPD) is the most commonly used clinical indicator of optic nerve function. The size of the pupillary defect can be measured by dimming the stimulus to the good eye by known amounts until the two eyes are balanced and no relative afferent pupil defect (RAPD) can be seen. This can be done clinically by holding a neutral density filter over the better eye and doing the swinging light test. The density of the filter needed to abolish the RAPD is recorded, in log units, as a measure of the relative afferent pupillary defect. Patients with unilateral loss of visual field were studied and the amount of RAPD was correlated with the amount of field loss as measured according to Trost *et al* (Arch. Ophthalmol. 97: 2175, 1979). The pupillary defect showed a better correlation with visual field loss than with visual acuity.

The details will be published in: Trans. Am. Ophthalmol. Soc., 1980.

Doc. Ophthal. Proc. Series, Vol. 26, ed. by E. L. Greve & G. Verriest

HEREDITARY DOMINANT OPTIC ATROPHY

EGILL HANSEN

(*Oslo, Norway*)

ABSTRACT

Hereditary dominant optic atrophy occurred in 5 patients from two families. In the first family a tritan colour defect was manifested with normal red-green matches in the anomaloscope. In family 2 a tritan defect was recorded together with a red-green defect of deuteranopic type. In this family deuteranomalous colour defects occurred in otherwise healthy members. The affected patients in family 2 had functioning blue sensitive receptors, though at a reduced level, as found by examination of increment thresholds against a yellow background. Static and kinetic perimetry performed under the same conditions showed great variability in the sensitivity of the blue mechanism in the visual field.

INTRODUCTION

Colour vision defects are of particular interest in the hereditary dominant optic atrophies serving here as a diagnostic criterion. In many cases showing only a slight impairment of visual acuity and reading capacity there may be significant colour defects. Most characteristically a tritan dyschromatopsia is found in this type of optic atrophy (4, 8, 11) although red-green deficiencies have also been described (2, 3, 13, 15). I report here findings in two types of patients with dominant optic atrophy where consideration is given to evaluate separate receptor mechanisms. It is of particular interest to see if the blue receptor mechanism can be identified in those patients with dominant optic atrophy and to what extent this type of receptor response can be measured in the visual field.

MATERIAL

Dominant optic atrophy was diagnosed in 4 patients and was highly suspected in one patient (case 2). The patients belonged to two families whose pedigrees are shown in Fig. 1. In family 1 comprising cases 1, 2 and 3 other affected persons were not known. In family 2 other members also had been examined. Those indicated by N have been found normal. Two males have been found deuteranomalous and have been indicated by DA. Another one, indicated by RG, was known to have a colour vision defect.

Case 1. A male, 16 years of age at the first examination had been partially sighted from

Doc. Ophthal. Proc. Series, Vol. 26, ed. by E. L. Greve & G. Verriest

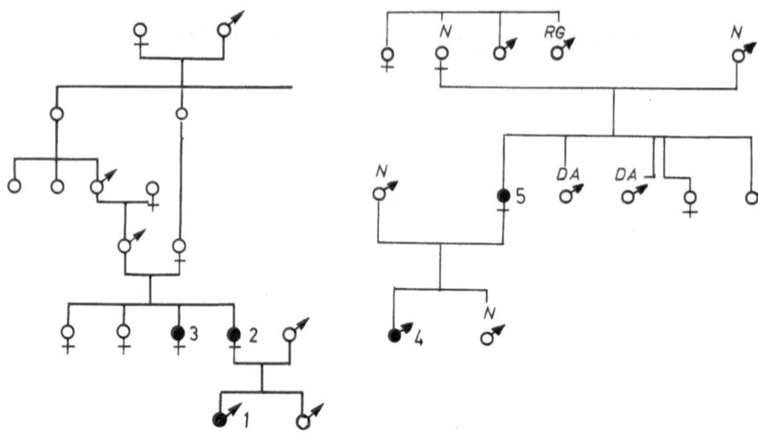

Fig. 1. Pedigrees of family 1 (left) and family 2 (right). N = normal, DA = deuteranomalous. RG = red-green defective, not examined. The cases of dominant optic atrophy are indicated by black.

childhood. Discrimination between blue and green had always been difficult. His visual acuity was 5/25 on the right eye and 5/20 on the left eye, emmetropic. Reading vision was good (Schiøtz 0.4 m). Normal pupillary reflexes were found. Ophthalmoscopy revealed a moderate pallor of the temporal discs. Dark adaptation was normal.

Case 2. A female, 50 years of age, is the mother of case 1. Routine examination revealed no abnormality except for the colour vision. Normal optic discs were found, and visual acuity was 6/6 on each eye.

Case 3. A female, 43 years of age, is the sister of case 2. This patient was examined at another eye department. She had always been partially sighted. A visual acuity of 6/12 was found on each eye. Some pallor of the optic discs was recorded.

Case 4. A male, had noticed deficient colour vision from early childhood when he was unable to distinguish between blue and green coloured toys. On admission to the hospital at the age of 8 years, his visual acuity was 5/50 on each eye. During 10 years of observation his visual acuity was unchanged. Reading vision was good. The optic discs were pale in the temporal parts. A dark adaptation record was normal.

Case 5. A female, 35 years at the first examination, is the mother of case 4. She had been partially sighted from about 10–15 years of age. She easily confused blue and green coloured clothes. No progression had been observed during a 10 year observation. Pallor of the optic discs was recorded from the first examination. Visual acuity was 6/30 on the right eye and 6/60 on the left eye. The dark adaptation course was normal.

METHODS

Colour vision examinations were carried out with the following tests: the Ishihara pseudo-isochromatic charts (11th ed.), the AO-HRR test, the Farnsworth's tritan chart (F-II), the Farnsworth's D-15 test and the Farnsworth-Munsell 100 Hue test, the tissue paper contrast charts of the Velhagen-Stilling test (21st ed.) and the Cohn's test (1905) besides a series of tissue paper contrast charts having been described earlier (6). The pigmentary tests were administered under two Macbeth Illuminant C lamps (about 300 lux). Anomaloscopic examinations were performed with a Nagel anomaloscope type I. Perimetric examination was performed in the usual way with a Goldmann perimeter.

Additional examinations of increment threshold against coloured backgrounds were performed in a modified Goldmann perimeter as has been described earlier (5, 7).

RESULTS

Colour vision

The Ishihara test and the Farnsworth's tritan chart were correctly read by *case 1*. Two screening charts for blue-yellow defects and for red-green defects were questionable by the AO-HRR test. With the F D-15 test he had some confusions in the blue-green and the purple region, i.e. a slightly tritan pattern. With the 100 Hue test he had 148 error scores predominantly about the red and in the blue-green part (Fig. 3). He had precise settings within the normal range by the anomaloscopic test (41–43.5/16). In *case 2* normal readings were recorded on the Ishihara test, the AO-HRR test and the F-II test. She failed the tissue paper contrast charts with blue and green backgrounds. With the 100 Hue test she had 106 error scores, predominantly in the red and blue-green part (Fig. 3). The anomaloscope settings were normal (40–42.5/16). *Case 3* was reportedly unable to read the Ishihara test. She performed the F D-15 test with a tritan-like confusion pattern (Fig. 2).

In *case 4* only a few figures could be seen on the Ishihara and the AO-HRR test, and no squares could be seen on the F-II chart. He failed a series of tissue paper contrast charts. On the F D-15 test he showed confusions of tritan type (Fig. 2) while a more irregular pattern was shown with the 100 Hue test (Fig. 3). His total error score was 354. His anomaloscope settings

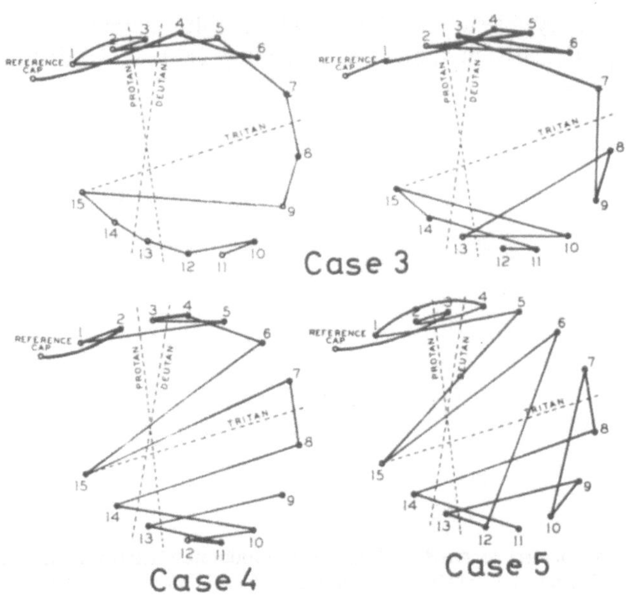

Fig. 2. The Farnsworth's D-15 test as performed by cases 3, 4 and 5.

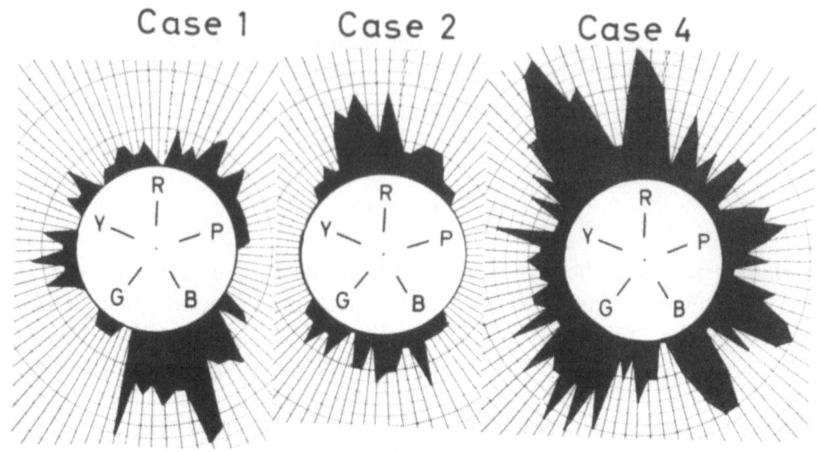

Fig. 3. 100 Hue test performed by cases 1, 2 and 4.

were of deuteranopic type (the yellow value matching the green was 18.5–24 and that of the red 9–11). *Case 5* failed the greater part of the Ishihara and the AO-HRR test charts as well as the Farnsworth's tritan chart. She passed none of the tissue paper contrast charts. The F D-15 test revealed an irregular tritan pattern (Fig. 2). The 100 Hue test was performed with great uncertainty giving a high error score (1003) with an irregular pattern. In the anomaloscope her settings were of deuteranopic type, red being matched with the yellow value 14–15 and green with yellow at 21.5–24.

Spectral sensitivity in white and coloured lights

Spectral sensitivity registered in the standard white illumination (case 1) was depressed, particularly in the short wave range (Fig. 4). Distinctly different

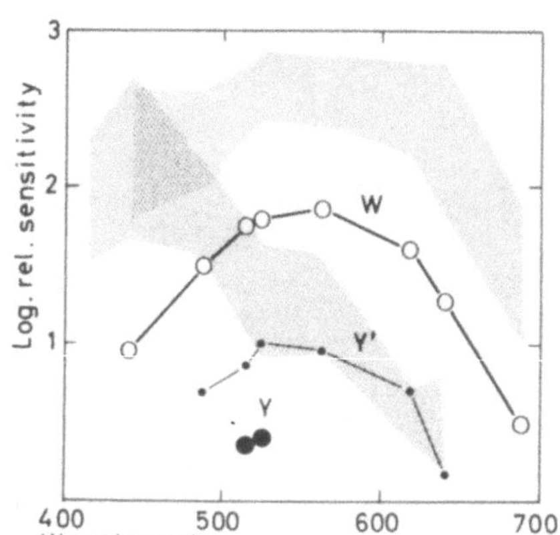

Fig. 4. Relative spectral sensitivity obtained by moderately narrow-banded interference filters in case 1 against a white background, 31.5 asb (W) and against a yellow background of high intensity, Wratten 22, 2900 lux (Y) and of greatly reduced intensity (Y'). Angular size of target 54'. Shaded areas indicate the normal variation (mean ± 2 SD).

response patterns were obtained with blue and purple backgrounds thus indicating red and green receptor activity, though at a reduced level. This is consistent with his normal anomaloscope matches. However, response to blue-violet stimuli in the yellow illumination indicating blue receptor activity could not be shown (Fig. 4).

In cases 4 and 5 no red and green mechanisms could be distinguished by selective chromatic adaptation, but only an unspecific response in the mid-wave range of the spectrum. This finding is consistent with their deuteranopic-like anomaloscope matches. On the other hand these patients could see the short-wave stimuli during adaptation to yellow light, their spectral sensitivity curves being consistent with a functioning blue receptor mechanism, though at a reduced level (Fig. 6).

Perimetric examinations

All patients had normal visual field limits by kinetic perimetry, even with the smallest isopters. Relative centro-coecal scotomas were demonstrated by kinetic perimetry (object size $1/4\,mm^2$, 0.1 relative intensity) in cases 4 and 5. However, the gratings of the Amsler's charts could be seen by both patients although case 4 did not see the upper temporal corners of the charts. Static perimetry demonstrated a low central threshold sensitivity, except for a high sensitivity at the fixation point of case 1. Case 5 had a clear reduction of threshold sensitivity paracentrally on the temporal side (Fig. 5).

Using a blue-violet target in the yellow illuminated sphere static perimetry curves were obtained showing the response of the blue mechanism (Fig. 7). In case 5 there was a significant loss of sensitivity on the temporal side, which was shown as a centro-coecal scotoma by the kinetic perimetry registration

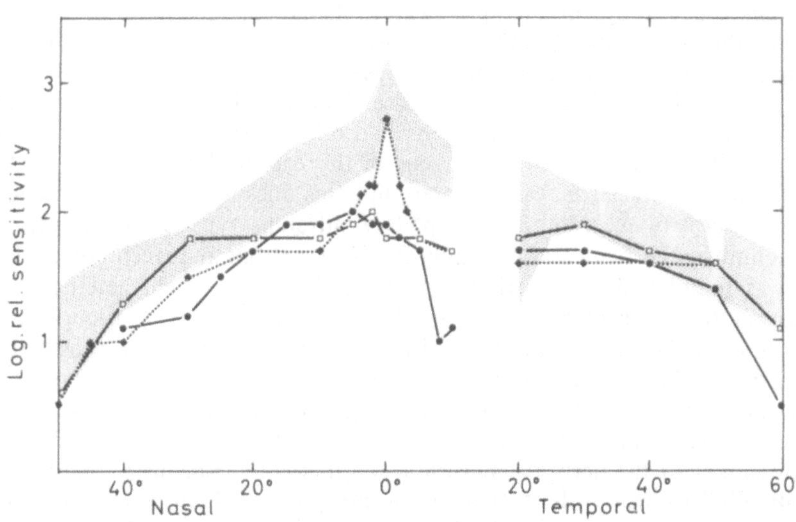

Fig. 5. Static perimetry recorded in 3 patients under standard illumination (31.5 asb). Object size II (13′ angular size). ♦ = case 1, □ = case 4, • = case 5. Shaded area indicates the normal variation (mean ± 2 SD).

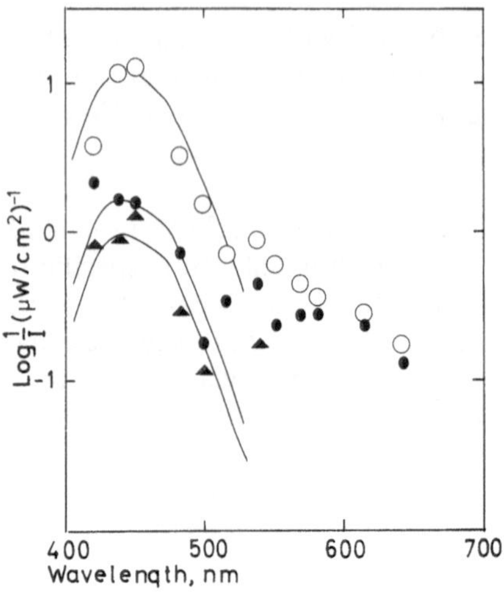

Fig. 6. Spectral sensitivity in yellow background light (low pressure Na-lamp at $\lambda =$ 589 nm, 500 lux) registered in case 4 at 5° temporal position (▲) and in case 5 at 5° nasal position (●). Open circles indicate the performance of a normal person at 5° eccentricity under the same conditions. Angular size of target 1°47′. The curves indicate the blue primary (17).

under the same conditions. The highest sensitivity of her blue receptors was indicated by the faint isopter showing an isolated nasal area suggesting an hemianopic border to the less sensitive area in the temporal half.

DISCUSSION

A tritan type of dyschromatopsia was a characteristic finding in all our patients though not particularly pronounced. In cases 1 and 4 confusions of green and blue was the first symptom observed, while a reduction of visual acuity was registered at a later stage. Case 1, in accordance with the classical description of dominant optic atrophy, had only a tritan defect and normal ability in discriminating red and green. In this case no blue sensitive mechanism could be traced as was expected, but this does not prove the absence of blue sensitive receptors. A completely different type of colour defect was found in the two cases of family 2 where a strong red-green colour defect was found besides the tritan defect. In these cases a characteristic response pattern of a blue receptor mechanism could be shown, though at a reduced level. As shown with the specific quantitative perimetry its sensitivity was manifested differently in the visual field.

In spite of the presence of the blue receptor mechanism there is a confusion of colours in the blue-green part of the spectrum. This could be due to abnormalities of the nerves as suggested by Alpern (1) reporting a completely colour blind subject with recessive optic atrophy in whom cone visual pigments were demonstrated in the fovea by densitometer analysis. I.e., there is a defect which is chiefly concerned with the visual channels rather than with the retinal pigments. This is supported also in the case of dominant optic

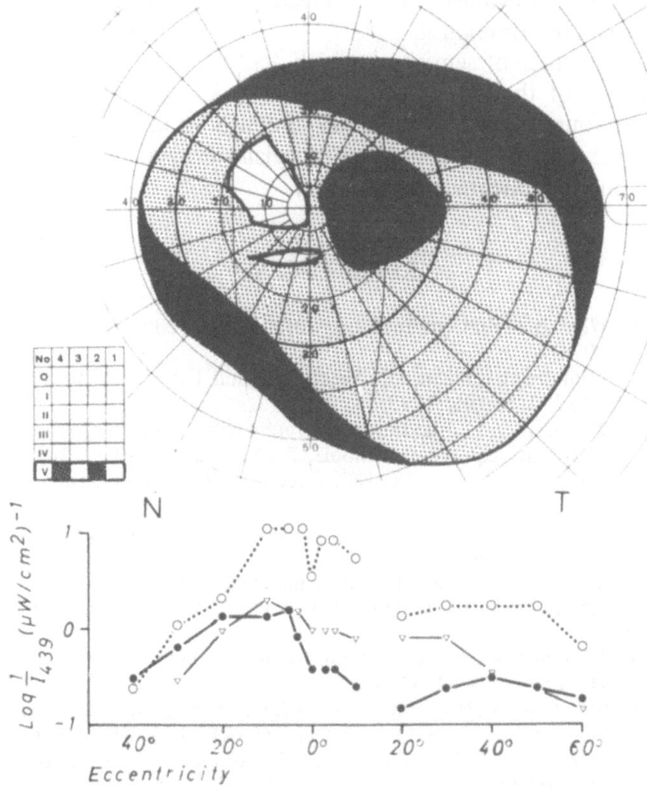

Fig. 7. Static perimetry against yellow background (low pressure Na-lamp, $\lambda = 589$ nm, 500 lux) registered in case 4 (▿) and case 5 (•). The performance of a normal person (43 years of age) is also indicated (○). A blue-violet target ($\lambda_{max} = 439$ nm) subtending 1°47′ angular diameter is used. For case 5 the kinetic perimetry record obtained under the same conditions is shown. The threshold value of the greater isopter is 5.37 $\mu W/cm^2$ and that of the smaller 0.49 $\mu W/cm^2$.

atrophy by the findings of a primary degeneration of the retinal ganglion cells together with loss of myelin and nerve tissue within the optic nerves, as reported by Johnston *et al.* (10).

In these cases having a strong red-green defect it might be, that the presence of blue receptors is not accidental. A relatively good function in the blue region of the spectrum was reported by Kok-van Alphen (13), Aulhorn and Grützner (3) and Völker-Dieben *et al.* (16) in their cases where red-green defects were predominant. Occurrence of deuteranopia in dominant optic atrophy has been reported (2, 9) as well as protanopia (3). In some pedigrees tritan defects could even be seen very infrequently (16).

Characteristically all our patients had a mild degree of visual impairment. This was the case in the patients with the deuteranopic type of defect also. Slightly affected cases of dominant optic atrophy could easily be confused with the congenital tritan defect as was pointed out by Krill *et al.* (14).

Cases 1 and 2 were obviously in this category with their slight affection and normal red-green discrimination.

A peculiar wryness of sensitivity which was most reduced in the temporal paracentral part of the visual field is in concordance with other reports (3, 12). This was found by static perimetry and also by kinetic perimetry using small and weak object lights, but was especially evident by the specific perimetry isolating the blue receptor function.

REFERENCES

1. Alpern, M. What is it that confines in a world without color? Invest. Ophthal. 13: 648–674 (1974).
2. Aulhorn, E. Dominant erbliche Optikusatrophie mit Farbsinnstörungen. Klin. Mbl. Augenheilk. 163: 248–249 (1973).
3. Aulhorn, E. & P. Grützner. Infantile optic atrophy with dominant mode of inheritance accompanied by an acquired protanopia. Progr. Neuro-Ophthal., 2nd Int. Congr., Montreal 1967, Vol. 2, pp. 128–132. Excerpta Medica Foundation, Amsterdam (1969).
4. Frey, R. G. Blaublindheit und dominant vererbte Optikusatrophie. Klin. Mbl. Augenheilk. 167: 577–580 (1975).
5. Hansen, E. The colour receptors studied by increment threshold measurements during chromatic adaptation in the Goldmann perimeter. Acta Ophthal. (Kbh.) 52: 490–500 (1974).
6. Hansen, E. Examination of colour vision by use of induced contrast colours. Acta Ophthal. (Kbh.) 54: 611–622 (1976).
7. Hansen, E. & T. Seim. Calibration of the Goldmann perimeter and accessories used in specific quantitative perimetry. Acta Ophthal. (Kbh.) 56: 241–251 (1978).
8. Jaeger, W. Dominant vererbte Opticusatrophie. Albrecht v. Graefes Arch. Ophthal. 155: 457–484 (1954).
9. Jaeger, W., D. Früh & H. J. Lauer. Types of acquired colour deficiencies caused by autosomal-dominant infantile optic atrophy. Mod. Probl. Ophthal. (Basel) 11: 145–147 (1972).
10. Johnston, P. B., R. N. Gaster, V. C. Smith & R. C. Tripathi. A clinicopathologic study of autosomal dominant optic atrophy. Amer. J. Ophthal. 88: 868–875 (1979).
11. Kjer, P. Infantile optic atrophy with dominant mode of inheritance. Acta Ophthal. (Kbh.), Suppl. 54, p. 147 (1959).
12. Kline, L. B. & J. S. Glaser. Dominant optic atrophy. The clinical profile. Arch. Ophthal. 97: 1680–1686 (1979).
13. Kok-van Alphen, C. C. A family with the dominant infantile form of optical atrophy. Acta Ophthal. (Kbh.) 38: 675–685 (1960).
14. Krill, A. E., V. C. Smith & J. Pokorny. Further studies supporting the identity of congenital tritanopia and hereditary dominant optic atrophy. Invest. Ophthal. 10: 457–465 (1971).
15. Ohba, N., M. Imamura & T. Tanino. Color vision in autosomal dominant hereditary optic atrophy. Acta. Soc. Ophthal. Jap. 79: 1213–1224 (1975).
16. Völker-Dieben, H. J., L. N. Went & E. C. De Vries-de Mol. Comparative colour vision and other ophthalmological studies in three families with dominant inherited juvenile optic atrophy. Mod. Probl. Ophthal. (Basel) 13: 277–281 (1974).
17. Walraven, P. L. A closer look at the tritanopic convergence point. Vision Res. 14: 1339–1343 (1974).

Author's address:
Egill Hansen, M.D.
Department of Ophthalmology
Rikshospitalet
Oslo 1, Norway

RESIDUAL FIELD CHANGES IN PATIENTS WITH IDIOPATHIC CENTRAL SEROUS RETINOPATHY

V. E. NATSIKOS, J. C. DEAN HART & E. R. RAISTRICK

(Bristol, Great Britain)

ABSTRACT

Although the merits of Amsler charting as a test for documenting the nature of central field changes in patients with acute central serous retinopathy are recognised, the value of this technique in detecting defects in retinal function after the oedema fluid has absorbed is less well established. It has been reported that static perimetry investigations, however, continue to reveal abnormal profiles in a high proportion of patients with a resolved retinopathy. In order to determine which of the two methods of investigation produced more information about the residual defects in central retinal function in such cases, static perimetric and Amsler chart testing were performed on 27 patients between 6 months and 5 years after they developed the disease, the condition having been diagnosed in the acute phase by fluorographic and biomicroscopic examination. 63% of cases retained abnormal static profiles, but 81% recorded defects on Amsler charting. The incidence of retinal changes was noted to be greater in patients where the oedema fluid resolved slowly. Needle shaped scotomata were most apparent on static perimetry testing if the meridian studied corresponded to that intersecting the site at which a focal breakdown of the choroido-retinal barrier had developed and the fovea.

INTRODUCTION

Although visual field changes can readily be detected in patients during the acute phase of idiopathic central serous retinopathy, the incidence of residual field changes found by various workers after the oedema fluid has absorbed has ranged from 10% to 100%. Investigators employing standard kinetic perimetric techniques have reported scotomatous defects close to fixation in 27% of patients with resolved central serous retinopathy (6), 50% (7) and 10% (4). Hache *et al.* (2), who examined such patients by static perimetry, noted abnormal profiles in all of the cases tested, but none of these with a satisfactory recovery of visual acuity plotted defects on the Amsler grid in the residual phase of the disease process, whereas distortions on the Amsler grid were recorded by 89% of cases assessed by Klein *et al.* (3).

Since the relative merits of static perimetry and Amsler charting remain unclear in evaluating any residual impairment of visual function in the central zone after the neural layers of the retina have become reapposed to the pigment epithelium in cases of resolved idiopathic central serous retinopathy, a study was initiated in an attempt to clarify this question.

Doc. Ophthal. Proc. Series, Vol. 26, ed. by E. L. Greve & G. Verriest

METHODS

Patients who attended the University Department of Ophthalmology, in the age group 20–50 years, with clear evidence of idiopathic central serous retinopathy, which was confirmed by biomicroscopic and fluorescein angiographic studies during the acute phase and who were re-examined regularly until the oedema fluid resolved, were recalled for static perimetric and Amsler charting studies at intervals ranging from 6 months to 5 years after the onset of their symptoms. No patient who was thought to have developed a recurrence of a serous maculopathy during this period, or who had evidence of an additional ocular or systemic disease process, was included in this study.

Amsler charting and static perimetry was carried out, using standard methods, and for the latter test a Goldmann perimeter model 940 was used. Two axes were plotted in the static perimetric studies, one along the 180°–0° meridian and the other selected by determining the axis joining the site of the focal breakdown of the choroido-retinal barrier noted on fluorescein angiography in the acute phase, to the fovea. This was determined by examining enlarged prints of fluorescein angiograms (Fig. 1) and the plot performed on the nearest corresponding standard meridian on the chart, which differs from that found on the angiogram by 90°.

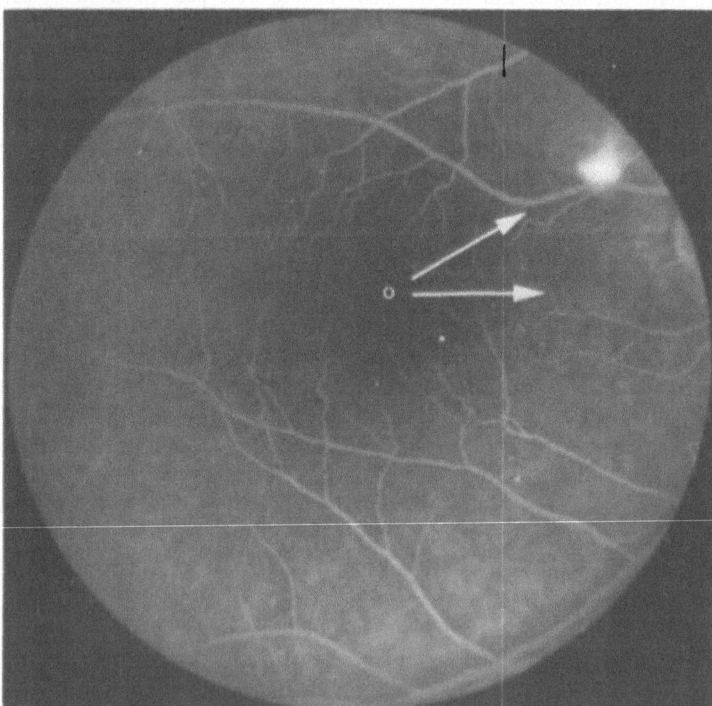

Fig. 1. Fluorescein angiogram of case with central serous retinopathy during the acute phase. Angle formed between line drawn through leaking site and fovea and horizontal axis is 30°, corresponding to the 120–300 meridian on a visual field chart.

RESULTS

27 patients were investigated, 23 males and 4 females, with a mean age of 40 years. All patients had a visual acuity of 6/12 or better at the time when visual field studies were performed.

Amsler grid test

Localised areas of metamorphopsia were plotted on the Amsler chart by 22 out of the 27 cases examined. In some the distortions recorded on the chart were observed to be close to fixation (Fig. 2), and in others at some distance away from this site (Fig. 3). No patient with a resolved central serous retinopathy plotted a partial scotoma, although such defects were frequently noted by patients during the acute phase of the disease.

Static perimetric investigations

17 out of the 27 patients examined were recorded as having paracentral needle shaped scotomata. These varied between 1° and 3° in width, and from a slight depression to quite dense cuts which approached the baseline of the static chart. In 11 cases residual paracentral scotomata were detected on the horizontal axis (Fig. 4). However, 6 others showed no abnormality on this meridian, but needle shaped defects became apparent when static profiles were plotted on the axis joining the site of the sealed breach in the choroido-retinal barrier to the fovea (Fig. 5).

The time taken for the serous fluid to absorb in cases of idiopathic central serous retinopathy examined in this study ranged from 2 to 11 months, with

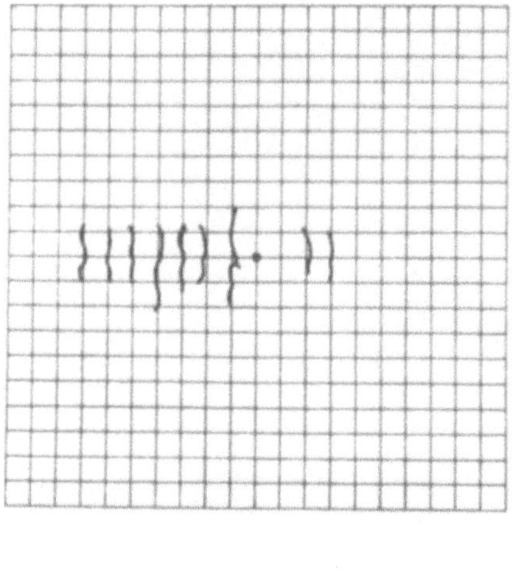

Fig. 2. Disturbances adjacent to fixation recorded on Amsler chart by case DS 6 months after the onset of symptoms.

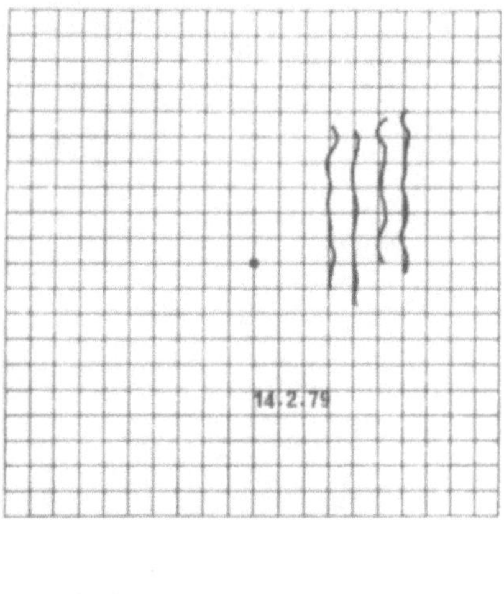

Fig. 3. Changes plotted on Amsler chart by case NE at 7 months from initial visual disturbance.

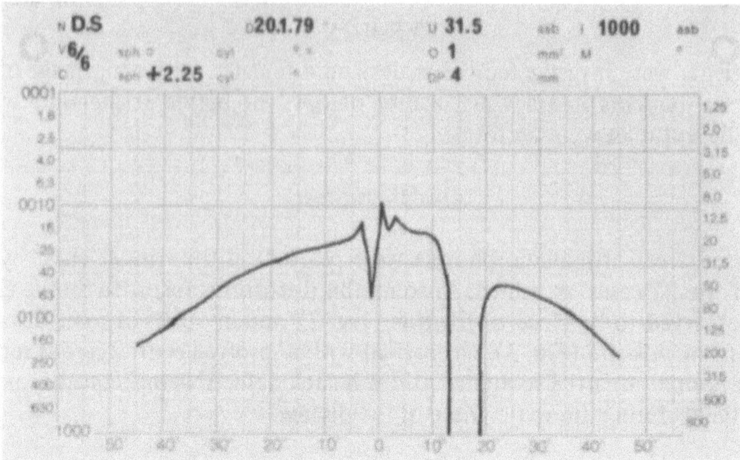

Fig. 4. Residual paracentral scotomata recorded by case DS on the 180°–0° axis 6 months after developing a central serous retinopathy.

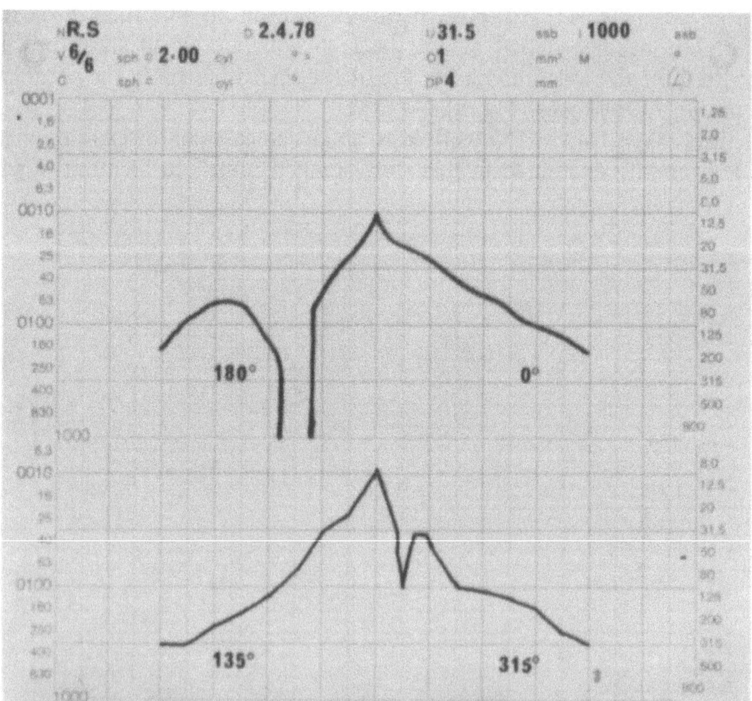

Fig. 5. Static profiles of case RS 18 months after developing macular oedema, showing no abnormality on the 180°–0° axis, but the presence of paracentral scotoma on the 135°–315° axis.

Table 1. Effect on field changes of time taken for fluid to absorb.

Duration of detachment	Number of patients	Defects on Amsler chart	Defects on static perimetry
Less than 4 months	11	6	3
4 months or more	16	16	14

a mean of 4 months. Of the 11 patients in whom detachments were observed to resolve in less than 4 months, 6 drew defects on the Amsler grid and 3 of these were noted to have static perimetric defects. Of the 16 patients whose detachment took 4 months or longer to settle, all continued to observe distortions on the Amsler grid and 14 retained abnormal static perimetric profiles (Table 1). No patients were found to have residual changes on static perimetric examination who did not record defects on Amsler charting.

DISCUSSION

As 81% of patients showed residual defects on the Amsler grid, whereas only 63% retained abnormal static perimetric profiles, it is clear that Amsler testing, which can be carried out quickly without recourse to any special technical expertise, is, in some ways, superior to static perimetry in evaluating the residual field disturbances in patients who have developed a central serous retinopathy. The reason why a high number of patients were noted to record disturbances on the Amsler chart, as opposed to perimetric testing, is probably because it is possible, by this method, to plot changes associated with persistent micropsia and metamorphopsia. It would appear, however, that the two forms of examination do not provide exactly comparable data about retinal function, as static perimetric testing reveals predominantly small paracentral lesions, whereas Amsler charting often indicates more widespread disturbances at the posterior pole.

Although no defect in retinal function was found overlying the site of the breakdown in the choroidoretinal barrier identified in the acute phase, it would appear likely that, in the majority of cases, the fluid separating the neural layers of the retina from the pigment epithelium tracks towards fixation, as perimetric studies performed on the axis joining the site of the initial breakdown of the choroidoretinal barrier to the fovea revealed that retinal function is more severely impaired along this meridian than on any other axis. Kroll and Machemer (5) showed that regeneration of photoreceptor outer segments appeared to occur more slowly in cones than in rods in animals in whom artificially detached retinae were reattached, so it seems that a persistence of cone malfunction in patients with resolved central serous retinopathy might well provide an explanation for the long standing paracentral field changes recorded on static perimetry testing. Support for this concept is provided by the fact that we found paracentral needle shaped scotomata in 27% of patients where the serous fluid cleared in less than 4 months, but when resolution was delayed beyond this time 85% of cases retained these defects. As Chisholm *et al.* (1) noted that recovery of central visual function in patients with successfully treated retinal detachments involving the macula depended on how long the retina had been detached, we suggest that similar, but more subtle, changes probably occur at the macula in patients with central serous retinopathy.

Although the majority of patients who have developed central serous retinopathy complain of little in the way of visual disturbances, it is also clear that those individuals requiring a high level of visual effort to carry out their jobs often continue to be aware that their sight remains defective. Such individuals are usually employed in the professions, or in printing, photographic or microengineering industries and, for these, the residual retinal disturbances may pose greater problems than has been previously thought likely.

ACKNOWLEDGEMENTS

We wish to thank the Department of Medical Illustration, University of Bristol, and Mr. J. Morgan for photographic services, and Mrs. M. Roach for secretarial assistance.

REFERENCES

1. Chisholm, I. A., E. McClure & W. S. Foulds. Functional recovery of the retina after retinal detachment. Trans. Ophthal. Soc. U.K. 95: 167–173 (1975).
2. Hache, J. C., G. Constantinides & P. Turut. Les aspects évolutifs de la choroïdite séreuse centrale. Bull. Soc. Ophthal. France 72(2): 257–260 (1972).
3. Klein, M. L., M. Van Buskirk, E. Friedmann, E. Gragoudas & S. Chandra. Experience with non-treatment of central serous retinopathy. Arch. Ophthal. 91: 247–250 (1974).
4. Kolin, J. & J. A. Oosterhuis. Pigment epithelium dystrophy in central serous detachment of sensory epithelium. Docum. Ophthal. 39: 1–12 (1975).
5. Kroll, A. J. & R. Machemer. Experimental retinal detachment and reattachment in the Rhesus monkey. Electron microscopic comparison of rods and cones. Amer. J. Ophthal. 68: 58–77 (1969).
6. Nørholm, I. Central serous retinitis (a follow-up study) Acta Ophthal. 47: 890–898 (1969).
7. Watzke, R. C., T. C. Burton & P. E. Leaverton. Ruby lazer therapy of central serous retinopathy. Trans. Amer. Acad. Ophthal. Oto. 78: 205–211 (1974).

Authors' addresses:
J. C. Dean Hart
University Department of Ophthalmology
Bristol Eye Hospital
Lower Maudlin Street
Bristol BS1 2LX
Great Britain

V. E. Natsikos
Kyvelis 6
Kifisia, Athens, Greece

VISUAL FIELD DEFECT CHARACTERISTICS IN CASES OF HYPERPROLACTINAEMIA

R. FULMEK & F. FRIEDRICH

(*Wien, Austria*)

ABSTRACT

A kinetic quantitative method of relative light-sense-perimetry was performed by means of Goldmann's perimeter during and after normal pregnancies of 14 women and in 25 amenorrhoic women with hyperprolactinaemia. Simultaneously with each visual field examination a blood sample was drawn and prolactin was estimated by RIA.

Visual field areas of 14 women in late pregnancy were compared with the visual field areas of the same women post partum. When low light intensities were used, 12 out of 14 women had significantly smaller visual fields during pregnancy as compared to the post partum period. No significant differences were found between early and late pregnancy despite significantly different prolactin values. The typical defect of late pregnancy was bitemporal upper quadrant depression.

A comparable visual field defect was found in 19 out of 25 women with the amenorrhea-hyperprolactinaemia syndrome. As 2 women were considered to have suprasellar extension of a prolactinoma in computer tomography the dysopia in the other patients and in late normal pregnancy could be explained by the pressure of the enlarged pituitary and its stalk on the optic chiasm from below and median. Visual field defects of minor degree in patients with amenorrhea-hyperprolactinaemia syndrome comparable to late pregnancy dysopia is found to improve after bromocriptin therapy and is not regarded as indication for neurosurgery.

INTRODUCTION

Since visual field defect in the amenorrhea-hyperprolactinaemia syndrome is an important factor, which may indicate neurosurgery, we compared visual fields of women with physiological hyperprolactinaemia as found in pregnancy with the visual fields of women with pathological hyperprolactinaemia.

METHOD

A kinetic-quantitative method of relative light-sense-perimetry by means of Goldmann's perimeter was used (1). 14 women with normal pregnancies had their visual fields examined by this method 2 to 3 times during pregnancy and in the post partum period. Visual field changes were quantitated by means of planimetry using Ott's planimeter. 25 women with amenorrhea-hyperprolatinaemia syndrome had their visual fields repeatedly examined,

Doc. Ophthal. Proc. Series, Vol. 26, ed. by E. L. Greve & G. Verriest

7 of them before and during bromocriptin therapy. Simultaneously with each visual field examination a blood sample was drawn and prolactin was estimated by RIA.

RESULTS

Visual field areas of 14 women in late pregnancy having serum prolactin levels of 206.5 ± 100.6 ng/ml were compared with the visual field areas of the same

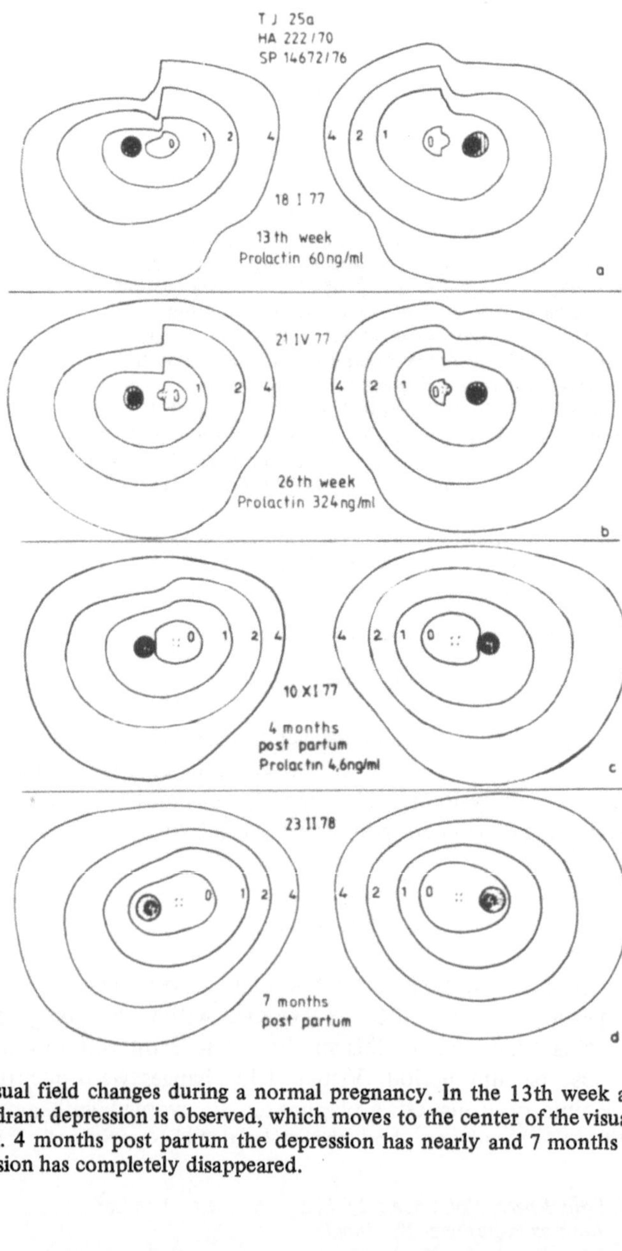

Fig. 1. Visual field changes during a normal pregnancy. In the 13th week a bitemporal upper quadrant depression is observed, which moves to the center of the visual field in the 26th week. 4 months post partum the depression has nearly and 7 months post partum the depression has completely disappeared.

women 3 months post partum with prolactin levels of 9.5 ± 6.5 ng/ml. Only in 3 of the 14 women a completely normal visual field was found in early pregnancy. Visual fields as measured utilizing high light intensities (periphery 4, midzone 2) were not significantly different during and after pregnancy. When low light intensities (central field 1, peak field 0) were used, 12 out of 14 women had significantly smaller visual fields during pregnancy as compared to the post partum period. No significant differences were found between early and late pregenancy despite of significantly different prolactin

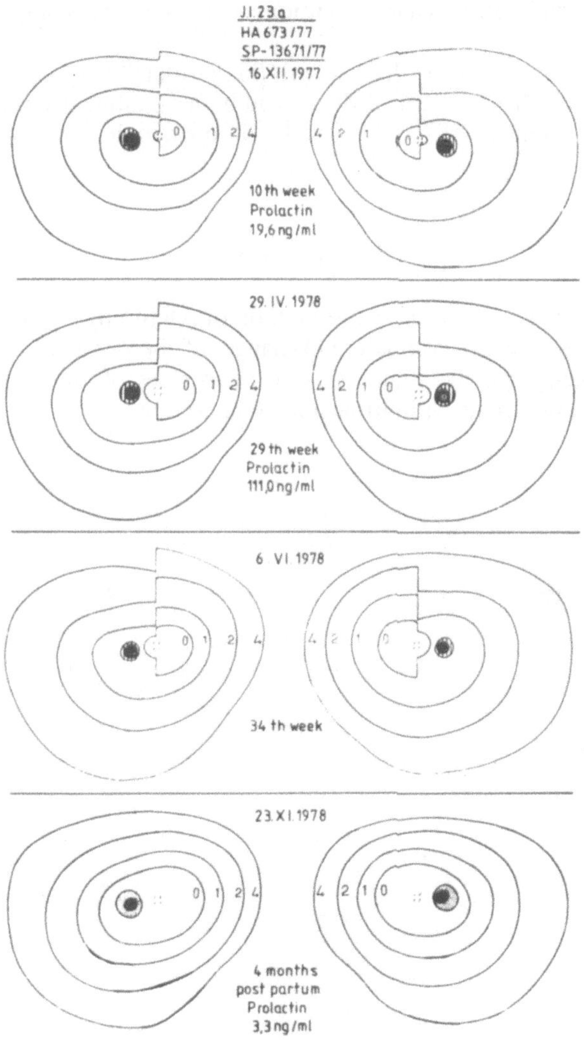

Fig. 2. Visual field changes during a normal pregnancy. Symmetric relative bitemporal upper quadrant depression. Complete bitemporal hemianopsia in the peakfield 0 with sparing of the macula. 4 months post partum a normal visual field is found.

values (early pregnancy 54.3 ± 60.7 ng/ml, late pregnancy 206.5 ± 100.0 ng/ml).

Two typical examples of the bitemporal upper quadrant depression (dysopia) found during normal pregnancy and restoration of the visual field in the post partum period are shown by Figs. 1 and 2.

Twenty-five women with amenorrhea-hyperprolactinaemia syndrome (prolactin 127.8 ± 81.4 ng/ml serum) had their visual fields examined. Only 3 had completely normal visual fields, while 19 women showed a typical bitemporal upper quadrant depression similar to the characteristic defect found during normal pregnancy. Only 2 of these women were considered to have a prolactinoma with suprasellar extension, diagnosed by computer tomography.

14 patients were treated with bromocriptin (Parlodel[R]) a prolactininhibitor. In 7 from these patients a control visual field under treatment was performed; 4 showed improvement of the visual field. Two examples are shown by Figs. 3 and 4.

DISCUSSION

By means of our kinetic-quantitative method of relative light-sense-perimetry by means of Goldmann's perimeter (1) changes of the visual field even during normal pregnancy can be found as well as in cases of amenorrhea-hyperprolactinaemia syndrome without demonstrable tumors.

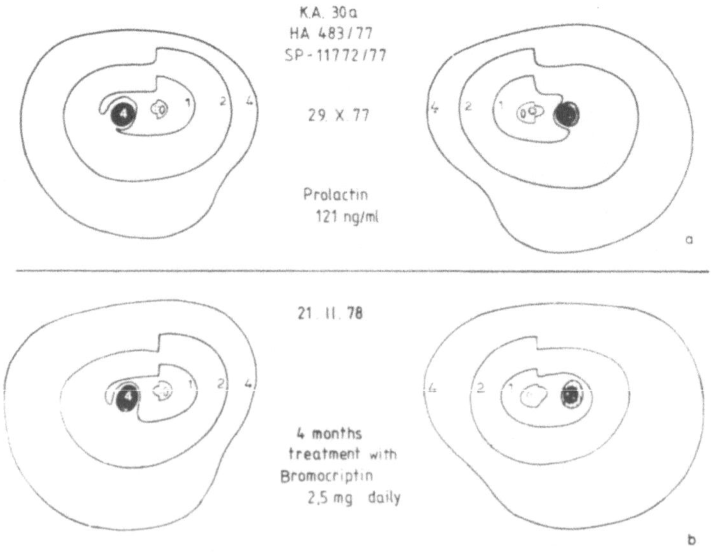

Fig. 3. This patient had no evidence of an intra- or suprasellar tumor. Prior to bromocriptin therapy a nearly symmetric and relative bitemporal upper quadrant depression is found. In the right peak field 0 a nasally expanding central relative scotoma is demonstrable; it disappeared during bromocriptin therapy.

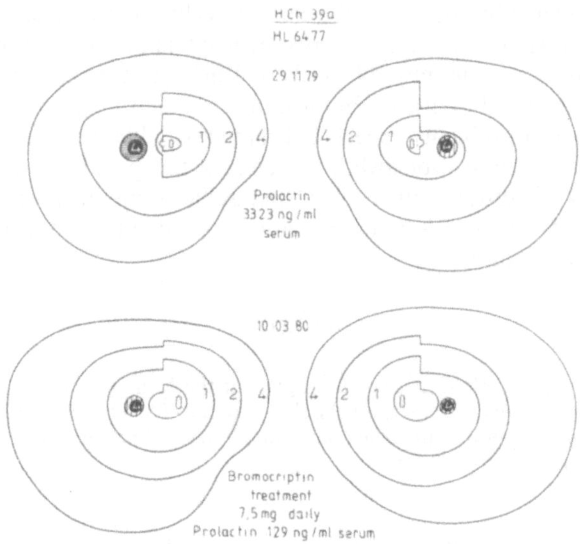

Fig. 4. This patient had evidence of a 3 cm suprasellar expanding prolactinoma in computer tomography. The visual field prior to the bromocriptin therapy shows the classical chiasmal lesion, with greater defects at the left side, caused by pressure on the anterior angle of the chiasm from below and median. The patient refused neurosurgery. A very impressive improvement of visual field for all light intensities occurred under bromocriptin treatment (7.5 mg/daily). At this time computer tomography showed shrinkage of the suprasellar tumor of about one third.

The improvement of the visual field post partum and during bromocriptin treatment in hyperprolactinaemic patients may suggest that in these cases the defects can be caused by pressure of the enlarged pituitary and its stalk on the optic chiasm from below and median.

REFERENCE

1. Fulmek, R. Vorschläge zur Vereinfachung und Standardisierung der quantitativ-kinetischen Lichtsinnperimetrie. Klin. Mbl. Augenheilk. 166: 326 (1975).

Authors' address:
Dr. R. Fulmek
I. Univ.-Augenklinik
Spitalgasse 2
A-1097 Wien
Austria

COMMENT BY F. DANNHEIM

(*Univ.-Augenklinik, Hamburg, F.R.G.*)

The search for minimal chiasmal lesions is one of perimetry's most exciting tasks. The results of manual perimetry, however, will never be free of an examiner's interpretation and bias. The high frequency of alterations in pregnancy termed "dysopsia" by the authors calls for a comparison with a group of normal subjects. An irregularity of isopters at the vertical meridian may be present even under physiological conditions, as for example described by Ehlers or Damgaard–Jensen. The planimetric quantification of field plots creates a number of problems, especially if based on a kinetic technique.

It nevertheless seems worthwhile to discuss the possibility of chiasmal involvement in conditions other than suprasellar tumours giving rise to a direct compressive type of lesion. The study presented here may be regarded as a first step in this direction.

References

1. Damgaard–Jensen, L. Vertical steps in isopters at the hemiopic border – in normal and glaucomatous eyes. Acta Ophthalmologica (Kbh.) 55: 111–122 (1977).
2. Ehlers, N. Demonstration of the hemiopic border in normal persons. Acta Ophthalmologica (Kbh.) 54: 198–202 (1976).

COMMENTS BY JOHN L. KELTNER AND CHRIS A. JOHNSON

(*Sacramento, Calif., U.S.A.*)

Drs. Fulmek and Friedrich have reported some rather surprising visual field findings in two groups of women. The first group of 14 women in late pregnancy exhibited bitemporal superior quadrant visual field depression. In the examples shown (Figures 1 and 2), the visual field loss appears to be rather extensive. No information is provided about post-partum neuro-radiologic studies to exclude pituitary tumors that may have been exacerbated during pregnancy. The second group consisted of 25 women with amenorrhea-hyperprolactinaemia syndrome, 19 of whom had bitemporal superior quadrant visual field depression. Two of the 19 women with bitemporal visual field loss were considered to have suprasellar extension of a prolactinoma, which accounts for their visual field defect. No information is provided about the neuro-radiologic studies for the remaining 17 patients with visual field loss. Thus, we are lacking essential neuro-radiologic information for both groups of women. Other aspects of the afferent visual pathway evaluation of these patients (e.g., visual acuity, color discrimination, color desaturation) are not presented. This makes if difficult to assess the significance of the visual field characteristics reported in this paper.

The authors indicate that the visual field defects in both groups of women were revealed by low light intensity visual field testing, but were not elicited by high light intensity visual field testing. Since the background luminance, target luminance, stimulus size and other test parameters are not specified, it is difficult to know what perimetric test procedures were employed in this study.

In summary, important psychophysical and neuro-radiological information is not reported for the two groups of patients tested in this study. Without this information it is hard to interpret these rather unexpected results. Further investigations incorporating more extensive correlations between visual field findings and neuro-radiologic testing, the use of control groups of women with normal visual fields and a "double-blind" experimental design, and replication studies by independent perimetric laboratories would be a useful adjunct to the present study of Drs. Fulmek and Friedrich.

CORRELATION BETWEEN THE STEREOGRAPHIC SHAPE OF THE DISC EXCAVATION AND THE VISUAL FIELD OF GLAUCOMATOUS EYES

HAJIME NAKATANI & NORIHITO SUZUKI

(*Osaka, Japan*)

ABSTRACT

By means of analysing the grating images on the ocular fundus, it became possible to draw the stereographic appearance of the ocular fundus. In glaucomatous eyes with visual field changes, the excavation started in the retinal area and the corresponding rim was destroyed. We suppose that the glaucomatous visual field changes are due to retinal ganglion cell and/or nerve fiber degeneration and that the papillary changes are the results of nerve degeneration in the retina.

INTRODUCTION

We have intended to develop a clinical method for measurement of the papillary excavation. Two years ago, at the International Symposium on Glaucoma in Japan, we reported that we were able to obtain a sectional plane of the ocular fundus by analysing the grating images on the ocular fundus. Using this method, it became clear that the diameter and the depth of glaucomatous papillary excavation became larger and its shape was transformed from triangle to trapezoid. Many profiles on ocular fundus were obtained by analysing grating images on the ocular fundus. Reconstructing these profiles, the stereographic appearance of the ocular fundus could be obtained. In this investigation, we studied the correlation between the stereographic shape of the excavation and the glaucomatous visual field.

METHOD

Vertical parallel, equidistant grating lines were projected onto the ocular fundus from either the nasal or the temporal side and the fundus was photographed in a routine manner (Fig. 1). The angle between these two directions was 0.1 radian. When the surface of the ocular fundus is in one level, the grating images on it should be straight (Fig. 2). On the other hand, when the surface of the ocular fundus is not in one level, the grating images on it should be distorted. That is, a phase shift of grating images should take place. By means of analysing the phase shift of all grating images on the ocular fundus,

Doc. Opthal. Proc. Series, Vol. 26, ed. by E. L. Greve & G. Verriest

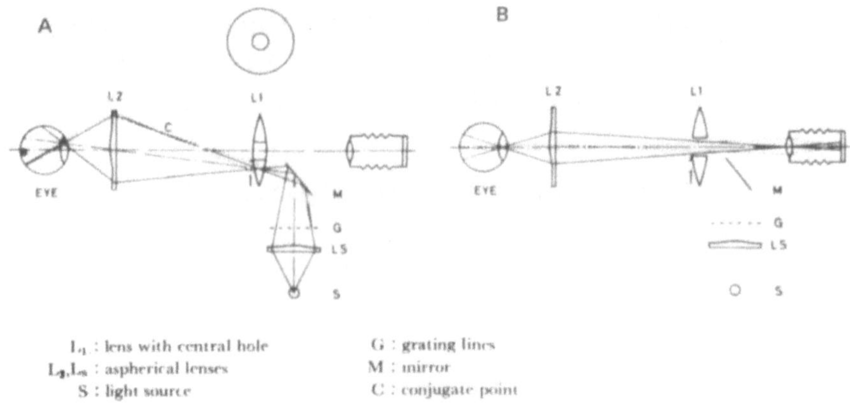

Fig. 1. (Fig. 1-a, 1-b) Principle of the optical system of the apparatus. Broken lines show the system of the grating image formation. Straight lines show the optical system of the light source.

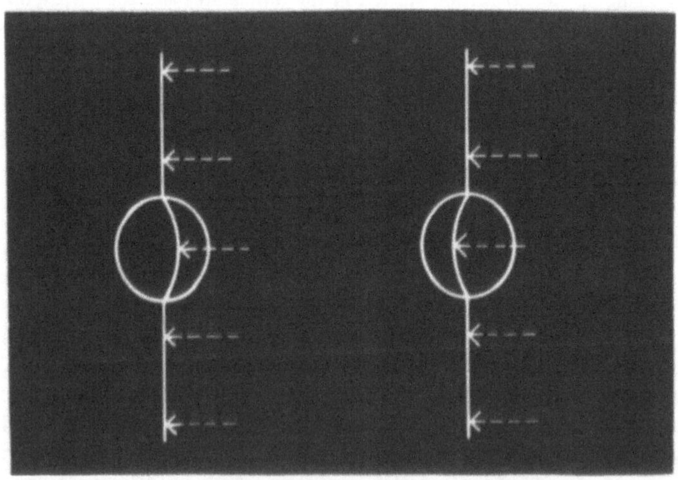

Fig. 2. The direction of the grating image on the surface of plane. Arrows show the light direction. Left is the grating image on a convex sphere. Right is the grating image on a concave sphere.

we are able to obtain profiles of the ocular fundus. Thus, we are able to obtain the stereographic shape of the ocular fundus by reconstructing these profiles.

RESULTS OF CLINICAL USE

Case 1. 30 years old, male, normal right eye

The ocular fundus of this case showed no abnormalities ophthalmoscopically and Fig. 3 demonstrates the ocular fundus with the grating images. Analysing

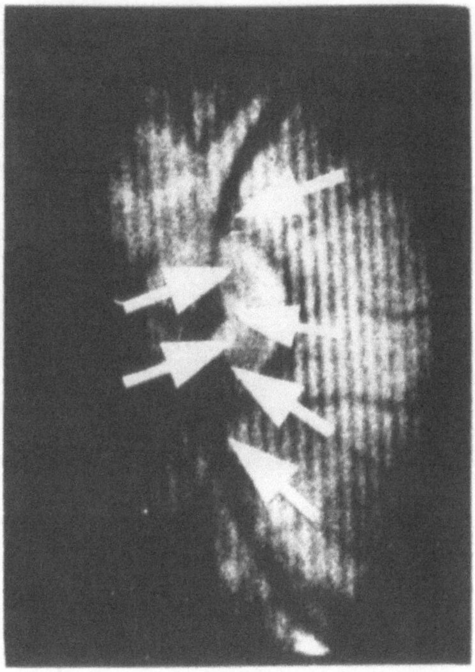

Fig. 3. The grating images on the retinal and papillary surface of case 1 (normal eye). Arrows show the grating image analysed.

the grating image shown with arrows (Fig. 3), we could obtain the vertical profile of the retinal and the papillary surface (Fig. 4). The center of the papilla was taken as zero and the papilla-retina borders are shown by arrows. Analysing all these grating images on the ocular fundus and reconstructing these profiles, we could obtain a stereographic drawing of the retinal and papillary surface as in Fig. 5. The physiologic excavation was located in the central area of the papilla and was cone shaped. The rim of the papilla and the retina were at the same level.

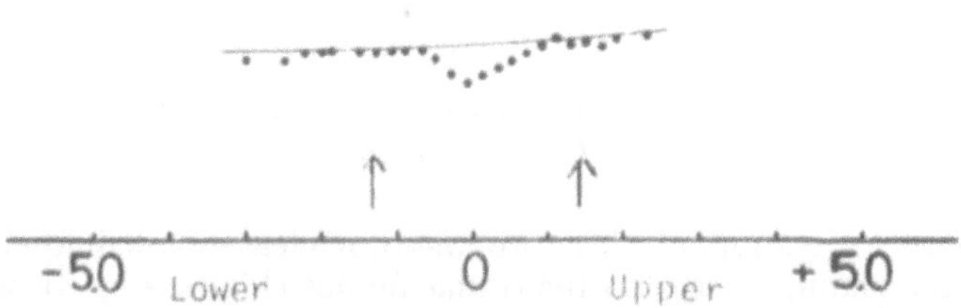

Fig. 4. The vertical sectional plane (profile) of retinal and papillary surface of case 1. Papillary center is 0. Arrows show papilla-retina border.

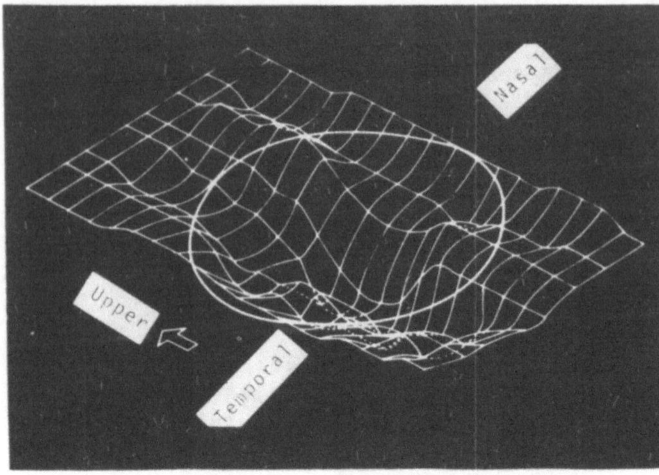

Fig. 5. Stereographic drawing of retinal and papillary surface of case 1 (normal eye). Circle shows papilla-retina border.

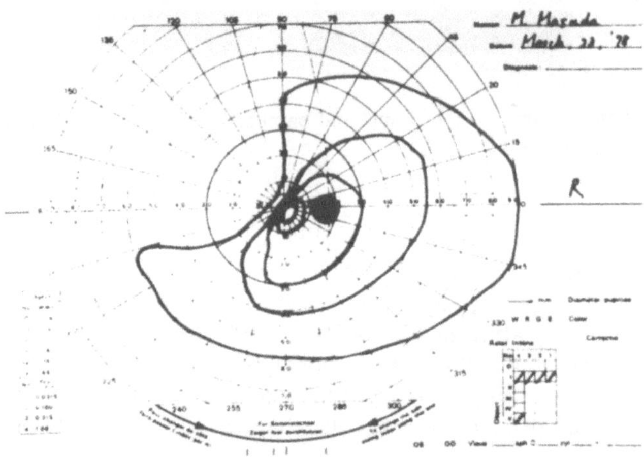

Fig. 6. The visual field of case 2.

Case 2. 57 years old, male, glaucomatous right eye with the visual field as shown in Fig. 6

The papillary excavation of this case was not clear ophthalmoscopically. Analysing the grating images on the ocular fundus (Fig. 7, Fig. 8), we could obtain a stereographic drawing of the retinal and papillary surface. The retinal surface was not smooth but wrinkled. The excavation started in the retinal area and the corresponding rim was slightly destroyed (Fig. 9).

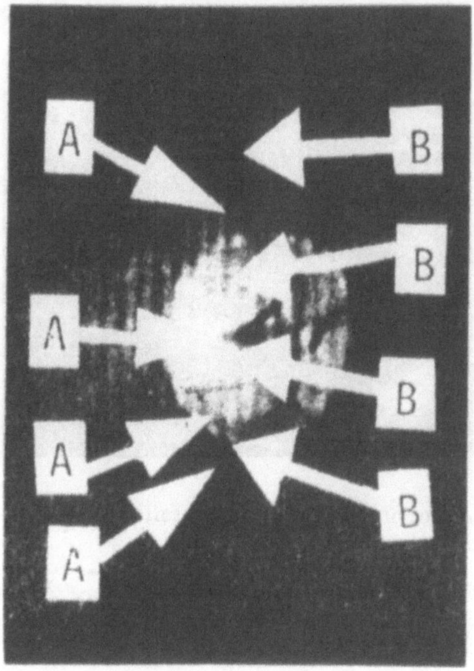

Fig. 7. The grating images on the retinal and papillary surface of case 2 (glaucomatous eye). Arrows show the grating image analysed.

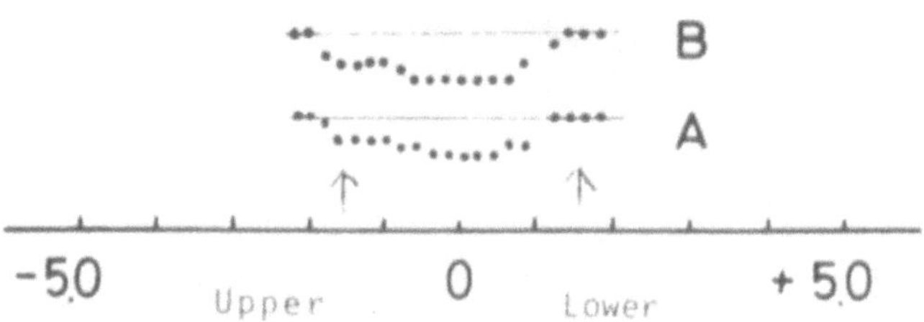

Fig. 8. The vertical profiles of retinal and papillary surface of case 2 (glaucomatous eye). Arrows show papilla-retina border.

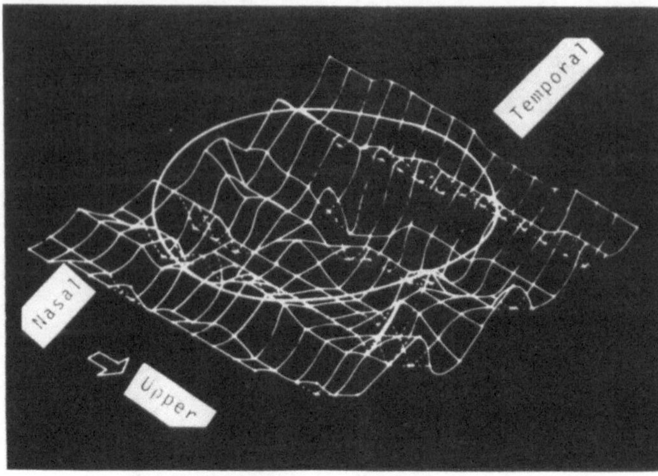

Fig. 9. Stereographic drawing of retinal and papillary surface of case 2.

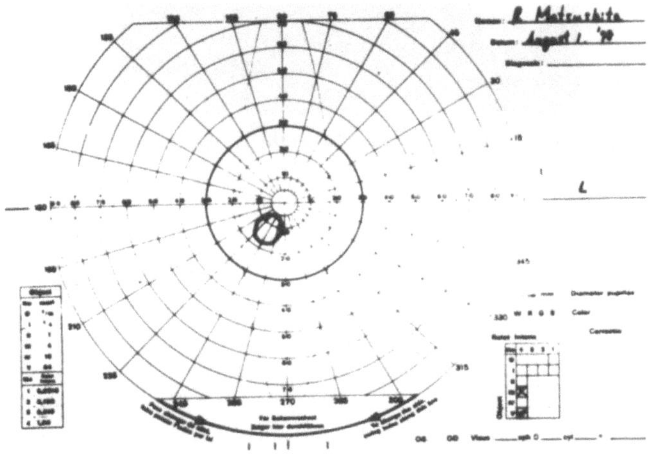

Fig. 10. The visual field of case 3.

Case 3. 45 years old, female, glaucomatous left eye with visual field as Fig. 10

Analysing the grating images on the ocular fundus (Fig. 11, Fig. 12), we could obtain a stereographic drawing of the retinal and papillary surface (Fig. 13). In this case, distinct retinal excavation was observed with the rim of the papilla extensively destroyed. However, the upper nasal rim and the corresponding visual field remained intact.

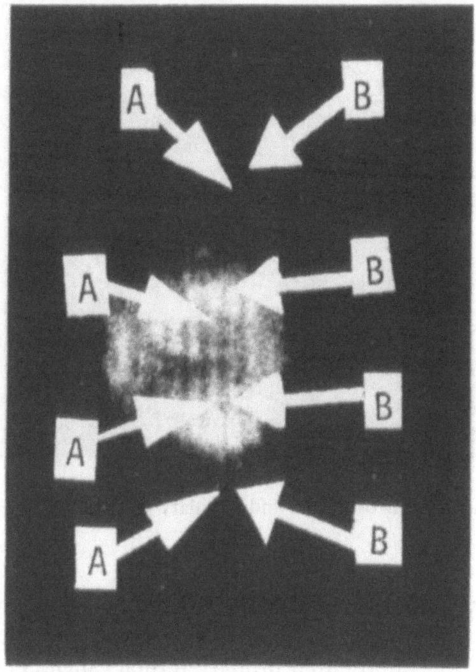

Fig. 11. The grating images on the retinal and papillary surface of case 3 (glaucomatous eye). Arrows show the grating images analysed.

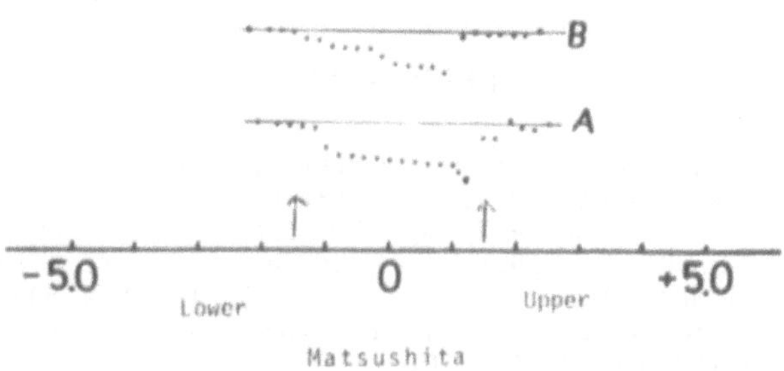

Fig. 12. Vertical profiles of retinal and papillary surface. Arrows show papilla-retina border.

COMMENTS

The apparatus

In this study, the grating images on the papilla became clearer than in our previous method. Analysing all grating images on the ocular fundus was very time-consuming in our previous method (about two hours). With the present method we could perform a rapid analysis by using a computer analyser (about fifteen minutes).

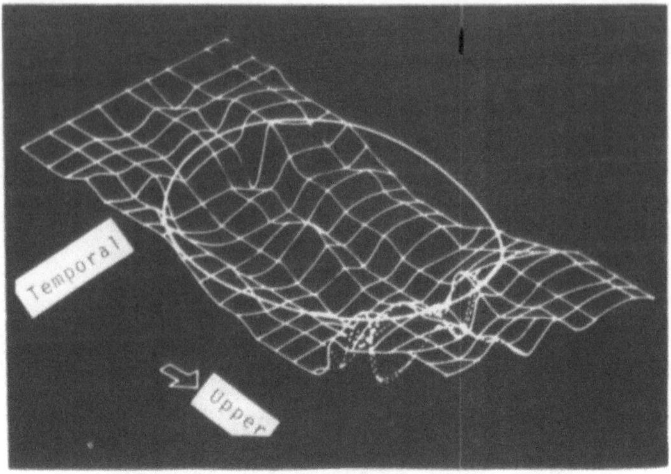

Fig. 13. Stereographic drawing of retinal and papillary surface of case 3.

In glaucomatous eyes with visual field damage, there were many wrinkles on the retina, the excavation started in the retinal area and the corresponding rim was destroyed. We suppose that primary retinal ganglion cell and/or nerve fiber degeneration due to increased intraocular pressure and secondary papillary changes occurs based on the results of this work and other works (1, 2, 3). In our opinion, glaucomatous visual field defects are caused by the nerve degeneration in the retina.

REFERENCES

1. Hoyt, W. F., L. Frisén, & N. M. Newman. Fundoscopy of nerve fiber layer defects in glaucoma. Invest. Ophthalm. 12: 814–829 (1973).
2. Nakatani, H., K. Maeda, K. Sumie, N. Suzuki, H. Satoh & S. Yokozeki. A profile on the surface of papillary excavation. Folia Ophthalm. Jap. 30: 412–418 (1979).
3. Nakatani, H., K. Maeda, K. Sumie, N. Suzuki, H. Satoh & S. Yokozeki. Correlation between the stereographic shape of the disc excavation and the visual field. Jap. Journ. of Clin. Ophthalm. 33: 197–201 (1979).

Authors' addresses:

Hajime Nakatani
Department of Ophthalmology
Osaka University Medical School
Fukushimaku
Osaka 553
Japan

Norihito Suzuki
Department of Applied Physics
Osaka University
Faculty of Engineering
Yamadakami, Suitashi
Osaka 565
Japan

THE FREQUENCY DISTRIBUTION OF EARLY VISUAL FIELD DEFECTS IN GLAUCOMA

M. COUGHLAN & A. I. FRIEDMANN

(London, Great Britain)

INTRODUCTION

A number of studies on the frequency distribution of early visual field defects in glaucoma have been carried out using different methods of perimetry. All workers agree that the earliest defects occur within the Bjerrum area, 5°–15° eccentricity (1–5). Controversy lies as to whether early temporal paracentral scotomas connected to the blind spot can occur as an early field defect in glaucoma.

In this paper we aim to investigate the frequency distribution of early visual field defects in glaucoma, using the Friedmann Visual Field Analyser Mark II, using white light. Likewise this study will enable us to determine which stimuli to use for further examination, like eccentric fixation.

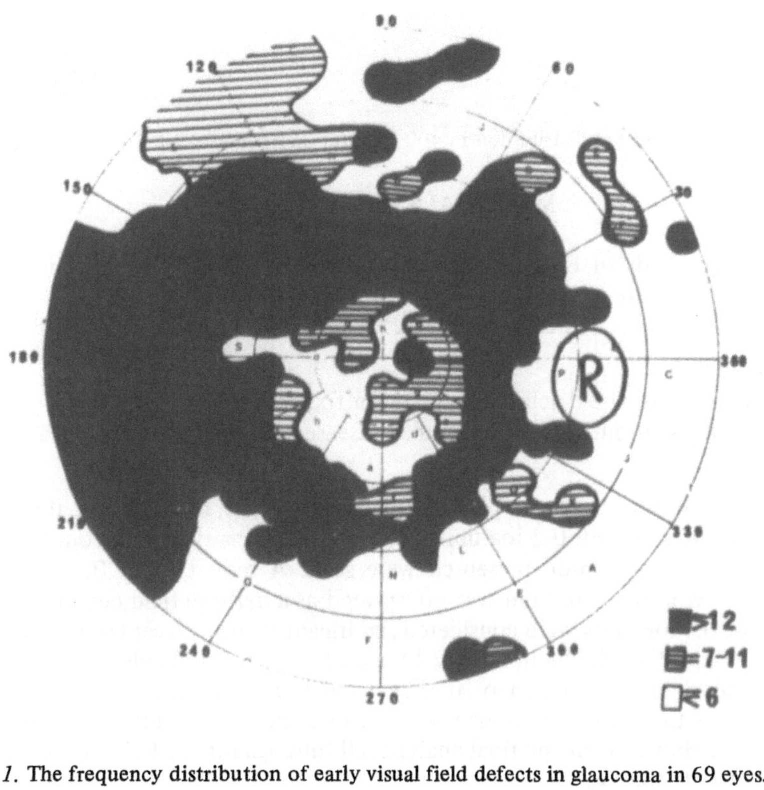

Fig. 1. The frequency distribution of early visual field defects in glaucoma in 69 eyes.

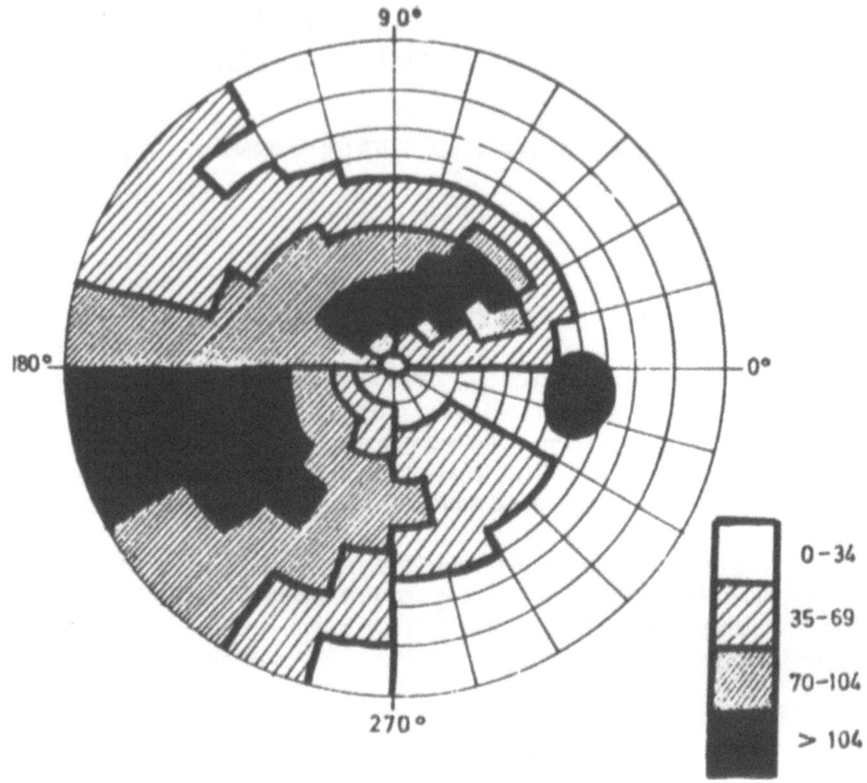

Fig. 2. The frequency distribution in 400 eyes (of 361 patients, 1953–1976) (Aulhorn, 1976).

MATERIALS AND METHODS

The visual fields of 69 eyes of 60 patients with open angle glaucoma, with early, but definite, visual field defects, were reviewed.

Patients included in this study were:

1. Good witnesses.
2. Patients with visual acuity adequate for fixation.
3. Patients without any other ocular disease that might obscure glaucoma field defects.

The working threshold was obtained for each patient, i.e. changing, if necessary, the threshold by 0.2 log units from the age density, until about half the total number of stimuli presented were seen. A reduction of 0.6 log units from the working threshold was interpreted as a definite field defect. Reductions of 0.4 log units were considered significant if they presented in a typical glaucoma pattern. Reductions of 0.2 log units were ignored unless they formed a typical glaucoma pattern or if they were found on repeated testing. The number of times each stimulus was missed was noted separately for right and left eyes. However, in the final analysis, all findings for the left eye were converted to the right eye.

OBSERVATIONS

In this study our observations are shown in Fig. 1.

1. High frequency distribution within the Bjerrum area, 5°–15° from fixation, superiorly and inferiorly, including 5°–10° between fixation and the blind spot. Nasally, it extends to 25° both in the upper and lower field.
2. Defects occurring temporally, close to the blind spot, both in the upper and lower field.
3. We also found defects occurring within 5° from fixation.

It is interesting to compare our findings with similar studies done in the past.

If we look at Aulhorn's results (Fig. 2) and take the two most frequently missed areas together, our findings correspond closely. We both agree that defects occur frequently 5°–15° from fixation and nasally extending to 25° both in the upper and lower field. However, our results differ in that, unlike Aulhorn, we find defects occurring close to the blind spot in the upper and lower field, and defects occurring close to fixation, but extending to the blind spot along the horizontal meridian.

A similar study was done by Furuno *et al.*, using the Friedmann Visual Field Analyser Mark I (Fig. 3). They noticed few independently occurring

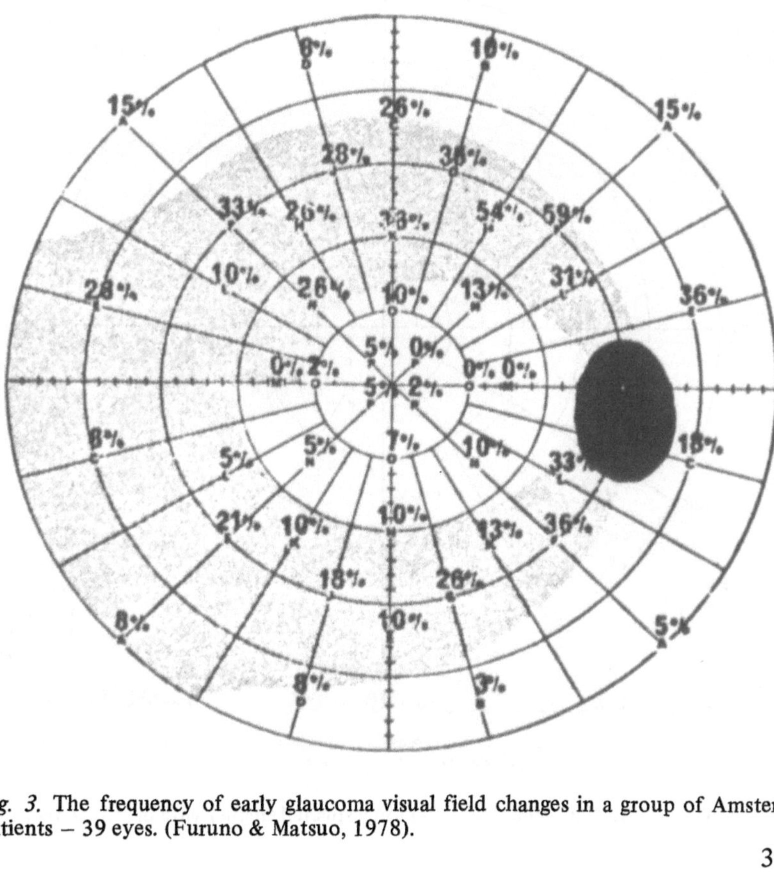

Fig. 3. The frequency of early glaucoma visual field changes in a group of Amsterdam patients – 39 eyes. (Furuno & Matsuo, 1978).

defects within 10° eccentricity. Their results are different from Professor Aulhorn's who, like us, found a high frequency within 10° eccentricity in the superior half of the visual field.

Similarly, we correspond fairly well with a study done in Amsterdam, except, one of their less frequently involved areas includes the lower nasal field, and some of their least frequently involved areas occur near the fixation. They also found no defects occurring between fixation and the blind spot.

Some of the differences in these results could be attributed to the different method of examinations employed. In the study done in Amsterdam and Shinzato's, the standard 46 hole front plate was used on the Friedmann Visual Field Analyser Mark I. Whereas, in our Mark II plate there are considerably more positions, especially near fixation and around the blind spot. However, it is interesting to note that, with Aulhorn's single stimulus and the Mark II plate, a very good correspondence is shown.

Finally, Fig. 4 is an illustration of an early glaucoma field defect occurring close to the blind spot superiorly and inferiorly, and on further investigation with eccentric fixation, demonstrate the extent of the defect. You will note

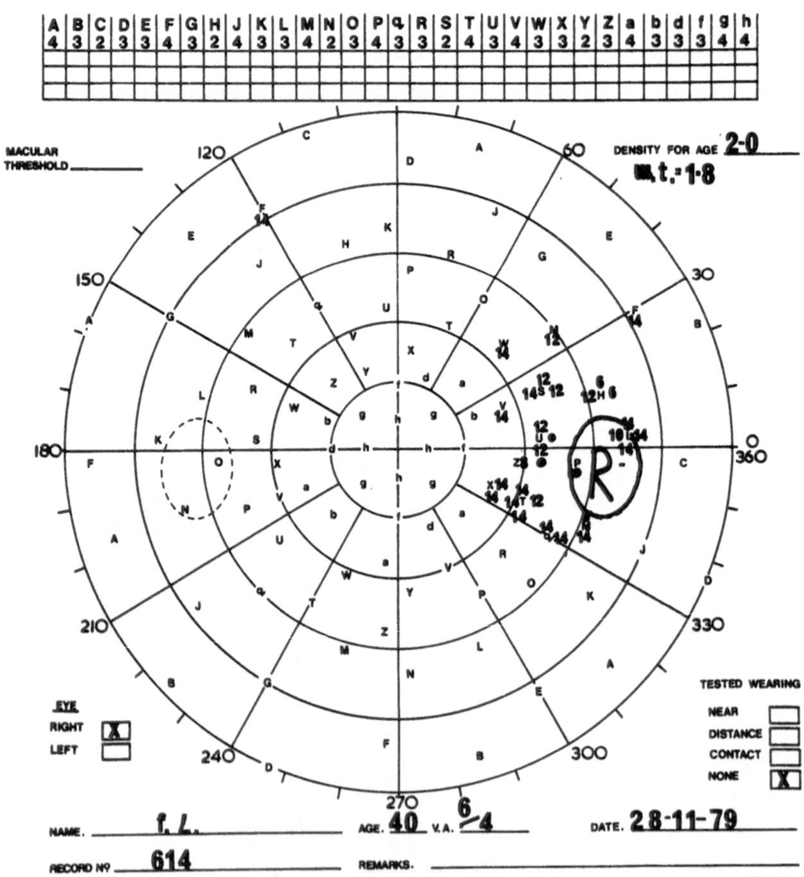

Fig. 4. Shows an early glaucoma field defect investigated further with eccentric fixation.

the working threshold is 1.8 log units and we can see reductions of 0.4 log units to 2.0 log units occurring in this area, close to the blind spot both in the upper and lower field. If we note that particular stimulus 'V', there are three other stimuli, all of which were seen at the working threshold. This also applies to the other stimuli in the defect.

It is hoped that studies like this will allow the clinician to decide which stimuli should be used for further investigation, like eccentric fixation, to detect the presence of early glaucoma field defects.

ACKNOWLEDGEMENT

We wish to thank Miss L. Howard and Mrs. P. Wright of the Courage Laboratory, Royal Eye Hospital for technical and secretarial services.

REFERENCES

1. Aulhorn, E. & H. Harms. Early visual field defects in glaucoma. Glaucoma Tutzing Symposium, ed. W. Leydhecker. Karger Basel, 151–186 (1967).
2. Drance, S. M.. Early visual field defects in glaucoma. Brit. J. Ophthal. 56: 106 (1972).
3. Furuno, F. & H. Matsuo. Early stage progression in glaucomatous visual field changes. Third International Visual Field Symposium, Tokyo. Doc. Ophthal. Proc. Series, Vol. 19: 247–253 (1978).
4. Kitazawa, Y., & O. Takahashi & Ohiwa. The mode of development and progression of visual field defects in glaucoma. A follow-up study. Third International Visual Field Symposium, Tokyo. Doc. Ophthal. Proc. Series, Vol. 19: 211–223 (1978).
5. Lichter & C. Standardi. Early glaucomatous visual field defects and their significance to clinical ophthalmology. Third International Visual Field Symposium, Tokyo. Doc. Ophthal. Proc. Series, Vol. 19: 111–118 (1978).

Authors' address:
Courage Laboratory of Ophthalmology
Royal Eye, St. Thomas' Hospital
London S.E.1
Great Britain

the working threshold ... 7.8 ... units and ... reductions of 0.4 ... [illegible]

[illegible]

ACKNOWLEDGEMENT

[illegible]

[illegible]

VISUAL FIELD INVESTIGATION IN CEREBROVASCULAR ACCIDENT

SYUJI MAEDA, SUMIO USUBA, KEN NAGATA & SHUICHI MATSUYAMA

(Hirosaki & Isezaki, Japan)

ABSTRACT

One hundred and thirty patients of cerebrovascular accidents were subjected to a visual field examination using a Static Campimeter and a Goldmann perimeter. Thirty seven cases of homonymous field defects were detected; right homonymous field defect in 12 and left one in 25 subjects. The clinical diagnosis in this series was as follows; 11 putaminal hemorrhage, 6 thalamic hemorrhage, 4 internal carotid artery occlusion, 7 middle cerebral artery occlusion, 5 posterior cerebral artery occlusion, 2 subcortical hemorrhage and 2 cerebral infarction of uncertain location.

In general, the main arterial branch occlusion revealed congruous visual field defects with steep margins, whereas cerebral bleeding showed various types of field defects.

Middle cerebral artery occlusion showed quadrantanopia of various degrees and thalamic hemorrhage showed small homonymous field defects within one quadrant.

Macular sparing is of little value in topical diagnosis in this series.

INTRODUCTION

Of the cerebrovascular accident (CVA) patients, 17–22% show homonymous hemianopia (2, 4). Visual field examinations in CVA patients are valuable not only in topical diagnosis of the lesions but also in estimation of their prognosis (2). Moreover, the field defects are not always noticed by patients themselves, and not knowing of them they may have some trouble in their life, for example, driving a car is much more dangerous. From these viewpoints, it seems evident that visual field examination is indispensable in CVA patients.

CVA can be classified as follows; infarction (carotid artery and vertebrobasilar artery), hemorrhage (putaminal, thalamic, subarachnoid, cerebellar and pontine). Of these lesions, internal carotid artery (ICA) occlusion, middle cerebral artery (MCA) occlusion, posterior cerebral artery (PCA) occlusion, putaminal hemorrhage (Put. H.) and thalamic hemorrhage (Th. H.) have a possibility to cause homonymous field defects.

In general, PCA occlusion produces an exact congruous homonymous field defect with more or less macular sparing (3, 5, 9). However, there are some controversies as to macular sparing and congruity. Smith (8) stated that PCA occlusion usually splits fixation rather than sparing it. Koerner (6), who precisely examined the patients of homonymous hemianopia with the Tübingen perimeter, concluded that sparing of foveal vision (averaged 1.5°) and incon-

Doc. Ophthal. Proc. Series, Vol. 26, ed. by E. L. Greve & G. Verriest

gruity were the rule in homonymous field defects. He also speculated that much of the congruence in earlier visual field studies were attributable to too much expectation by the examiner.

As to the cerebral hemorrhage, there have been only a few reports about its field defects. Fisher (1) stated that in putaminal hemorrhage (Put. H.) homonymous field defects were common, on the other hand, in thalamic hemorrhage (Th. H.) the homonymous field defects were shown at the time of the onset but cleared up early.

Although several authors have studied the visual field defects of CVA patients they have often adopted the confrontation method, where thorough visual field testings, as quantitative perimetry, are required.

MATERIAL AND METHOD

One hundred and ninety six patients who were admitted to the Mihara Memorial Hospital with a diagnosis of CVA were studied, in August 1979. Tumors or head injuries were eliminated from this study.

Each subject had undergone a series of neurological examinations including CT scanning. Prior to the visual field testing, examination of the anterior segment of the eyes and ocular fundus was performed in all subjects. Then, the visual field was examined with the use of a Static Campimeter (Takada Co. Japan) for screening. Those who had been selected by the screening or had been detected for some ocular abnormalities were subjected to quantitative perimetry with the Goldmann perimeter.

The correlation between the site and type of the lesion and the type and extent of the visual field defects was investigated.

RESULTS

Sixty one cases of ocular disease, such as cataract, retinal bleeding and papilledema etc., were detected before the screening of the visual field defect was made. We were not able to complete the field examination in 66 patients of the 196 subjects, because of their poor comprehension or conscious disturbance. We could investigate the visual field in the remaining 130 subjects.

Of 130 subjects, 56 cases were detected to have a visual field defect; 37 cases revealed homonymous defects (Table 1) and 19 other types of defects (6 retinal bleeding, 3 glaucoma, 5 opaque media and 5 miscellaneous). The relation between the intracranial lesion and the homonymous field defects is shown in Table 2. Left homonymous defects were twice as many as right homonymous defects. There was no case of bilateral homonymous hemianopia.

In 16 cases a homonymous hemianopia had been found with the confrontation test at the time of CVA onset. In the present study, however, only 9 cases of them revealed homonymous field defects and the remaining 7 cases (3 Put. H., 2 ICA occlusion, 1 Th. H. and 1 postoperative aneurysm) were regarded as normal.

The correlations between the lesion and the type of homonymous field defect are shown in Table 3.

Table 1. Subjects.

	Numbers	Average age	Homonymous field defects
Male	90	56	31
Female	40	59	6
Total	130	57	37

Table 2. Lesions and homonymous field defects.

Diagnosis	Number	Homonymous defect	(R, L)
Put. H.	24	11	(4,7)
Th. H.	17	6	(2,4)
MCA occlusion	20	7	(1,6)
ICA occlusion	13	4	(1,3)
PCA occlusion	5	5	(2,3)
LSA occlusion	19	1*	(1,0)
cerebral aneurysm	8	2**	(0,2)
subcortical hematoma	6	2	(1,1)
V-B insufficiency	8	0	(0,0)
subdural hematoma	2	0	(0,0)
brain infarction (location unknown)	16	2	(1,1)
ACA occlusion	2	0	(0,0)
Total	140***	37	(12,25)

* Complicated with PCA occlusion.
** Complicated with Th. H. and Put. H. respectively.
*** This number exceeds real number 130; because in some patients the lesions are duplicated.

Table 3. Diagnosis and topography of visual field defects.

	Number	1/2	1/4	Smooth*	Steep*	Congruity		Macula	
						+	—	sparing	splitting
Put. H.	11	4	4	2	6	6	2	1	2
Th. H.	6	0	2	4	2	2	4	0	0
MCA	7	0	7	1	6	6	0	0	0
ICA	4	2	0	2	2	3	0	1	1
PCA	5	4	0	0	5	5	0	1	3
Sub. H.	2	0	2	0	2	2	0	0	0
Infarct.	2	0	0	1	1	0	2	0	0

Sub. H. = subcortical hematoma; Infarct. = brain infarction (location unknown).
* Isopter slop at the margin of the field defects.

1. Complete hemianopia or quadrantanopia. Of 37 cases of homonymous field defects, 10 (27%) showed complete hemianopia. Among them 4 were cases of PCA occlusion (Fig. 1A). Fifteen cases (40%) showed homonymous quadrantanopia. All of the 7 cases of MCA occlusion showed quandrantanopia (Fig. 1B). Two cases of Th. H. showed quadrantanopia. But their field defect may be not so much a quadrantanopia as a sector defect (Fig. 1C).

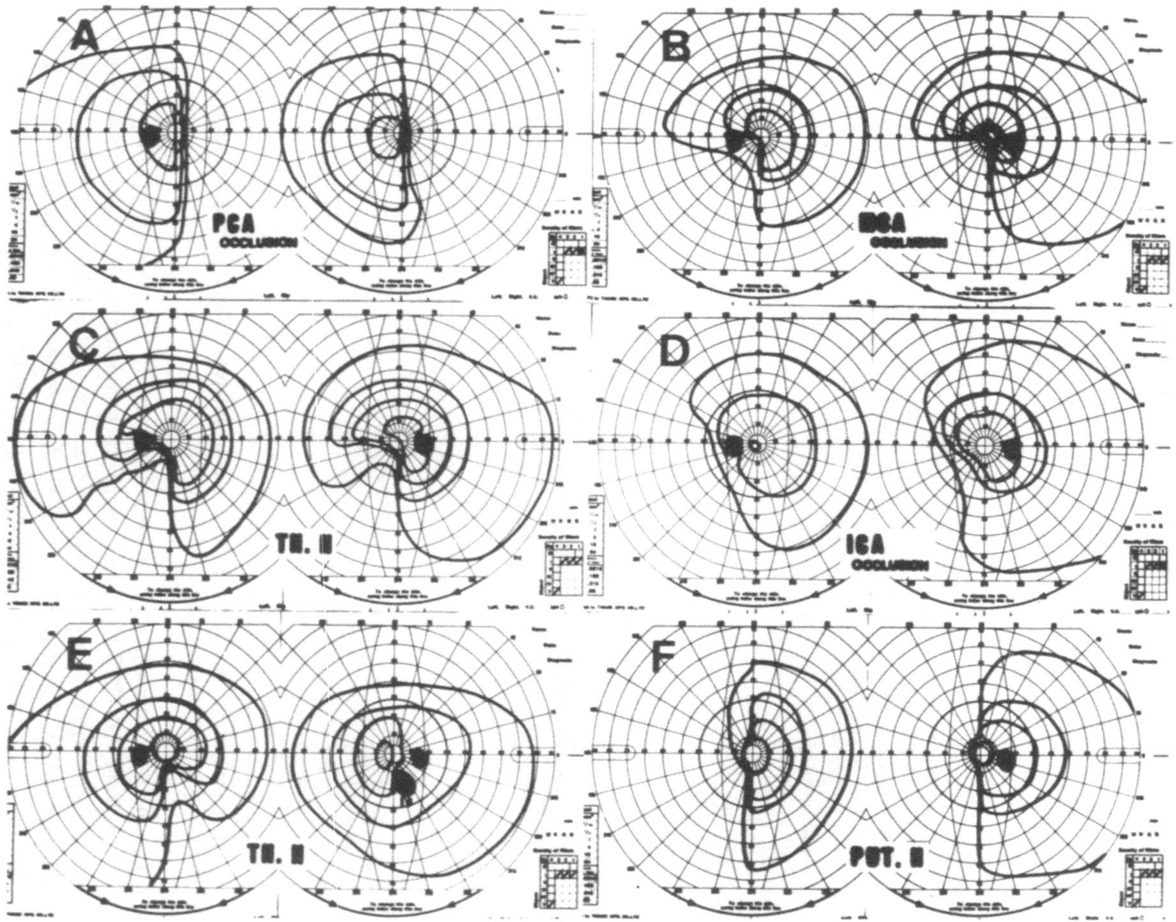

Fig. 1.
A. Visual fields of the case of left PCA occlusion showing right complete homonymous hemianopia with macular splitting.
B. Typical visual fields of the case of right MCA occlusion showing left inferior homonymous quadrantanopia.
C. Visual fields of the case of right thalamic hemorrhage showing left inferior homonymous quadrantanopia or homonymous sector defects.
D. Visual fields of the case of right ICA occlusion showing left homonymous field defects. They are wide defects extending to two quadrants. Note gently sloping margin of the field defects.
E. Visual fields of the case of left thalamic hemorrhage. Note incongruous homonymous field defects. Small defect is the rule in the thalamic hemorrhage.
F. Visual fields of the case of right putaminal hemorrhage showing left complete homonymous hemianopia with macular sparings.

2. Margin of the field defect. It seems that the boundary between invaded field and remaining field is generally steep in PCA and MCA occlusion, in contrast with the fact that it often is gently sloping in ICA occlusion (Fig. 1D) and cerebral bleeding.

3. Congruity. In general, cerebral arterial occlusion tended to show congruous field defects. On the other hand, many cases of cerebral hemorrhage, especially Th. H. (Fig. 1E), showed incongruous field defects.

4. Macular sparing. Ten cases of complete homonymous hemianopias were available for assessment. There was no correlation between macular sparing and the type of the lesion. Fig. 1F is a case of Put. H. showing a macular sparing.

5. Superior dominance or inferior dominance. With reference to the dominance of the field defect; superior or inferior, the former was found in only 2 cases, and the latter was found in 22 cases.

DISCUSSION

One hundred and thirty patients of CVA were investigated for visual field defect using Static Campimeter and Goldmann perimeter.

Among them, 37 cases (28%) were detected to have homonymous field defects. Our detecting rate of 28% differs from Isaeff's data (4). He detected 17% of homonymous field defects out of 322 CVA patients by the confrontation test. The disparity may be attributed to the method of screening.

As we have studied only stable cases, our detecting rate should also differ from that of early stage cases. Actually, 7 out of 16 cases, who had been diagnosed as having homonymous hemianopia at the time of the early stage of CVA by the confrontation test, were not picked up in this study. Supposedly, this improvement may be a result of restoration of cerebral edema and absorption of bleeding. Then, it should be noticed that a considerable number of cases might have shown homonymous field defects in the early stages.

The number of left homonymous field defects was about twice as many as that of the right one. It seems that some of the disturbance of the dominant hemisphere may cause an aphasia and may make it difficult to carry out the visual field examination. This presumption, however, conflicts with Lanshe's report (7). He stated that visual field defects could not be charted easily, if the lesion was in the nondominant parietal lobe.

Correlations between the type of the lesion and the shape of the field defects were as follows:

1. ICA occlusion. The field defects cover over two quadrants with gently sloping borders and extend to complete hemianopia. They are roughly congruous. Peripheral field is more vulnerable than central field.

2. MCA occlusion. Inferior homonymous quadrantanopia is the rule. They also show congruous field defects with steep vertical meridians.

3. PCA occlusion. All cases of PCA occlusion showed dense homonymous field defects. Definite macular sparing is not necessary in complete hemianopia.

4. Thalamic hemorrhage. As a rule, the field defects are limited within one quadrant. They are often incongruous and show a variety of shapes. Peripheral field is more vulnerable than central.

5. Putaminal hemorrhage. They may cause various types of field defects, as well.

6. Lenticulo-striate artery occlusion (Basal ganglionic small infarction). They may not cause any field defects.

We have no idea about subcortical hemorrhage and cerebral infarction without definite location, because they are too few for assessment.

Occlusion of the MCA, which nourishes the parietal lobe region, may disturb the superior part of the optic radiation and cause inferior homonymous quadrantanopia. In this series, with exception of one case of superior quadrantanopia, all the remaining cases of MCA occlusion showed inferior quadrantanopia.

Our cases of ICA occlusion did not show quadrantanopia but a broader field of defects within two quadrants. It is thought that ICA occlusion causes the ischemia of the area of MCA and of anterior choroidal artery, and then it subsequently develops into such a broad field of defects.

Hitherto, thalamic hemorrhage has been said to present homonymous hemianopia in the early stage of CVA and disappear later (1). The author, however, detected 6 cases of homonymous field defects out of 17 thalamic hemorrhages in this study. As the defects were small within one quadrant, if one examined them by the confrontation test, they should have been overlooked.

Many thalamic hemorrhages in this study showed incongruous field defects. Supposedly, some of the Th. H. may affect the lateral geniculate body, which lies adjacent to the thalamus, and may cause the incongruous field defects.

Cerebral hemorrhage may cause various types of cerebral damage according to the extent of the lesion. On the other hand, cerebral infarction, in which the cerebral damage is limited to the drainaged area of the involved vessels, may show uniform symptoms. In this way, cerebral infarction showed a uniform type of field defects while cerebral hemorrhage showed various types.

As we did not use a more accurate perimeter such as a tangent screen or Tübingen perimeter, we could not assess precisely the well-known macular sparing. Nevertheless, definite macular sparings were shown in 3 cases in this study. No significant correlations between the location of the lesion and the macular sparing could be found in this study.

ACKNOWLEDGEMENT

The authors would like to thank Dr. H. Mihara for his kind permission and support of this study at the Institute of Brain and Blood Vessels, Mihara Memorial Hospital.

REFERENCES

1. Fisher, C. M. *et al.* Acute hypertensive cerebellar hemorrhage: diagnosis and surgical treatment. J. Nerv. Ment. Dis. 140: 38 (1965).
2. Haerer, A. F. Visual field defects and the prognosis of stroke patients. Stroke 4: 163 (1973).
3. Huber, A. Röntgen diagnosis vs visual field. Arch. Ophthalmol. 90: 1 (1973).
4. Isaeff, W. B. Ophthalmic findings in 322 patients with a cerebral vascular accident. Ann. Ophthal. 6: 1059 (1974).
5. Kaul, S. N. *et al.* Relationship between visual field defect and arterial occlusion in the posterior cerebral circulation. J. Neurol. Neurosurg. Psychiatry, 37: 1022 (1974).
6. Koerner, F. & H. L. Teuber. Visual field defects after missile injuries to the geniculo-striate pathway in man. Exp. Brain Res. 18: 88 (1973).
7. Lanshe, R. K. Ocular manifestations of strokes. Int. Ophthal. Clin. 8: 337 (1968).
8. Smith, J. L. Homonymous hemianopia. Am. J. Ophthalmol. 54: 616 (1962).
9. Tate, Jr. G. W. & J. R. Lynn. Principles of interpretation of the visual field. In: Principles of quantitative perimetry. Grune & Stratton, New York, p. 191 (1977).

Authors' addresses:
S. Maeda, M.D., S. Usuba, M.D. & S. Matsuyama, M.D.
Department of Ophthalmology Hirosaki University
School of Medicine
5 Zaifucho, Hirosaki 036
Japan

K. Nagata, M.D.
Institute of Brain and Blood Vessels
Mihara Memorial Hospital
Isezaki
Japan

REFRACTION SCOTOMATA AND ABSOLUTE PERIPHERAL SENSITIVITY

LUCIA R. RONCHI & LUIGI BARCA

(*Florence, Italy*)

ABSTRACT

By comparing the absolute thresholds recorded 10° nasally, in the dark-adapted retina, for two different stimulus durations (10 and 400 ms), an index (Δ) of temporal integration is obtained. Δ is found to depend on target size u as well as on stimulus wavelength. A peculiar 'tuning' phenomenon, denoting maximal time integration is found when u is about 6 min of arc, in the middle of the spectrum, and about twice at the blue end.

INTRODUCTION

One of the outstanding characteristics of peripheral vision, often referred to in clinical perimetry, is its large spatio-temporal summation, evident at most in the dark-adapted state. As an additional proof, we may quote the insensitivity to defocus (7), shown, for instance, in Fig. 1.

Now, recent research has put into evidence the so-called non summation across small areas (10), and the rod-cone interaction under other-than-steady stimulation, in scotopic vision (2). Personally, we are interested in absolute threshold. We find (8) that temporal summation is independent of wavelength, when test field size is as large as 2°. On the other hand, it is found to be wavelength dependent (6, 9) for test fields subtending at the eye 4 to 6 min in Fig. 2, where (left insert) the philosophy of our procedure is also displayed. Briefly, we recorded the radiance-time relationship for monochromatic stimuli, at absolute threshold, at a given retinal eccentricity (10° nasally). We assumed as an index (Δ) of integrative capacity the log difference of liminal radiance-time products (L · t) for two different stimulus durations, say, t = 400 ms and t = 10 ms, that is:

$$\Delta = |\log(L \cdot t)_{400} - \log(L \cdot t)_{10}|.$$

The smaller Δ, the more active the time integration process.

According to classical beliefs (11), Δ should be independent of stimulus wavelength, at absolute threshold.

Our small-field findings (6, 9) sould contradictory. As a matter of fact, we cannot apply the distinction between the spatio-temporal integrative properties of luminosity channel and of opponent-color channels (3) at absolute

Doc.Ophthal. Proc. Series, Vol. 26, ed. by E. L. Greve & G. Verriest

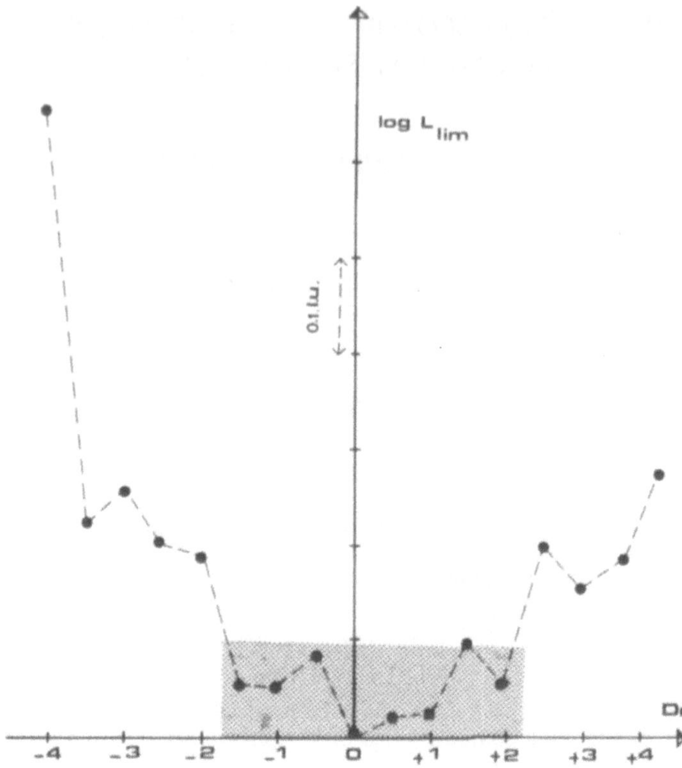

Fig. 1. Log absolute threshold luminance versus the degree of defocus, in diopters. Eccentricity, 10° nasally, $u = 3$ min of arc, $t = 400$ ms, $\lambda = 593$ nm. The blurring lens is placed close to the eye, perpendicularly to the line joining the target to the pupil, while the fixation light is left to the naked eye.

threshold, where cones are currently assumed to be silent, unless some subliminal influences on rod threshold are suggested (1, 2).

Therefore, it seemed worthwhile to record further experimental data, in order to throw some light on this complex problem. In the present experiment we deal with the dependence of Δ on target size u, once fixed stimulus wavelength, at a given retinal eccentricity (10° nasally). Looking at Figure 2, one might expect that the plot where Δ is displayed versus u is flat in some spectral regions, while it shows a rising trend in other regions. Indeed, the response pattern found by us is more complicated, as is described in the following paper.

MATERIALS AND METHOD

The experimental set-up is the same as that used in previous experiments (6, 9). A circular test spot of variable size and intensity is flashed at the wanted retinal location, on a dark-background. Light emitted by an incandescence

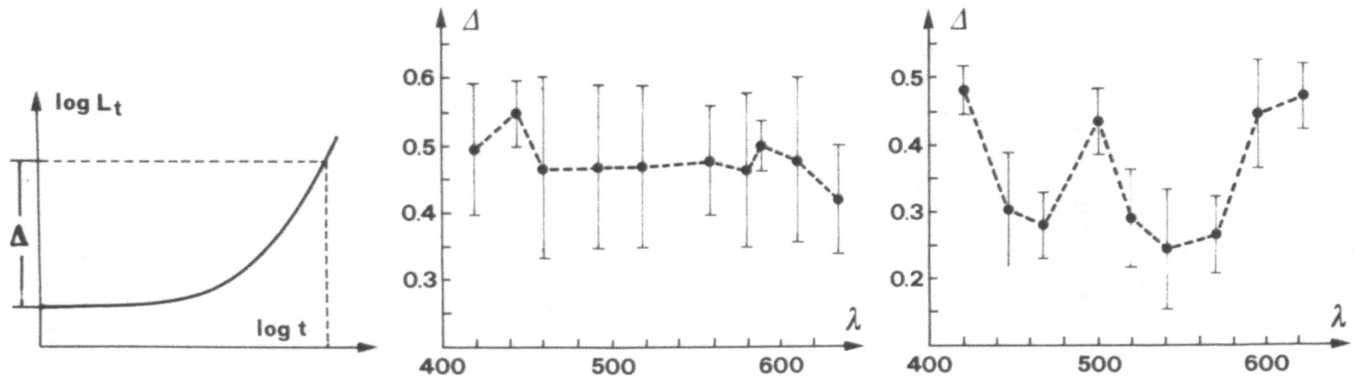

Fig. 2. A general view of the findings of our previous experiments. Left, a schematized luminance-time relationship, and the definition of quantity Δ. In the middle, the wavelength dependence of Δ for a 2 deg diam test-field. To the right, the said dependence for a 4 min of arc test field.

lamp (2800°K) is rendered monochromatic through Balzer interference filters, and next focused on the shutter plane.

The observer, after 30 min dark-adaptation is given a fixation target, consisting of a LED source, green in some sessions, red in others.

Once fixed stimulus size (u), duration (t) and wavelength (λ), absolute threshold is recorded by the use of constant stimuli method, and estimated through Probit Analysis. Target size is varied from 2.5 to 36′. For every u value, ten estimates of Δ were obtained. Average and standard deviation were then computed for each sample of such data.

Three normal highly skilled observers took part in the sessions. However, a more complete data set was obtained with observer OND. Therefore, this observer's data are presented to describe the results of the present work.

EXPERIMENTAL FINDINGS AND DISCUSSION

Fig. 3 shows how the u-dependence of Δ varies across the spectrum. Now, looking for a feature common to every plot, we might argue that there is a

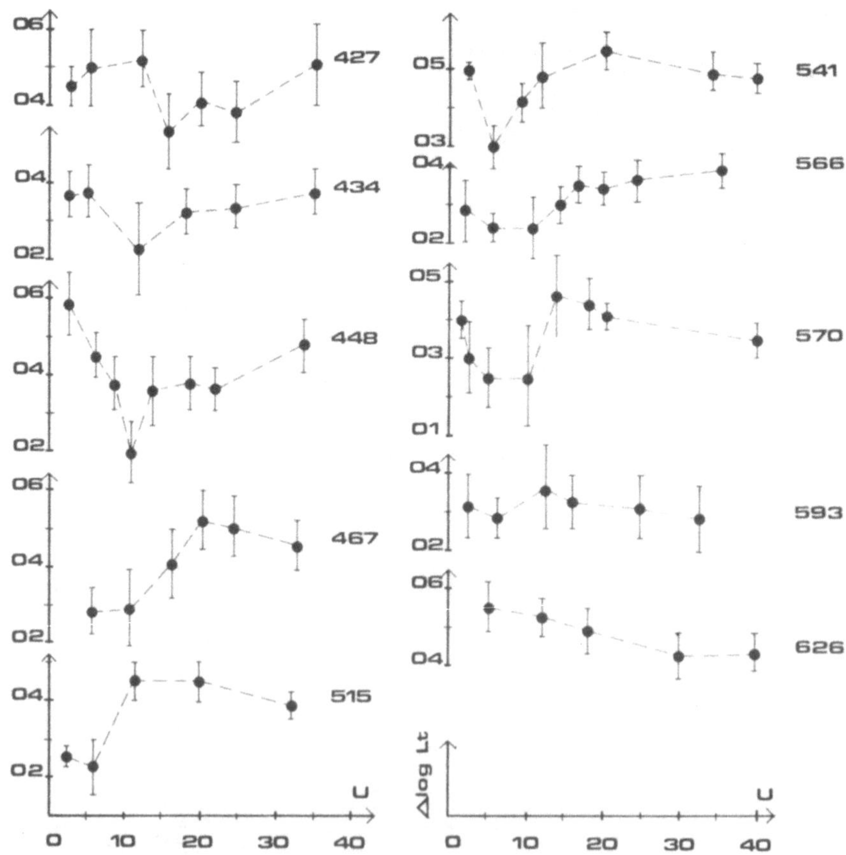

Fig. 3. Quantity Δ, defined in the text, is plotted versus test spot size (u) in min of arc. Label denotes the wavelength. Bars denote the standard devaition.

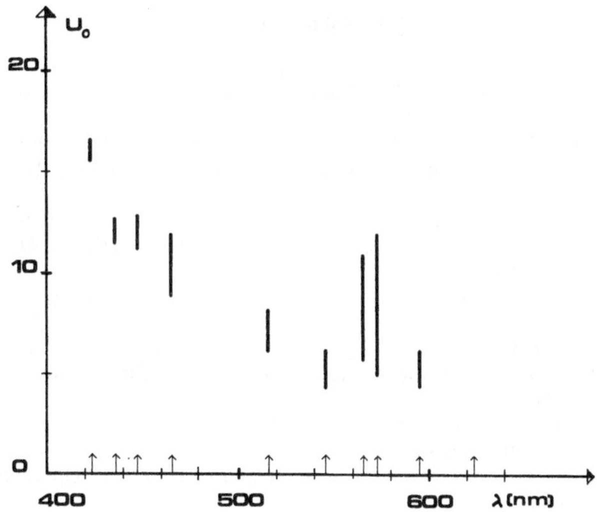

Fig. 4. Target size (or range for target size), in minutes of arc, where Δ is minimum (see Fig. 3), and hence time summation is maximal, plotted versus stimulus wavelength.

peculiar target size (let us denote it by u_0) where Δ attains its minimum. In other words, we are looking for an optimal target size where temporal integration is effective at most, in line with the known non-independence of spatial and temporal summation, recently discussed by Owens (4).

As is shown in Fig. 4, u_0 is wavelength dependent. No data are produced for $\lambda = 626$ nm (see Fig. 3), although one could guess that u_0 is very small, in this spectral region. We applied the Student-*t* to test the significance of the Δ difference estimated for the assumed u_0 value, at every wavelength. The significance (at the 0.05 confidence level) is attained at all the tested wavelengths, except for 434 and 593 nm.

In addition, in agreement with previous findings (5) we have once more confirmed that our results are not a mere artifact due to eye chromatic aberration, called into play by the differences in spectral composition of fixation light and test field light, respectively.

In conclusion, we might assume that temporal integration becomes optimal when target size is large enough to avoid non summation effects (10). However, the understanding of u_0 dependence on wavelength, found by us is other-than-immediate, unless some inferences are made about the lack of homogeneity of time constant of receptor population mediating the absolute threshold response.

In perimetric tests where large and long-lasting stimuli are used, the above effects are of but little relevance. On the other hand, they are likely to play a role, e.g. in dynamic perimetric tests, relying upon local spatio-temporal integrative properties. Under these conditions, if brief and small stimuli are used, one should consider that a short of 'tuning' occurs around 6′ size, in the middle of the spectrum (around 12′ at the blue end). In this connection, it seems likely that the lack of adequacy of dioptric correction could avoid the optimization of performance, even if classical considerations about peripheral Ricco's area would not lead to suspect it.

REFERENCES

1. Foster, D. H. Rod- and cone-mediate interactions in the fine-grain movement illusion. Vision Res. 17: 123–127 (1977).
2. Frumkes, T. E., M. D. Sekuler, M. C. Barris, E. H. Reiss & L. M. Chalupa. Rod-cone interaction in human scotopic vision. I. Temporal analysis. Vision Res. 13: 1269–1282 (1973).
3. King-Smith, P. E. & D. Carden. Luminance and oppoent-color contributions to visual detection and adaptation and to temporal and spatial integration. J. Opt. Soc. Am. 66: 709–717 (1976).
4. Owens, W. G. Spatio-temporal integration in the human peripheral retina. Vision Res. 12: 1011–1026 (1972).
5. Ronchi, L. & G. Molesini. The scotopic luminance-time relationship and its possible dependence on the chromatic aberration of the eye. Brit. J. Physiol. Opt. 28: 162–168 (1973).
6. Ronchi, L. Dependence of peripheral sensitivity on exposure time. Mod. Probl. Ophthal. 13: 98–102 (1974).
7. Ronchi, L. & G. Molesini. Depth-of-focus in peripheral vision. Ophthalm. Res. 7: 152–157 (1975).
8. Ronchi, L. & L. Barca. Experiments on absolute threshold for monochromatic stimuli. Rev. Sens. Disabil. 32: 3–9 (1978).
9. Ronchi, L. & S. Stefanacci. Some remarks on time-integrative properties of the dark-adapted retina. Optica Acta 25: 265–267 (1978).
10. Scholtes, A. M. W. & M. A. Bouman. Psychophysical experiments on spatial summation at threshold level of the human peripheral retina. Vision Res. 17: 867–873 (1977).
11. Sperling, H. G. & C. L. Jolliffe. Intensity-time relationship at threshold for spectral stimuli in human vision. J. Opt. Soc. Am. 55: 191–199 (1965).

Authors' addresses:

Prof. Lucia Rositani Ronchi, Ph.D.
Istituto Nazionale di Ottica
6 Largo E. Fermi
I-50125 Florence
Italy

Luigi Barca, M.D.
Clinica Oculistica dell'Università
Viale Morgagni, Careggi
I-51000 Florence
Italy

SCREENING OF VISUAL FIELD DEFECT AMONG HEALTHY ADULTS

A preliminary trial of population survey of ocular disease

SYUJI MAEDA

(*Hirosaki, Japan*)

ABSTRACT

Mass screening for visual field defect was performed on 1,811 supposedly healthy persons. Static Campimeter was used for screening and Goldmann perimeter and Tübinger perimeter for thorough field examination.

21 patients (1.2%) were detected to have definite field defects. Diagnosis of these 21 patients were classsified as follows; 9 intracranial lesions, 6 retino-choroidal lesions, 4 glaucomas and 2 cases of unknown origin. The time taken for the screening was about 3 min for both eyes.

This study indicates that screening of visual field defect can contribute very much to preventive medicine, especially to the early detection of intracranial lesions.

INTRODUCTION

The visual field examination is an important part of ophthalmological examinations and is of particular help in topical diagnosis of many neurological lesions in visual pathways. The early detection of field defects is of great value for the detection of some ocular diseases and intracranial lesions. However, there are some difficulties in the early detection of field defects. Frequent unawareness of field defects is one of the most important causes, and intricacy of procedure of examination is another.

A number of visual field screening tests have been carried out by many investigators (1, 2, 3, 4, 5, 6, 7). Most of them studied it for the early detection of glaucoma.

This paper reports the result of mass screening of visual field defects in subjects composed of supposedly healthy persons. For this purpose, the author used a Static Campimeter (Takada Co. Tokyo), which was developed to refine the Friedmann Visual Field Analyser (8).

The aims of this study were as follows:

1. To know the proportion of visual field defects in a population of supposedly healthy adults.
2. Detection and etiologic distribution of intraocular and intracranial diseases referring to visual field defects.
3. Evaluation of visual field screening.
4. Possibility of practical use of visual field screening.

Doc. Ophthal. Proc. Series, Vol. 26, ed. by E. L. Greve & G. Verriest

Table 1. Age and sex in the subjects studied.

Age	15–19	20–29	30–39	40–49	50–59	60–64	Total
Male	343	420	245	290	35	3	1336
Female	222	133	61	33	26	0	475
Total	565	553	306	323	61	3	1811

MATERIAL AND METHOD

The visual field was examined in 1,811 adults who were engaged in their daily work without any complaint about their eyes. The sex and age distribution were shown in Table 1. The age averaged 28 years. Visual field was examined in two steps: (1) screening of field defects (SFD), and (2) accurate field examination (AFE). Static Campimeter (Takada Co. Japan) was used for SFD. Each subject was dark adaptated for ten minutes or more in a dark room, and then the visual field was examined, while wearing the required correction for near sight (30 cm).

Each subject was investigated with a neutral density filter, set at its own dial position (1.2 to 1.8 log units) according to age. If one failed twice, the procedure of the test was repeated and reexamined cautiously to prevent a false positive. Any people in whom visual field defects had been detected were subjected to AFE i.e. a quantiative perimetry using Goldmann type perimeter and/or Tübinger perimeter.

RESULTS

It was shown that reliable visual field examinations can be carried out in a short time (2 to 3 minutes per two eyes). Of this series 48 subjects (2.7 percent) were diagnosed as 'failed' during a mass screening program with the Static Campimeter and referred to further accurate visual field examination using Goldmann type perimeter and/or Tübinger perimeter. As the result of the accurate examination, 21 subjects (1.2 percent) revealed definite visual field defects. The other 27 subjects were thought to be false positive. As many of them had hyperope or high graded myope, incomplete correction was the most suspected cause of the false positive.

Visual acuity was better than 20/25 in 21 subjects having visual field defects. Although case 8 complained of headaches and asthenopia, and case 14 complained of blurred vision, the other 19 did not have any complaints.

Sex, age, type of the visual field defects and the result of ophthalmological and neurological examinations were summarizedly shown in Table 2. Among 21 subjects which revealed visual field defects, intracranial disorders were detected in 9 cases, glaucoma in 4 cases and intraocular diseases of other types in 6 cases.

The average age was 33 years in the cases of intracranial disorders and 32 years in the cases of glaucoma. On the other hand, it was 41 years in the group of retino-choroidal disorders. Eighteen were male and 3 were female.

Table 2. Type and cause of visual field change detected by visual field defect screening.

Case No.	Sex	Age	Visual field defect	Cause
1	M	59	Rt. homonymous defect	Cerebral A-V malformation
2	M	19	Rt. homonymous defect	unknown
3	M	29	Rt. homonymous defect	unknown
4	M	24	Lt. homonymous defect	Cerebral atrophy
5	M	45	Lt. homonymous defect	Cerebral atrophy susp. Cerebral aneurysm
6	M	34	Bitemporal scotoma	Sellar lesion
7	M	28	Bitemporal scotoma	susp. Cerebral aneurysm*
8	M	44	Lt. paracentral scotoma	Sellar lesion
9	F	24	Rt. nasal contraction	Sellar lesion
10	M	44	Bilat. arcuate scotoma	Glaucoma*
11	M	30	Rt. temporal contraction	Glaucoma*
12	M	35	Rt. paracentral scotoma	Glaucoma*
13	M	19	Rt. inf. sector defect	Glaucoma
14	M	49	Lt. arcuate scotoma	Branch obstruction of central retinal vein*
15	M	49	Rt. paracentral scotoma	Retinal atrophy*
16	M	20	Rt. paracentral scotoma	Retinal atrophy*
17	M	46	Lt. inf. contraction	Retinal pigment epithelial detachment*
18	F	52	Bilat. anular scotoma	Pigmentary degeneration of the retina*
19	F	27	Dislocated blind spot	Dislocation of the optic disc*
20	M	53	Rt. paracentral scotoma	unknown
21	M	58	Lt. paracentral scotoma	unknown

* Case revealed ophthalmoscopic changes.

CT and radiographic examinations of the skull showed pathological findings corresponding to the defects of visual field in five of seven cases having homonymous hemianopia or bitemporal scotoma.

Case 1 revealed almost complete right homonymous hemianopia. But no other neurological abnormalities were detected in this case. On plain film of the skull, shadows supposing calcification were found on the left parietal and occipital lobes. On CT scanning, this part was strongly enhanced by contrast media. A-V malformation was most suspected. Case 2 and 3 were cases of incomplete right homonymous hemianopia, but no abnormality was found on CT, skull plain film and brain radioisotope scanning. Case 4 was a case of left inferior homonymous quadrantanopia with slight congruity (Fig. 1). A low density area suggesting enlargement of sulcus calcarinus was found in the right occipital lobe (Fig. 2). Case 5, a 45-year-old male, revealed incongruous left superior homonymous quadrantanopia. CT scan revealed enlargement of Sylvian fissure and sulci in the right temporoparietal region. High density spots were enhanced along the Willis arterial circle and in the frontal lobe. Cases 10, 11 and 12 had glaucomatous field defects and glaucomatous cuppings of the discs corresponding to the field defects. Intraocular tension was in normal range. Case 13 showed glaucomatous field defect (Fig. 3) and intraocular hypertension; R. 27 mmHg, L. 23 mmHg. However, neither glaucomatous cupping of the disc nor degenerative change of retinal nerve fibers was

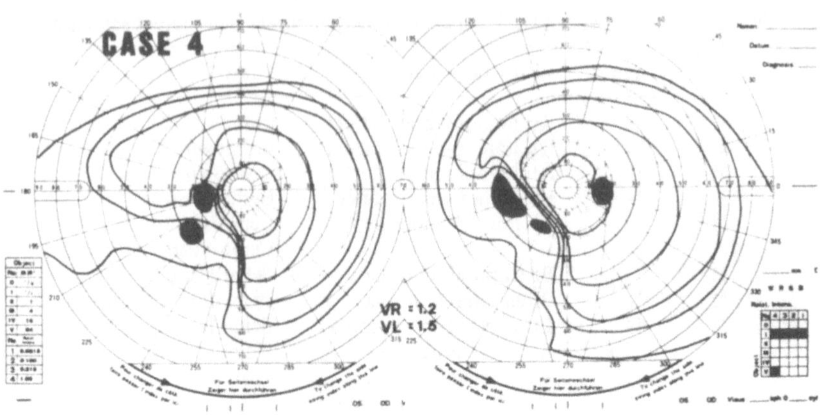

Fig. 1. Visual fields of the case of cerebral atrophy showing left inferior homonymous field defects.

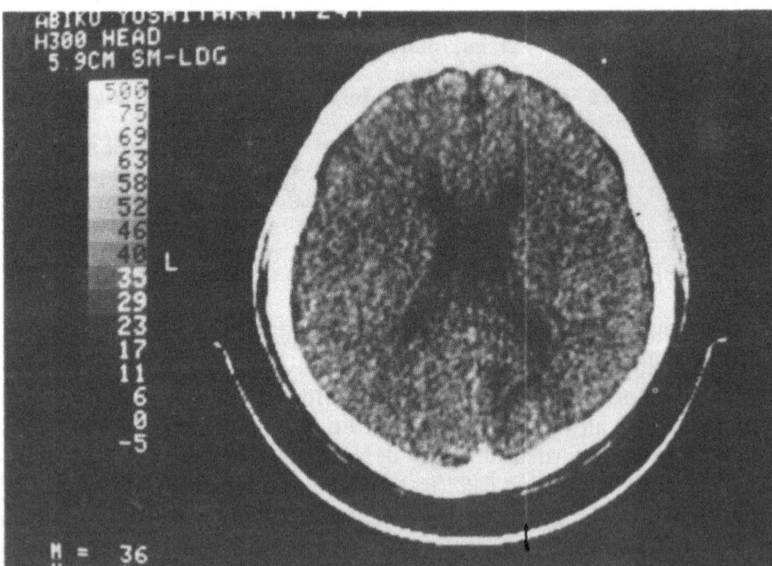

Fig. 2. CT scan film of the same case in Fig. 1. Low density area is shown in the right occipital lobe. It is thought to be due to enlargement of the calcarine sulcus.

found in this case. Each case of retinal lesion showed field defects corresponding to the lesions in the fundus. Case 19 was a case in which Mariotte's blind spot was found to be more nasally than usual. There was no change in size or shape of the isopters surrounding it. An abnormal location of the optic disc in the left eye was recognized by ophthalmoscopy. Case 20 and 21: Unilateral small paracentral scotomata was found. However, no abnormal finding was obtained. Micro-infarction in the optic disc was a possible cause of the defects.

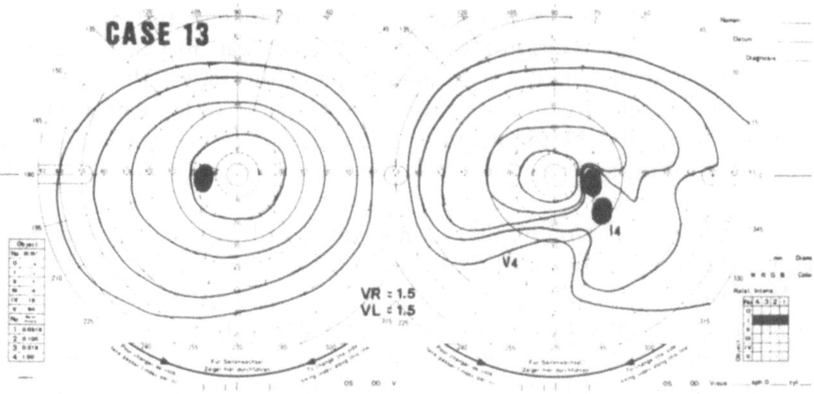

Fig. 3. Visual fields of the case of primary open angle glaucoma. The right field signifies a nerve fiber bundle defect.

DISCUSSION

As Cassidy and Havener (1) described, reduced visual acuity is of remarkable value as a screening test for the detection of refractive errors or opacities of the transparent media. On the other hand, retrobulbar lesions which affect mainly visual field are hardly detected in their early stage of minimal changes, because patients are unaware of the visual field defects. Therefore, there was a necessity for the establishment of a rapid screening method.

The results of the investigations of the different authors vary considerably and this may be caused by difference of the composition of the groups investigated, and the condition of the examinations, as previously stated by Greve and Verduin (4). According to Graham and Hollows (3), the proportion of subjects where field defects were accounted for was 13 percent of the 1,339 subjects aged 40–74 years. The screening was done with the use of Friedmann Visual Field Analyser. Robertson (7) carried out visual field screening in 5,630 employees in seven industrial plants using Harrington's Multiple Pattern Field Screener. Of these 258 (4.6%) were recorded as abnormal. Linfield (6) studied also visual fields of industrial employees using Friedmann Visual Field Analyser and detected 20 persons (1.9%), of 1,078 employees who were more than 35 years of age.

The proportion of visual field defects are higher than those of our own series. Our own investigation can be best compared with that of Greve and Verduin with respect to age distribution and composition of the group. They studied healthy 1,834 subjects with normal visual acuity and the age was between 20 and 60 years. 34 cases (1.9%) of field abnormality including 3 cases of homonymous hemianopia were recognized by the screening. The proportion in our series (1.2%) very much resembles their proportion. From these results, the proportion of field defects among healthy subjects may be accounted for 1 to 2 percent.

Etiological survey in relation to the field defect of suspected intracranial lesion has not been sufficiently studied in previous investigations.

We recognized some intracranial lesions corresponding to field defects in 9 of our series. The average age in these 9 cases was 30 years, and this is almost equal to that of the total population of this series. This means that such an intracranial lesion exists from a younger age of life and it does not progress so rapidly. Motor neuron disturbances are not so rare (1.3/1000 persons) at birth, and they are not overlooked because motor palsy makes characteristic figures.

However, if the lesion localizes in the visual pathway, it can course without being noticed by the patient's family and even himself.

Moreover, on the other hand it is said that such a lesion, in either case of haemorrhage or infarction, is altered to granulation tissues in the course of time and under such a condition it is no longer confirmed by CT scan. Such cerebral lesions at birth were most suspected in cases 2, 3 and 4 which showed no definite change except visual field defects in spite of neurological and radiological examinations. All lesions of this type do not always remain benign. Intracranial A-V malformation and aneurysm was suspected in cases 1, 5 and 7. Usually, the existence of these vascular abnormalities are noticed first after the appearance of cerebral nerve disturbances following intracranial haemorrhage from ruptured vessels. Early detection of the abnormalities is a matter of life-and-death for the patients. The fact that we could detect the cases among healthy subjects, by field screening, in their silent state of the disorders, reveals the necessity and availability of the screening.

In three cases (cases 6, 8 and 9), a destructive figure of bone was suggested surrounding the Turkish saddle on X-ray film, though no abnormal findings were given by other examinations. These cases must be cautiously followed up.

All of the subjects with field defects in the series had good central acuity and none of them was aware of visual field defect before the screening test. This fact may lead to postulate that screening of field defects should be always included in the periodic health examination program. Furthermore, 11 subjects revealed no ophthalmoscopic change.

Screening by Static Campimeter can be well carried out in a short time (2 to 3 min per two eyes). This is a merit of this method.

As to false negative, it was not studied in the present study.

ACKNOWLEDGEMENT

I am very grateful to Prof. Shuichi Matsuyama for his kindly direction throughout this study.

REFERENCES

1. Cassidy, V. & W. H. Havener. Evaluation of a screening procedure in the detection of eye disease. Arch. Ophthal. 61: 589–598 (1959).
2. Friedmann, A. I. Serial analysis of changes in visual field defects, employing a new instrument, to determine the activity of diseases involving the visual pathways. Ophthalmologica 152: 1–12 (1966).

3. Graham, P. A. & F. C. Hollows. The Ferndale glaucoma survey. In: Glaucoma, epidemiology, early diagnosis and some aspects of treatment, L. B. Hunt, ed., pp. 24–44 & 103–115. London, Livingstone (1966).
4. Greve, E. L. & W. M. Verduin. Mass visual field investigation in 1834 persons with supposedly normal eyes. Albrecht v. Graefes Arch. klin. exp. Ophthal. 183: 286–293 (1972).
5. Harrington, D. O. & M. Flocks. The multiple-pattern method of visual field examination. Arch. Ophthalmol. 61: 755–765 (1959).
6. Linfield, P. B. Industrial screening for the early detection of glaucoma. Ophthalm. Optician 17: 1044–1058 (1970).
7. Robertson, L. T. Use of the Harrington multiple-pattern field screener in industry. Trans. Amer. Acad. Ophthal. Otolaryng. 60: 806–811 (1956).
8. Shinzato, E. Quantitative perimetry using new developed Static Campimeter – discussion on normal eyes. Acta Soc. Ophthalmol. Jpn. 82: 167–174 (1978).

Author's address:
Department of Ophthalmology
Hirosaki University
School of Medicine
5 Zaifucho
Hirosaki 036
Japan

GRIDS FOR FUNCTIONAL SCORING OF VISUAL FIELDS

BEN ESTERMAN

(*New York, N.Y., U.S.A.*)

ABSTRACT

The scoring of peripheral vision is an assessment of visual *function*. Yet, until recently all scoring was erroneously based on a field's *size* rather than its *usefulness*. This was corrected by the invention of a relative value scale in the form of a grid which scores different parts of the field in proportion to their functional value to the patient.

The grid is designed for either the full field (perimeter) or the paracentral field (25°) (tangent screen). It consists of 100 units, each unit worth 1%. A simple count of units which are not obscured by contraction or scotoma yields a direct score in percent of the normal functional field.

In the decade since the grid was approved by the American Committee on Optics and Visual Physiology it has gained increasingly wide use in the U.S. It has proven to be accurate, fast, inexpensive, easily reproducible, and can be used by untrained personnel. It scores irregular isopters and scotomata *within* the field as easily as ordinary *peripheral* contraction.

The grid is adaptable to all sizes of field charts used by the different kinds of perimeters and tangent screens, whether manual, automatic or computerized.

THE PROBLEM

The scoring of visual fields is, by definition, an assessment of *function*, an expression of the patient's visual capability to perform within his environment. Yet, prior to 1967, existing methods of scoring were limited to those based on area alone. (Table 1) Most of us who gave the matter thought were uneasy about this system. It didn't work well. It didn't really express function. Patients turned up with scores that were totally unrealistic in relation to their disability. (Fig. 1, A & B shows two such fields with identical scores by the old method but obviously dissimilar in their usefulness for a human patient: Fig. 1, C & D).

At a meeting of the International Perimetric Society in 1979 (1) it was concluded that 'we are faced with a major problem – to specify loss within a field – where loss is other than simple contraction'. It was recalled that the I.P.S. had been charged by the Concilium Ophthalmologicum Universale with development of a standard for measuring field loss – and to do it soon.

In 1967 a new system was devised in the form of grids (2, 3) which included *function* as a main criterion (Figs. 2 & 3). It proposed the thesis, which was soon generally accepted, that human activity in modern society made

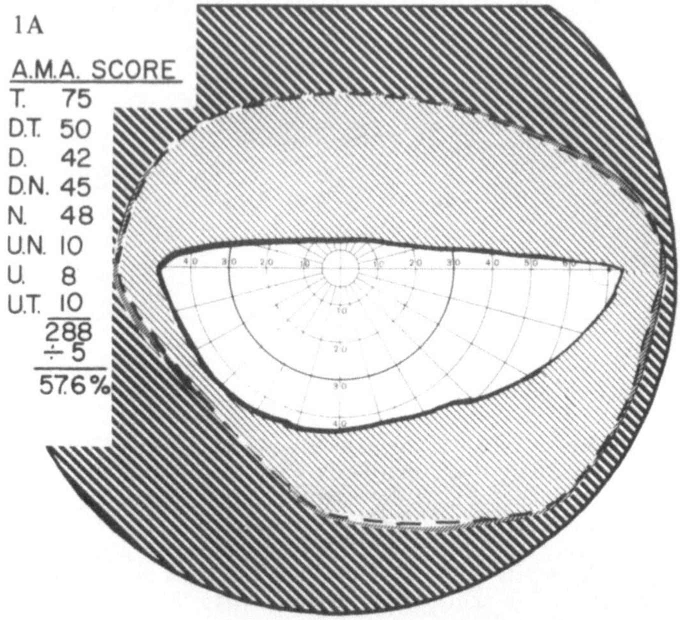

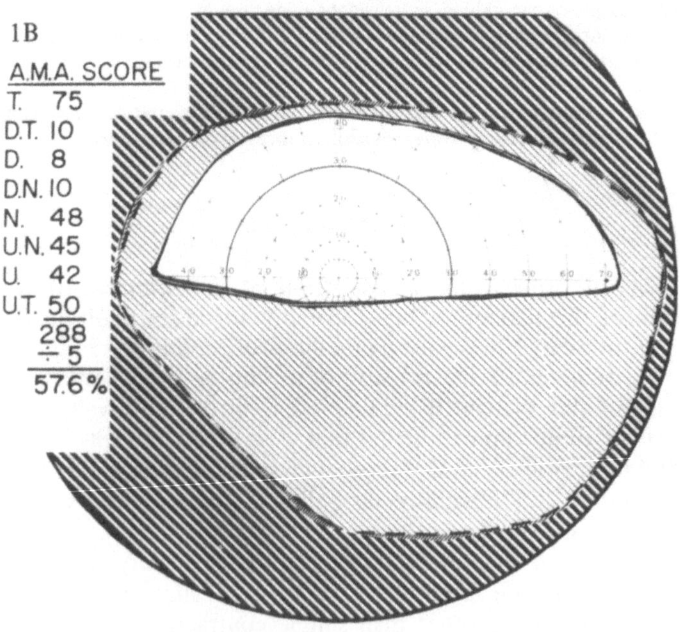

Fig. 1. A. Loss of *upper* field. B. Loss of *lower* field.
By *old* method, area scores are an identical 58%, totally unrealistic from a functional point of view.

1C

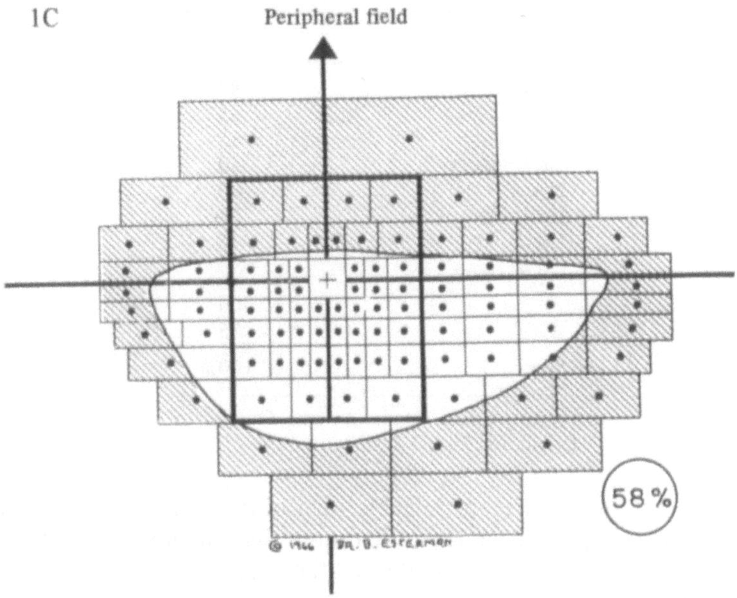

1D

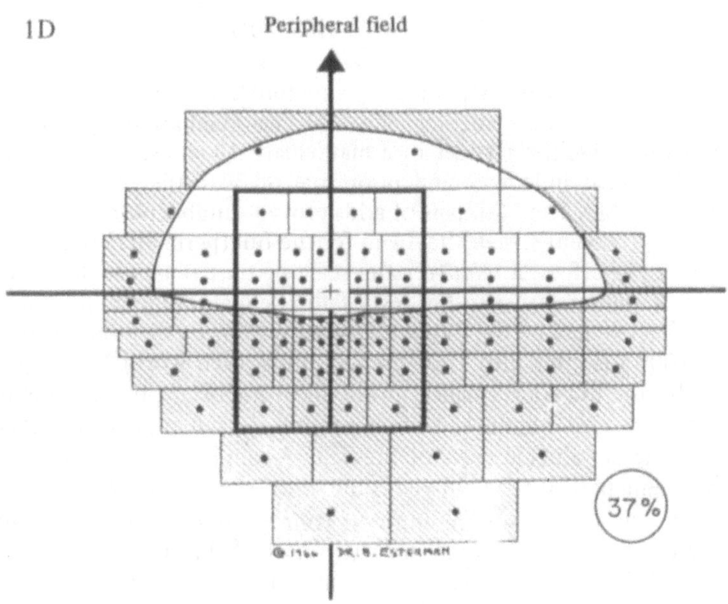

Fig. 1. C. & D. Grid scores, by *new* method are 58% and 37% functionally realistic.

Table 1. Minimal normal extent of visual field from point of fixation.

	Degrees
Temp	85
Dn & Temp	85
Dn	65
Dn & Nas	50
Nas	60
Up & Nas	55
Up	45
Up & Temp	55
	500
	÷ 5
Score	100%

From: Amer. Med. Assoc., Guides to Evaluation Visual System.

certain parts of the field more valuable than others – the paracentral area more than the periphery; the lower half more than the upper; and the area along the horizontal meridian more than all the other meridia.

MATERIAL AND METHODS

A three year study included perimetric and functional evaluation of three hundred patients in the glaucoma clinic of the Manhattan Eye, Ear and Throat Hospital, plus the services of a mathematician and statistician, simple experienced clinical judgment and prior trial of 34 earlier grids, soon discarded as unsuitable. The 35th pair of grids proved suitable both for the intermeridate (25°) (tangent screen) field and for the full (perimeter) field.

This grid is, in effect, a *relative value* scale because it assigns, to each part of the field, a value relative to the rest of the field and to its importance for the visual effectiveness of the patient. It achieves this by dividing the normal standard (100%) isopter into 100 *UN*equal units, each worth 1% (Figs. 2 & 3). Naturally, the units are smallest in the most important parts of the field; they increase in size (while each unit retains its value of 1%) becoming largest in the least valuable parts of the field. A simple count of the 1% units within the seeing part of the field yields the direct score in percent.

Advisedly, the central area is omitted from scoring because it is already adequately expressed by the Snellen scale. The test object used as a standard is of sufficient size and brightness to be easily detected by a patient of average intelligence and alertness (1/2° white for the perimeter – as in the former A.M.A. standard; for the tangent screen, 2 mm white at 1 meter). This does not, by any means, rule out smaller or fainter stimuli used, *in addition*, for more delicate diagnostic plotting, static or dynamic. But for scoring, a workable stimulus must obviously be uniform and would, along with what constitutes a normal (100%) isopter, be determined by each country or by a world organization.

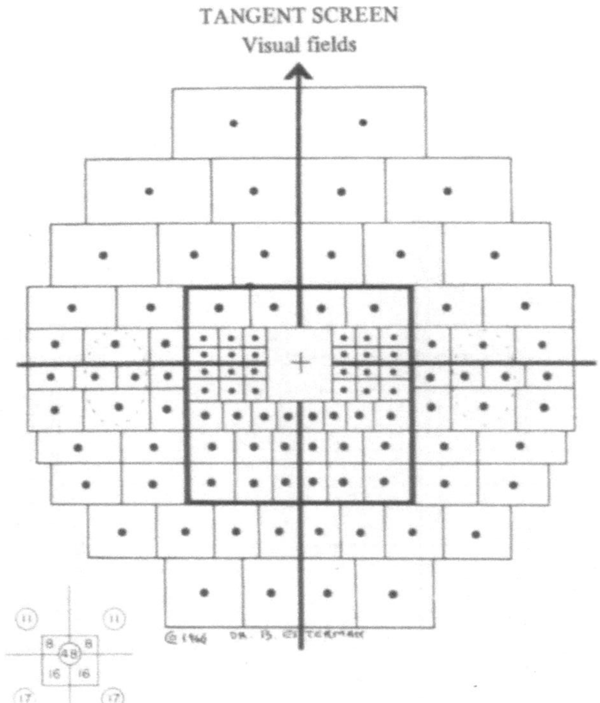

Fig. 2. Grid for Tangent Screen (25°) Field.
The central area is not scored because it is expressed by the Snellen score. There are 104 units, of which 4 are elminated by either normal blind spot. Of the remaining 100 units, each unit scores 1%. The central dot in each unit makes counting easier. Dots to be counted must lie wholly within the seeing field. Small inset grid at lower left speeds the scoring by counting in *blocks* of units, as indicated by numerals.

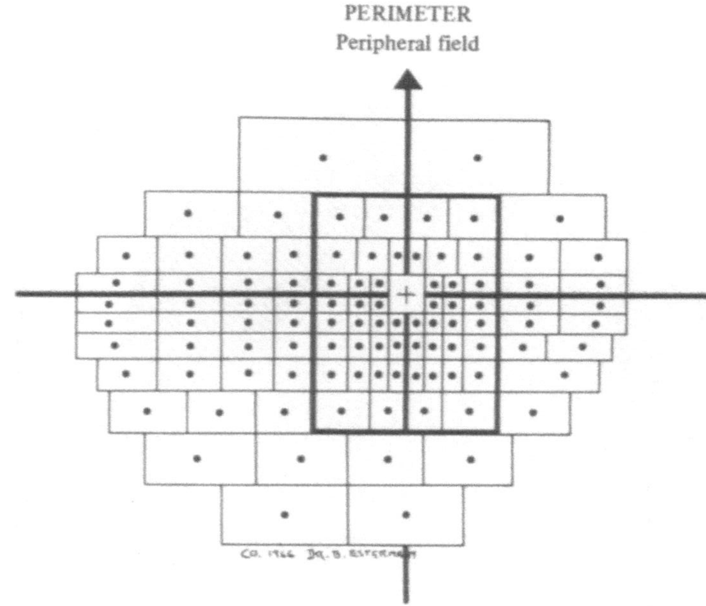

Fig. 3. Grid for Peripheral (Perimeter) Field fits exactly within the Normal (100%) isopter. Each of the 100 units scores 1%. HEAVY rectangle encloses 50 units (50%) merely to speed counting. Opposite eye's grid would be a mirror image of this.

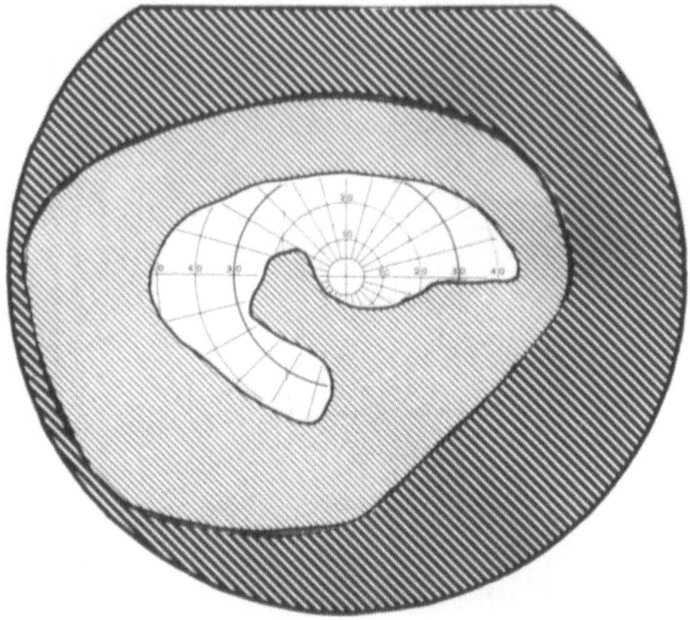

Fig. 4. Late Glaucoma. A difficult contour to score by old method.

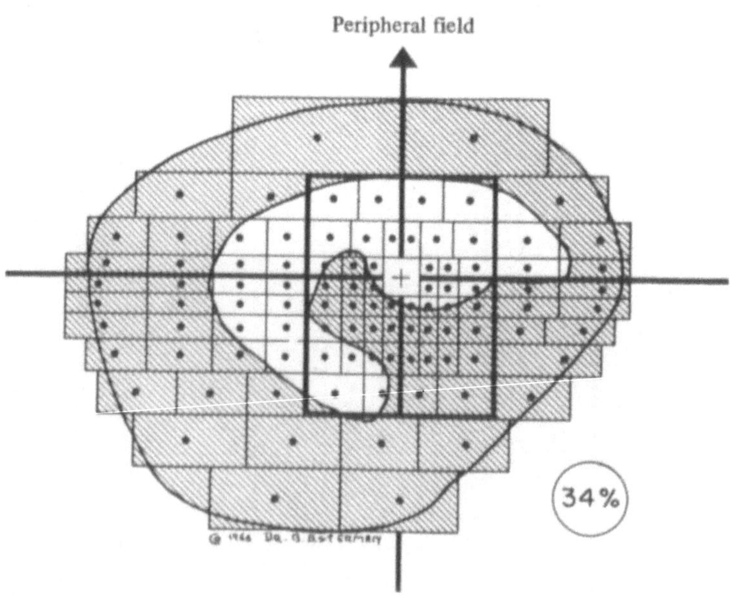

Fig. 5. Same field, easily scored by grid:

Within the central rectangle	=	21
Outside of central rectangle	=	13
	Score	34%

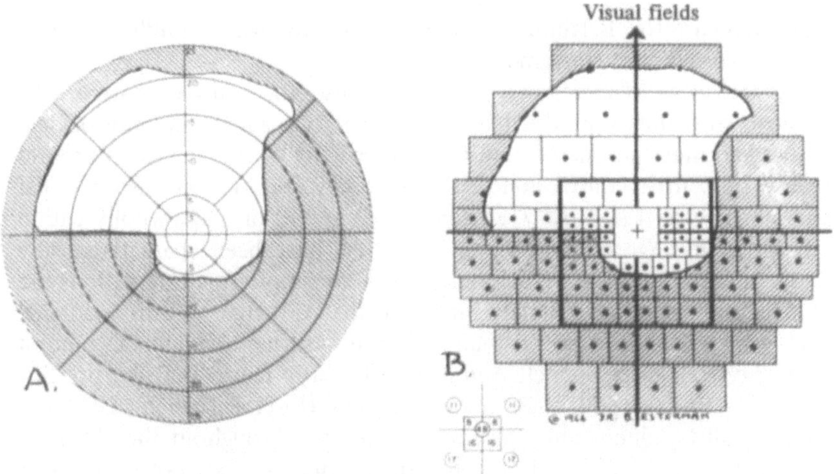

Fig. 6. Tangent Screen Field: A. Advanced glaucoma
B. Within the central rectangle = 28
Outside of central rectangle = 11

Score 39%

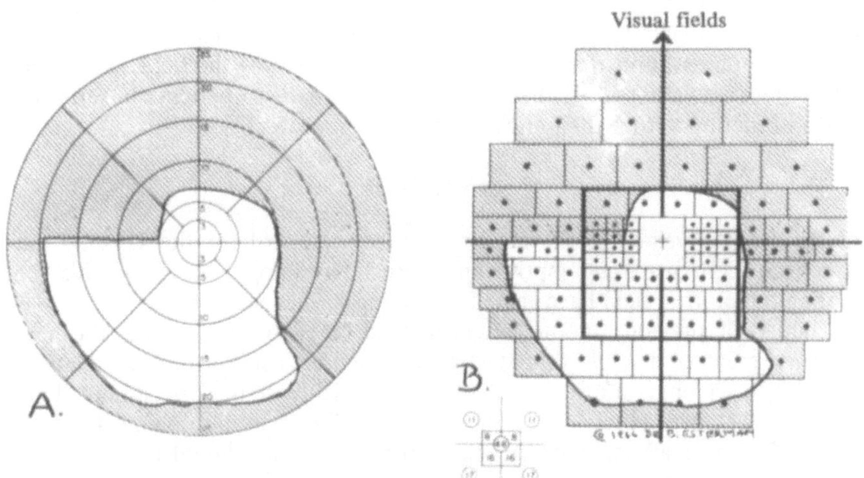

Fig. 7. A. Same field as Fig. 6 in area, but inverted:
B. Central rectangle: 48 − 5 = 43
Outside of rectange 13

Score 56%

Compare with Fig. 6. Greater functional value is reflected in its higher score.

DISCUSSION

Two years after publication, the grid was approved by the American Committee on Optics and Visual Physiology, which consists of representatives of the American Academy of Ophthalmology, the Association for Research in Vision, the American Medical Association and the American Ophthalmological Association. They recommended to the A.M.A. that the new scale be made the official standard for the U.S.A. More recently it has been adopted as the official standard for Belgium and the French now use a simplified, more approximate version of the same.

After ten years of increasingly widespread use, the grid has proved to be functional, workable, reproducible, and adaptable to almost all kinds of field charts and to most perimeters and tangent screens. With equal ease, it scores not only concentric contraction of the periphery (Fig. 1), but also irregular contractions (Figs. 4 & 5; 6 & 7) scotomata of any size or shape wholly within the field, even ring scotomata – all of which have been characteristically difficult to score by the old method. It is so simple (no calculations are needed because these are already built into the grid) that an untrained aide can score a plotted field in less than a minute – saving the valuable time of more highly trained personnel. And it is sufficiently cheap that, by printing 30,000 at a time, the Manhattan Eye and Ear Hospital (which distributes them to oculists, clinics and government agencies throughout the U.S.) has been able to sell them for eight cents apiece and use the profit to fund a lectureship.

Most important, prior to publication, its accuracy was tested by twenty of the senior ophthalmologists at the same hospital, doing 2000 scorings of 50 diverse fields. Agreement came within 10% of the actual score 1862 times out of 2000, a very satisfactory correspondance (93%) for a test susceptible to much human inaccuracy. Still better, most of these opthalmologists volunteered the observation that use of the grid, after plotting the field, gave them a heightened awareness of what that field loss meant to patients in terms of human function within their environment.

SUMMARY

In the 10 years since they were approved as standard for the U.S. by the American Committee on Optics and Visual Physiology, the new grids for scoring the plotted field have gained increasingly wide acceptance.

Unlike all previous methods which were based on area alone, the new system's greatest asset is that it stresses *function*, using a built-in relative-value scale which requires no calculation or highly trained personnel. It is accurate, fast, reproducible and cheap. It is easily adaptable to any size field chart, to almost all tangent screens or perimeters and should be a valuable adjunct to the newer automated perimeters.

REFERENCES

1. Research Group on Standards of the International Perimetric Society, Bonn, F.R.G., March 20, 1979.
2. Esterman, B. Grids for scoring visual fields. I: Tangent. A.M.A. Arch. Ophth. 77: 780 (June 1967).
3. Esterman, B. Grids for scoring visual fields. II: Perimeter. A.M.A. Arch. Ophth. 79: 400 (Apr. 1968).

Author's address:
Ben Esterman, M.D., F.A.C.S.
130 Central Avenue
Lawrence, N.Y. 11559
U.S.A.

A PROCEDURE FOR THE COMPUTER CODING OF VISUAL FIELDS

S. S. HAYREH, R. F. WOOLSON & J. A. KOHLER

(Iowa City, Iowa, U.S.A.)

ABSTRACT

Perimetry is of great diagnostic significance in the evaluation of visual function. In order to summarize statistically the visual field information we have developed and tested a procedure for computer coding and retrieving the peripheral visual fields as well as the size, shape, orientation and location of scotomata with the use of a mechanical instrument. These data are manually transcribed onto a computer-coded data form for calculation of numerical data and computer plotting of fields. In this paper these numerical data are compared to ratings of the fields made by three clinicians in our clinical studies. The fields are ranked from worst to best by each clinician on each of eight characteristics: central scotoma with I/2e, I/4e and V/4e; overall assessment of central scotoma; peripheral field with I/2e, I/4e and V/4e; and overall assessment of peripheral field. The rankings are compared between pairs of raters in addition to being compared to the numerically-derived data. Generally, the rankings agreed quite closely with the numerical data. Various details of these reliability studies are discussed.

INTRODUCTION

In a recent paper (2) we have discussed in detail a procedure for coding visual field data for automated statistical data analysis. This procedure involves the use of an instrument which we term a 'scotometer', whose construction and method of use is fully explained in the earlier paper (2). The scotometer was developed in order to convert visual fields plotted on a Goldmann perimeter into a digital form so that the data could be analyzed and stored by a computer. Essentially, this instrument is a device which facilitates the recording of the key mathematical and geometrical aspects of elliptically-shaped scotomata. A scotoma is defined in this paper as an area of the visual field in which no visual function can be detected and which is totally surrounded by an area possessing some detectable visual function for a target with a given object size and intensity. A central scotoma is one that includes the central point of the chart. The scotometer was designed on the premise that every scotoma can be approximated to an elliptical shape. The only exceptions we permitted were arcuate defects. This scotometer, we have found, does facilitate the determination of the key geometrical descriptors of each elliptical scotoma. The five characteristics which are easily read from the scotometer are: the major and minor axes' half-lengths, the angle of rotation that the major axis makes

Doc. Ophthal. Proc. Series, Vol. 26, ed. by E. L. Greve & G. Verriest

with the horizontal meridian, and the two coordinates of the center of the ellipse.

The scotometer consists of a baseplate (150 mm square) and a freely rotating wheel (135 mm diameter) on top of the plate (see Fig. 1 in Trost *et al.*, 2). Using the scotometer, it is easy to record the five characteristics of any scotoma. A technician then records the observed five figures on a computer-ready data form. A typical data form which we have used in our studies is seen in Fig. 1[2]. Other aspects of the visual field such as the peripheral field coordinates and the coordinates of any arcuate defects are also recorded on this data form. The data forms which we are currently using in our studies of the ocular vascular occlusive disorders allow for a peripheral field coordinate at each 15 degree increment from 0 to 345 degrees. Arcuate defects are recorded in each thirty degree sector from 0 to 360 degrees, i.e. 0–30 degrees, 30–60 degrees, . . . , 330–360 degrees. For the most part we have found this method of recording peripheral field data and arcuate defect data to be satisfactory. Additionally, we have found that the approximation of a scotoma by an elliptical shape generally approximates the plotted scotoma on a visual field chart. Of course, this may not be true for visual field data for other diseases.

The goal in this paper is to determine how well two simple numerical figures computed from the data in Fig. 1[2] agree with an ophthalmologist's subjective ratings of the fields.

MATERIALS AND METHODS

Sixteen patients with an initial diagnosis of venous stasis retinopathy (VSR) were selected for this exercise. Most of the patients were in their sixties and had been receiving either prednisone or placebo treatment for the disorder. For each patient-visit, three targets were used in plotting the field; I/2e, I/4e and V/4e. Each of these patients was a participant in a clinical study in which his fields were plotted at five different times. These times were: 1) the time of treatment assignment, 2–5) one, three, six and twelve months respectively after treatment began. We refer to these as visits 1, 2, 3, 4 and 5 respectively in the sequel. For eight patients all five visits were available, for six patients four visits were available, while only three visits were available for the remaining two patients.

The fields for a given patient were erased of all patient identification information and were then arranged in a random order. Three persons were then asked to rank the fields for a given patient on each of eight characteristics. The characteristics rated were:

Central Scotoma with I/2e
Central Scotoma with I/4e
Central Scotoma with V/4e
Overall Assessment of Central Scotoma
Overall Assessment of Field with I/2e
Overall Assessment of Field with I/4e
Overall Assessment of Field with V/4e
Overall Assessment of Field

A rater would rank the visual fields by assigning a value of 1 through 5 to each field; a value of 1 is assigned to the worst field, and a value of 5 to the best field. The raters independently ranked each patient's set of fields in this manner. Two of the raters, R_1 and R_2, were board-certified opthalmologists with expertise in ocular vascular occlusive diseases. The third rater, R_3, was a research assistant who had initially assisted in the development of the field coding process.

In addition to these subjective rankings of each field, eight summary numbers were computed from the computer coded data. The first three summary numbers were the areas of the central scotoma for each of the three isopters; these quantities were computed via

$$\text{I.} \quad A = ls\pi \quad \text{where } A = \text{area of the scotoma}, \; l = \text{long axis length}, \; s = \text{short axis length}.$$

To provide an overall figure for central scotoma, a weighted average (A_0) of the three areas, $A_{I/2}$, $A_{I/4}$ and $A_{V/4}$, was computed via

$$\text{II.} \quad A_0 = 0.6\, A_{I/2} + 0.3\, A_{I/4} + 0.1\, A_{V/4}.$$

The remaining four quantities were also area figures. Three were the areas of the field in which there was detectable vision (T) for each isopter, I/2e, I/4e and V/4e. These areas, $T_{I/2}$, $T_{I/4}$ and $T_{V/4}$, were computed in the following manner:

a. Compute the area of each 15° circular sector of the field (P_i) via $P_i = (\pi r^2/24)$ where r is the distance from the point of fixation on the chart to the outer boundary of the isopter.

III. b. Sum the twelve areas by adding $P_1 + P_2 + P_3 + \ldots + P_{12} = P$ ($\Sigma_{i=1}^{12} P_i = P$).

c. Subtract from P the areas of the central scotoma, other scotoma and arcuate defects.

d. This figure is the area of detectable vision for the isopter (T).

Denoting these areas by $T_{I/2}$, $T_{I/4}$ and $T_{V/4}$, the overall field area (T_0) was computed via

$$\text{IV.} \quad T_0 = 0.6\, T_{I/2} + 0.3\, T_{I/4} + 0.1\, T_{V/4}.$$

In the remainder of this paper we focus on the two simple numerical figures, A_0 and T_0. The principle question is simply how well do A_0 and T_0 agree with the raters' rankings of the fields?

STATISTICAL PROCEDURES

For each patient's set of fields the central scotoma assessment and the overall field assessments were analyzed separately. The values of A_0 and T_0 were ranked from worst to best for each patient. These rankings, R_0, were then compared to the subjective rankings via Spearman's correlation coefficient (1). In addition, the raters were compared against one another via Spearman's correlation coefficient. For two sets of rankings on a patient, say $B_1, \ldots, B_5$

Table 1. Summary of patient visit data and reliability tests.

Patient	Rating scheme	Visit 1	Visit 2	Visit 3	Visit 4	Visit 5		Reliability R_1 vs R_0	R_2 vs R_0	R_3 vs R_0	R_1 vs R_2	R_1 vs R_3	R_2 vs R_3
1	A_0	0	442	160	0	0	D_{CS}	1.5	1.5	0	0	1.5	1.5
	T_0	5803	5685	5892	6682	6564	D_O	0	2	2	2	2	0
2	A_0	0	0	0	0	0	D_{CS}	0	0	0	0	0	0
	T_0	5789	5515	5780	6781	6481	D_O	10	6.5	10	2.5	0	2.5
3	A_0	15	0	8	312	45	D_{CS}	20	20	20	0	0	0
	T_0	3879	4305	4853	5943	6329	D_O	2.5	2	2	0.5	2.5	2
4	A_0	769	37	60	53	195	D_{CS}	2	2	6	0	2	2
	T_0	3568	4394	3600	3259	2987	D_O	5	8	2	11	5	6
5	A_0	101	371	506	335	268	D_{CS}	2	2	2	0	6	6
	T_0	4150	2027	5146	2696	2488	D_O	6.5	12	14	2.5	7.5	2
6	A_0	28	0	0	0	0	D_{CS}	0	0	0	0	0	0
	T_0	4930	6984	6972	7203	6469	D_O	10.5	5	6	4.5	3.5	5
7	A_0	0	28	47	15	32	D_{CS}	10	10	10	0	0	0
	T_0	4870	5150	5159	3040	2741	D_O	2	8	6	2	2	2
8	A_0	200	131	19	68	38	D_{CS}	16.25	15.5	20	5	7	5.5
	T_0	3334	4741	3028	5256	4275	D_O	2	2	2	0	0	0
9	A_0	40	0	32	34	–	D_{CS}	6.5	8	8	0.5	0.5	0
	T_0	4316	5054	3395	2968	–	D_O	2.5	2.5	0	0	2.5	2.5
10	A_0	–	99	299	240	152	D_{CS}	8	2	0	6	8	2
	T_0	–	4409	3157	3216	4016	D_O	8	5	0	5	8	5

11	A_0	34	34	19	11	–	D_{CS}	0.5	0.5	0.5	0	0	0
	T_0	2849	2142	1200	3409	–	D_O	8	2	0	6	8	2
12	A_0	92	30	22	17	–	D_{CS}	2	2	6	0	2	2
	T_0	4190	5116	4225	4942	–	D_O	0.5	0.5	2	0	0.5	0.5
13	A_0	0	28	0	0	–	D_{CS}	1.5	6	1.5	8.5	3.5	6
	T_0	4778	5078	5654	5401	–	D_O	2.75	3	0	10.5	0.75	6
14	A_0	0	212	720	586	–	D_{CS}	2	0	2	2	6	2
	T_0	5077	4293	1967	3008	–	D_O	2	2	0	0	2	2
15	A_0	55	19	166	–	–	D_{CS}	2	2	2	0	0	0
	T_0	3217	4012	4611	–	–	D_O	3.5	2	0	0.5	2.5	2
16	A_0	11	17	11	–	–	D_{CS}	1.5	1.5	0.5	0	2	2
	T_0	3719	3959	6463	–	–	D_O	2	2	3	0	1	1
Summary – D_{CS} $\chi^2(32)$								64.19	67.74	68.34	101.57	83.95	89.99
Summary – D_O $\chi^2(32)$								59.94	58.29	78.85	75.65	69.69	72.81

Notes

A_0 and T_0 are the values of the areas of central scotoma and peripheral fields respectively, as described in the text (See II and IV).

R_0, R_1, R_2, and R_3 are the rankings of the objective data, rater 1, rater 2 and rater 3 respectively.

D_{CS} and D_O are D computed values for the rankings on the central scotoma and peripheral fields respectively as described in the text (See V).

and $C_1, \ldots, C_5$, we computed the statistic D by summing the squares of the differences between the rankings.

$$\text{V.} \qquad D = \Sigma_{i=1}^{5} (B_i - C_i)^2$$

and under the hypothesis of no association between the rankings, determined its P-value from the tables of Spearman's correlation coefficient. Then summing $-2 \log_e$ (P-value) across patients, a chi-square statistic with 32 degrees of freedom arose for testing the hypothesis of no correlation between the rankings. The actual test statistic was then the standard normal deviate Z which arose by computing

$$\text{VI.} \qquad Z = \frac{X^2 - 32}{8}$$

where X^2 is the chi-square statistic computed across the sixteen patients.

RESULTS

The left half of Table I shows the numerical rankings of the central scotoma and peripheral field for each patient. It should be noted that in the case where two or more scales were tied, the mid-rank was used. For example, in patient 1 in Table I, A_0 values for the five visits were 0, 442, 160, 0 and 0 respectively. Thus in order of ranking of these visits, their score would be 1 for visit two, 2 for visit 3, while the other three visits have a tied ranking because of identical scores. The visits with tied ranking would normally have scored 3, 4 and 5. Since the actual score for these three visits was the same, we assigned an average score (mid-ranking) to each of these three visits by summing up the total normal score (i.e. $3 + 4 + 5 = 12$) and dividing it by the number of these visits, i.e., three; this then gives a rank of 4 for the visits 1, 4, and 5. Thus the final ranks for visits 1, 2, 3, 4 and 5 in this patient would be 4, 1, 2, 4 and 4 respectively. Similarly, the same procedure was used for computing mid-ranks for tied subjective rankings from the individual raters.

The right half of Table 1 shows the degree of differences (D_{CS}, for differences in central scotoma and D_O for differences in peripheral field rankings) between all possible pairs of rankings (R_0 through R_3) for each patient. It can be seen that the subjective ratings (R_1 through R_3) agreed quite closely with the ranks of the numerically derived data. For central scotoma the Z-values computed via (VI) were 4.024, 4.468 and 4.543 for raters 1, 2, and 3 respectively when compared to the numerical data rankings. The comparable Z-values for the overall field assessments were found to be 3.493, 3.286 and 5.856 respectively. When compared to the standard normal curve, each of these six statistics is highly statistically significant ($P < 0.001$ for each statistic). In a similar manner the tests for the agreement between pairs of subjective ratings are also strongly indicative of concordance or agreement between the subjective ratings.

DISCUSSION

From these data it appears that the two simple visual field measures, A_0 and T_0, correlate quite highly with the rankings of visual fields made by ophthalmologists. This suggests that these two quantities may be useful in the longitudinal analysis of visual field data. With the use of a computer these figures would be easier to track longitudinally than a continual subjective assessment on the part of an ophthalmologist.

A further study was also performed to see how well the quantity T_0 correlates with an ophthalmologist's ratings across patients. For this study one field was selected at random from each of the sixteen patients' array of fields. The two ophthalmologists, R_1 and R_2, then ranked the fields from 1 to 16 on the basis of the overall field assessment. These rankings were then compared to the computed values of T_0. In Fig. 1 the raw data are plotted and the correlation coefficient determined. Each of the three pairwise coefficients is significant at $P < 0.001$, indicating that inter-patient rankings of fields also correlate highly with the numerical figure T_0.

While further work is certainly required, these data do offer the hope that these simple numerical figures may be valuable in the assessment of visual fields.

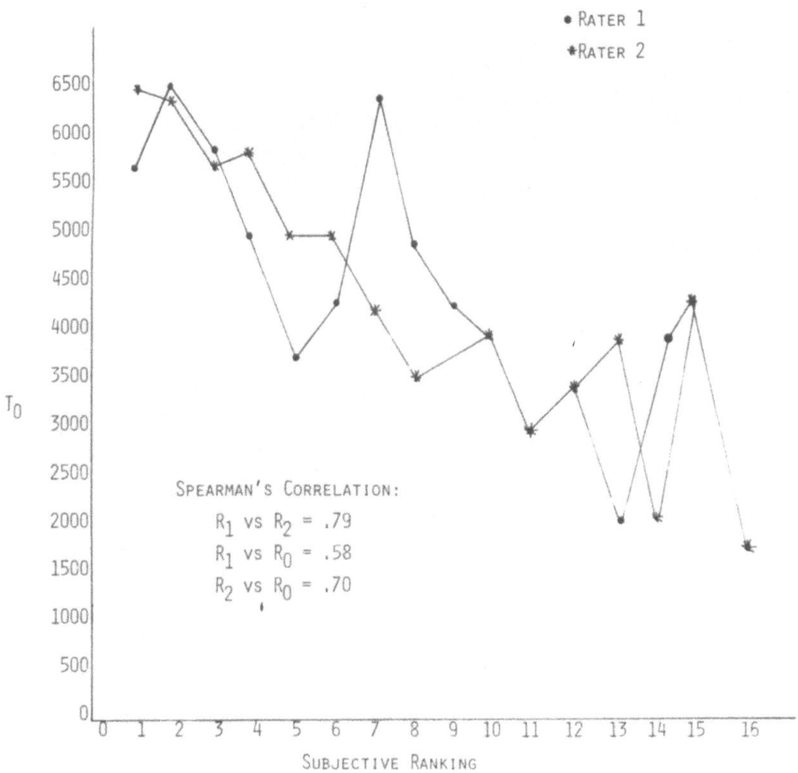

Fig. 1. Relationship between raters' subjective rankings and the measure, T_0.

REFERENCES

1. Hollander, M. & D. A. Wolfe. Nonparametric statistical methods. New York: John Wiley and Son, Inc. (1973).
2. Trost, D. C., R. F. Woolson & S. S. Hayreh. Quantification of visual fields for statistical analysis. Arch. Ophth. 97: 2175–2180 (1979).

This study was supported by National Eye Institute Grant No. EY01151.

Authors' address:
Dr. S. S. Hayreh
Department of Ophthalmology
University of Iowa
Iowa City, Iowa 52242
U.S.A.

RELATIONSHIP BETWEEN FUNDUS DENSITOMETRIC ANALYSIS AND PERIMETRY

M. ZINGIRIAN, M. ROLANDO & F. CARDILLO PICCOLINO

(*Genoa, Italy*)

ABSTRACT

Comparisons of glaucomatous perimetric defects and ophthalmoscopical changes of the optic disc and of the peripapillary area have already been reported by other authors. These studies are generally based on subjective evaluations that greatly reduce the reliability of the results. The elaboration of red free light photograms and angiograms by an image processor offers an objective method of evaluating disc pallor and hypofluorescence. The correlation between these findings and visual field defects are shown.

INTRODUCTION

The correlation between perimetric defects and morphologic and angiographic findings in the papillary area has been previously studied (1–9). Subjective interpretations, on photographic findings, have certainly influenced the data up until now. In the present study, the relationship between visual field defects and the following factors has been evaluated by an objective method:

- Disc pallor.
- Fluorescein injection defects in the optic disc.
- Fluorescein injection defects in the peripapillary choroid.

MATERIAL AND METHOD

Black and white photographs were taken in red free light and fundus fluoroangiographic studies were performed on 15 normal and 15 glaucomatous eyes. The glaucomatous eyes had perimetric defects in one quadrant.

In order to obtain a uniform illumination of the papillary area the fundus camera was centered exactly on the disc. The wide angle (45°) lens guaranteed a good focusing of all the papillary planes.

The photographic and the angiographic negatives, taken in the arteriovenous phase, were displayed on a monitor. An image processor selected, on each photogram, up to 10 levels of grey and assigned an arbitrary colour to every single level (10).

The method allowed for an objective evaluation of the photograms.

The colour scale made this evaluation easier as a consequence of the

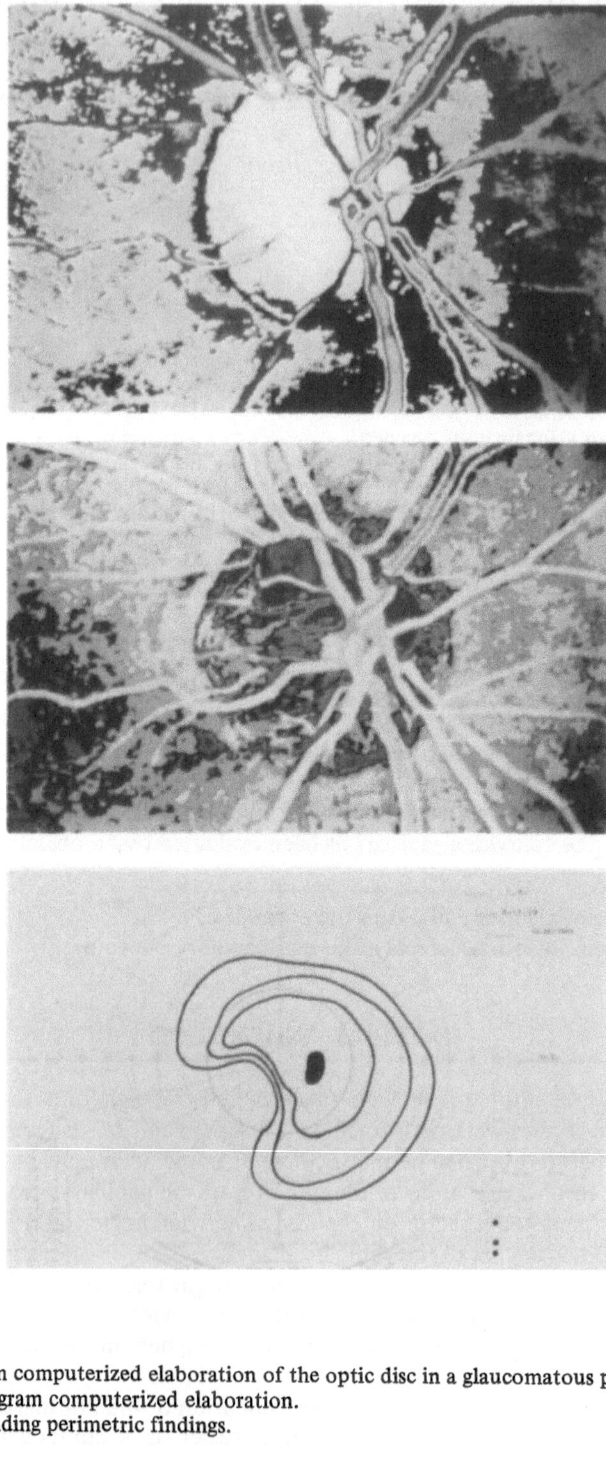

Fig. 1.
A. Photogram computerized elaboration of the optic disc in a glaucomatous patient.
B. The angiogram computerized elaboration.
C. Corresponding perimetric findings.

chromatic and intensity graduations. The visual field examination in each subject was performed using the Goldmann perimeter (background luminance = 31.5 asb) with the kinetic method.

RESULTS

Normal eyes

In 11 cases, an area of major pallor corresponded to the central portion of the disc; in 4 cases, it also corresponded to a part of the rim. In 3 cases, hypofluorescent areas were seen, not exceeding 1/4 of the disc surface. The localization of these areas did not correspond to pale zones of the disc. In 3 cases there were wide areas of peripapillary background hypofluorescence.

Glaucomatous eyes

In all cases examined, areas of pallor were seen both in the central portion and at the rim of the disc. The pale areas were located in one or more sectors of the rim. In all cases, limited areas of hypofluorescence were present in different sectors of the disc. In each case a good correspondence between hypofluorescence and pallor zones could be observed. In 7 cases, choroidal filling defects were found in the peripapillary area. The pale areas and rim fluorescence defects were not always correlated with a visual field defect. When pallor and hypofluorescence were present in the same district of the papillary rim there was always a perimetric defect in the corresponding sector (Fig. 1a, b, c). In no case could a correlation between choroidal injection defects and perimetric alterations be detected.

DISCUSSION

From the results of our studies, the following conclusions can be drawn:

- Papillary rim pallor and zones of papillary and peripapillary hypofluorescence do not necessarily seem to be correlated with visual field defects when they exist as isolated signs.
- Pallor and hypofluorescence, concomitant in the same portion of the disc, must be considered as a significant index of the existence of a visual field defect, probably due to a severe vascular disturbance.
- Both these signs can be evaluated in a reliable and objective way only when the photograms are analyzed by a quantitative densitometric method.

REFERENCES

1. Begg, I. S., S. M. Drance & H. Goldmann. Fluorescein angiography in the evaluation of focal circulatory ischemia of the optic nervehead in relation to the arcuate scotoma in glaucoma. Canad. J. Ophthal. 7: 68–74 (1972).

2. Blumenthal, M., K. A. Gitter, M. Best, M. Galin & H. Toyofuku. Peripapillary choroidal circulation in glaucoma. Arch. Ophthal. 86: 31–38 (1971).
3. Bonnet, M., T. Baserer & J. D. Grange. Angiographie fluoroscénique de la papilla dans l'hypertension oculaire et le glaucome. J. Fr. Ophtalmol. 2: 239–246 (1979).
4. Cardillo Piccolino, F., M. Zingirian & G. C. Parodi. The electronic image analysis in retinal fluoroangiography. Ophthalmologica 179: 142–147 (1979).
5. Hayreh, S. S. Colour and fluorescence of the optic disc. Ophthalmologica 165: 100–108 (1972).
6. Hitchings, R. A. & L. G. Spaeth. Fluorescein angiography in chronic simple and low tension glaucoma. Brit. J. Ophthal. 61: 126–132 (1977).
7. Hoskins Jr., H. D. & E. C. Gelber. Optic disk topography and visual field defects in patients with increased intraocular pressure. Amer. J. Ophthal. 80: 284–290 (1975).
8. Oosterhuis, J. A. & N. Grtzak-Moorein. Fluorescein angiography of the optic disc in glaucoma. Ophthalmologica 160: 331–351 (1970).
9. Schwartz, B., J. C. Reiser & S. L. Fishbein. Fluorescein angiographic defects of the optic disc in glaucoma. Arch. Ophthal. 95: 1961–1974 (1977).
10. Tsukahara, S., S. Nagataki, M. Sugaya, S. Yoshida & Y. Komuro. Visual field defects, cup-disc ratio and fluorescein angiography in glaucomatous optic atrophy. Adv. Ophthal. 35: 73–93 (1978).

This study was supported by a grant from the Consiglio Nazionale delle Ricerche, Roma, Italy.

Authors' address:
University Eye Clinic
Viale Benedetto XV
I-16132 Genoa
Italy

THE NORMAL PERICOECAL AREA
A static method for investigation

M. ZINGIRIAN, G. CALABRIA, E. GANDOLFO & G. SANDINI

(Genoa, Italy)

ABSTRACT

A careful perimetric assessment of the pericoecal area is quite important since it is often considered the site of earlier glaucomatous defects. The results of such examination by means of classical techniques are however made unreliable by several factors as the presence of the blind spot, the coecal funnel, the angioscotomata, peripapillary chorioretinal degenerations, especially found in myopic eyes, etc. . . . . For these reasons we analysed the distribution of the luminance threshold in the pericoecal area of normal subjects, using single static stimuli, closely arranged around the blind spot. Special attention was paid to the convenience of presenting data in a numerical or in a graphical form (grey scales, colour scales, multiple static profiles, etc. . . .).

INTRODUCTION

Inter-individual variability of the light sensitivity in the pericoecal area is well known (1, 2, 3). An accurate static analysis of this area in normal subjects and a densitometric evaluation of the results has allowed us to obtain further information on the physiological distribution of luminance threshold around the blind spot.

MATERIAL AND METHOD

20 normal emmetropic right eyes in 20 subjects, whose ages ranged from 20 to 30 were examined using the Goldmann perimeter (background luminance = 31.5 asb) by the following procedure.

105 stimuli positions evenly arranged in the pericoecal area (as shown in Fig. 1) were statically analyzed. For each position the target I of the Goldmann's series ($1/4\,mm^2$) was presented three times for each luminance level. The target luminance was initially subliminal and then gradually increased by steps of 0.1 L.U., until the threshold was reached. We considered threshold the luminance level perceived at least twice for every three presentations.

The results of each examination and the mean values derived from all individual measurements in each position were plotted on suitable graphs. Five representation methods were used: numerical scales (Fig. 2), proportional surfaces (Fig. 3), grey scales (Fig. 4), conventional colour scales (Fig. 5) and multiple static profiles (Fig. 6).

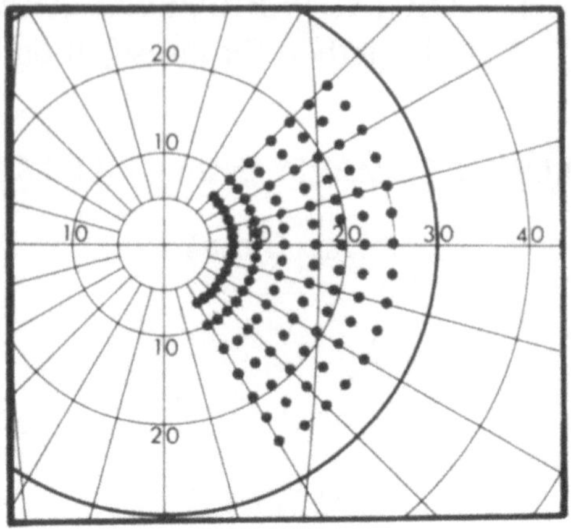

Fig. 1. Stimuli distribution in the pericoecal area.

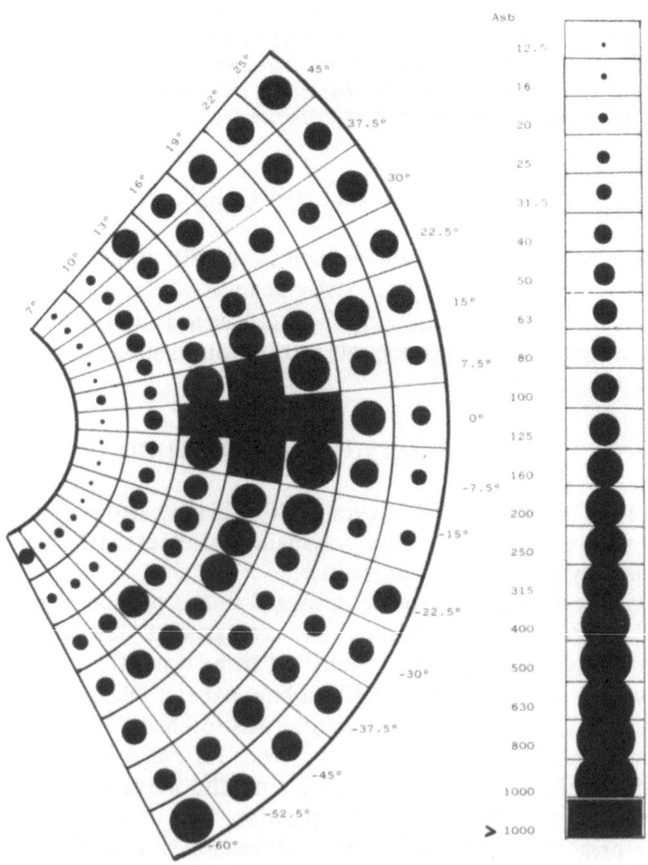

Fig. 3. Proportional surfaces.

PERICOECAL VISUAL FIELD

Name: CARLO TRAVERSO
Age: 26
Day: Sept.14th,1979
Diagnosis: Normal
Right Eye

Object = 1/4 mm^2

ECCENTRICITY

MERIDIANS	7°	10°	13°	16°	19°	22°	25°
45°	16	20	80	63	80	80	125
37 5°	16	25	50	80	50	100	80
30°	16	40	40	125	63	50	100
22.5	12.5	40	25	63	50	63	80
15°	12.5	31.5	50	125	100	125	80
7.5°	20	25	200	ABSOL.	200	63	40
0°	12.5	40	ABSOL.	ABSOL.	ABSOL.	125	40
-7.5°	12.5	25	160	ABSOL.	400	80	31.5
-15°	12.5	31.5	63	125	315	40	31.5
-22.5°	12.5	40	63	160	63	40	80
-30°	12.5	25	40	160	40	50	63
-37.5°	16	20	50	50	63	80	80
-45°	20	20	100	63	50	100	100
-52.5°	16	20	40	80	50	63	80
-60°	31.5	20	31.5	40	63	50	160

Fig. 2. Numerical scale.

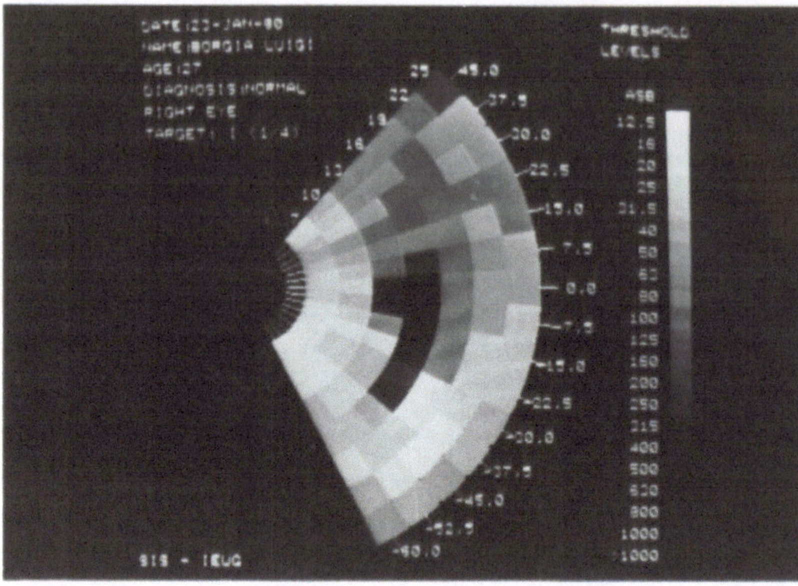

Fig. 4. Grey scale.

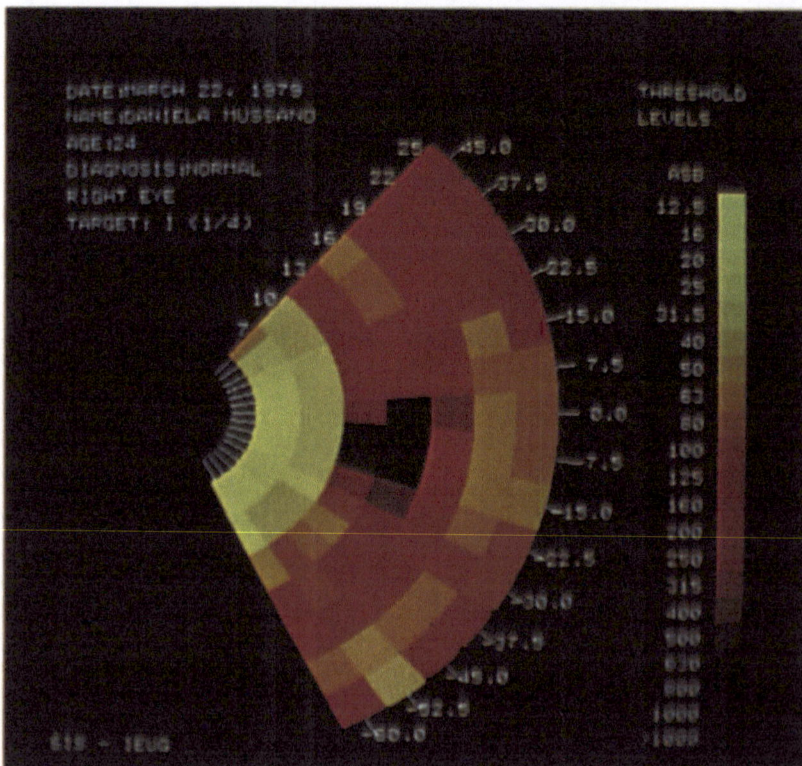

Fig. 5. Conventional colour scale.

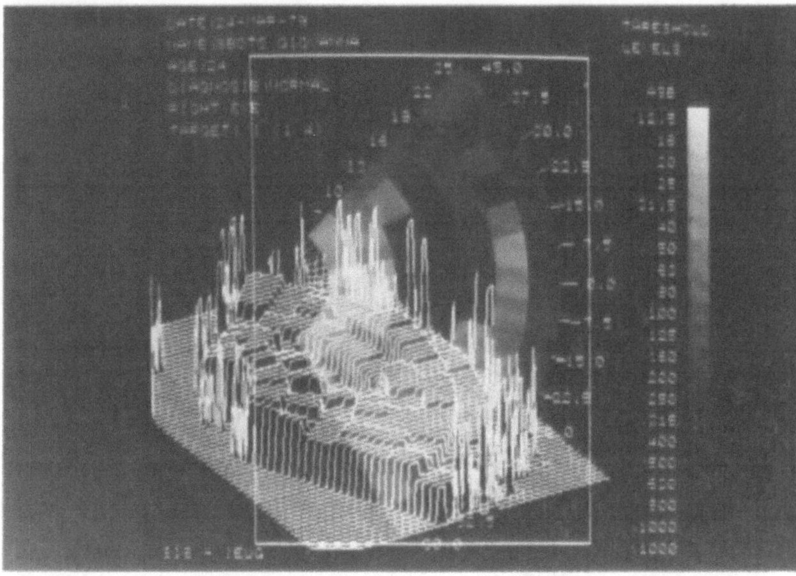

Fig. 6. Multiple static profiles.

The most indicative results were obtained from the grey scales and from the conventional colour scales representations. In the latter the density and chromatic gradations made the distribution threshold more easily interpreted. This kind of representation required previous data storage in an image processor and a subsequent reproduction on the visual display. The procedure also allowed us to obtain an equidensitometric evaluation of the results, i.e. the extraction of the stimuli positions corresponding to the same threshold level or to a limited interval of levels.

RESULTS

1. *Individual threshold distribution*

Every pericoecal graph shows in the middle portion three to six positions where the sensitivity is completely lost. These positions correspond to the absolute density nucleus of the blind spot. Around these positions some high threshold points clearly reveal their relationship with the relative density ring of the blind spot. Above and below the blind spot the gradient appears very irregular as a consequence of localized sensitivity depression in single points or in groups of confluent points. These confluent points tend to arrange themselves primarily along the parallels, but not necessarily those parallels that cross the blind spot (Fig. 7). If a limited interval of grey levels is isolated from the total data of one examination, we can observe more accurately how discontinuous the sensitivity gradient is from the central to the peripheral border of the pericoecal area (Fig. 8).

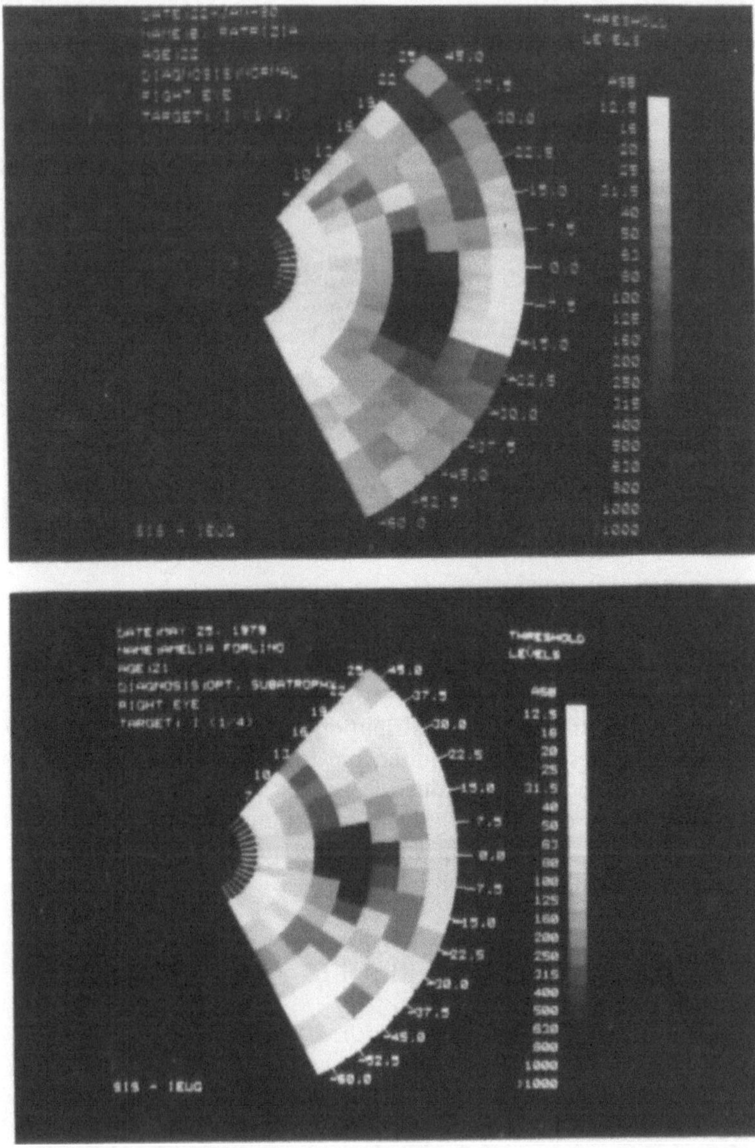

Fig. 7. Pericoecal threshold distribution in four normal right eyes (grey scales representation).

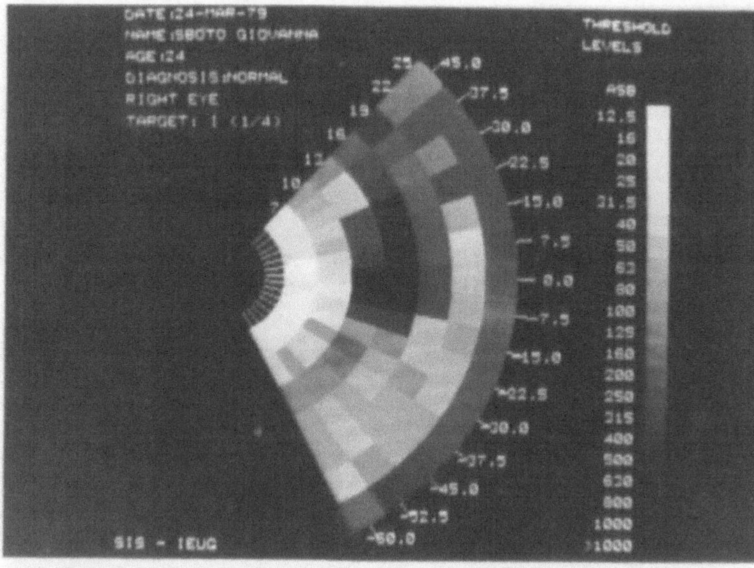

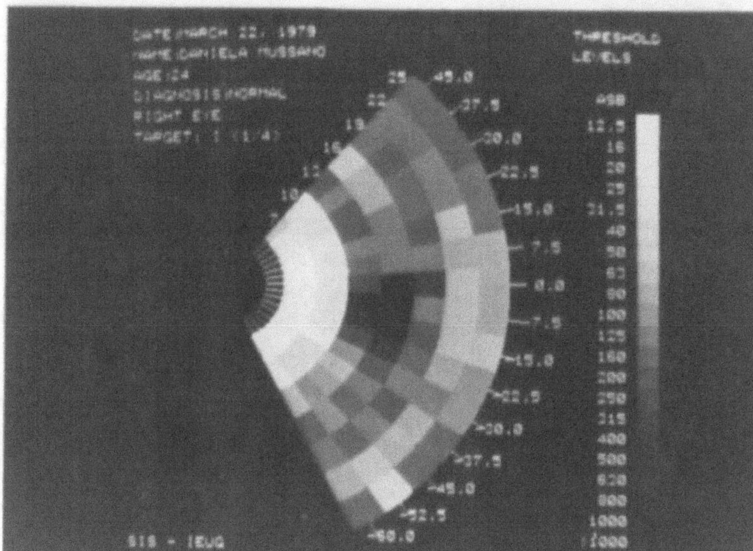

Fig. 7 (continued).

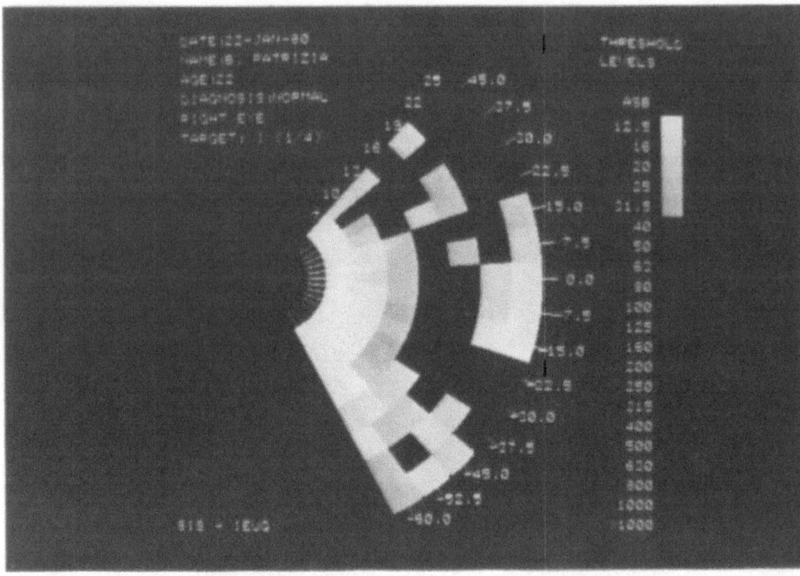

Fig. 8. Pericoecal area of a normal eye. A limited interval of grey levels was isolated.

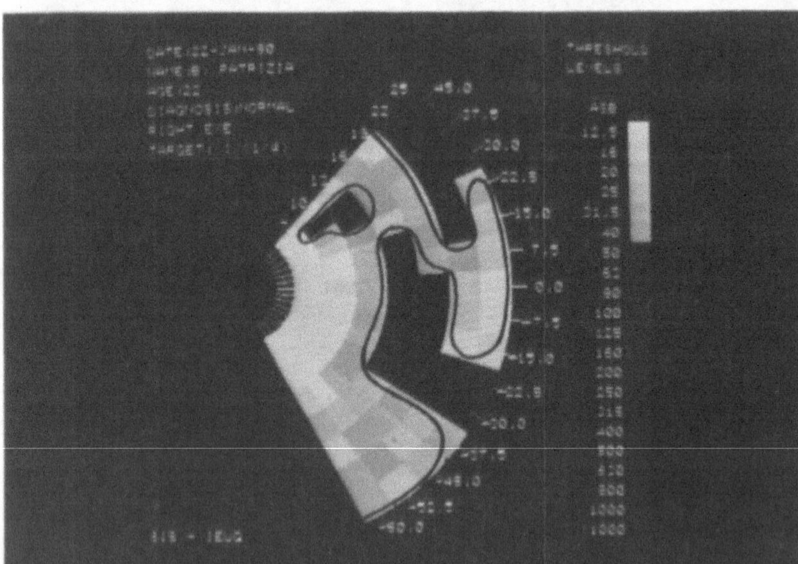

Fig. 9. Isopteric-like reproduction of light sensitivity in the pericoecal area (the same case as in Fig. 8).

Finally, the representation of all grey levels above a selected luminance enables us to obtain isopteric-like reproductions of the irregular threshold distribution above and below the blind spot (Fig. 9).

In reference to the individual gradient, the localized maximum sensitivity fall detected in the pericoecal area was 1.0 L.U.

2. *Mean threshold distribution*

The mean results derived from the examination of 20 normal eyes are displayed in Fig. 10 (grey scale). Due to inter-individual variations, only three positions of the diagram correspond to the absolute nucleus of the blind spot and three to its relative density ring. Above and below the blind spot an area of irregular sensitivity depression occupies the peripheral two thirds of the pericoecal area. Below the blind spot the points of low sensitivity are more concentrated in the middle portion and along the peripheral border of the pericoecal area with a strip of higher sensitivity in between. The mean localized sensitivity reduction is 0.3 L.U. with a s.d. of 0.2. The localized maximum sensitivity fall is 0.6 L.U. Isopteric reconstructions, based on equidensitometric analysis, indicate the shape and the maximal extension of the areas of reduced sensitivity (Fig. 11).

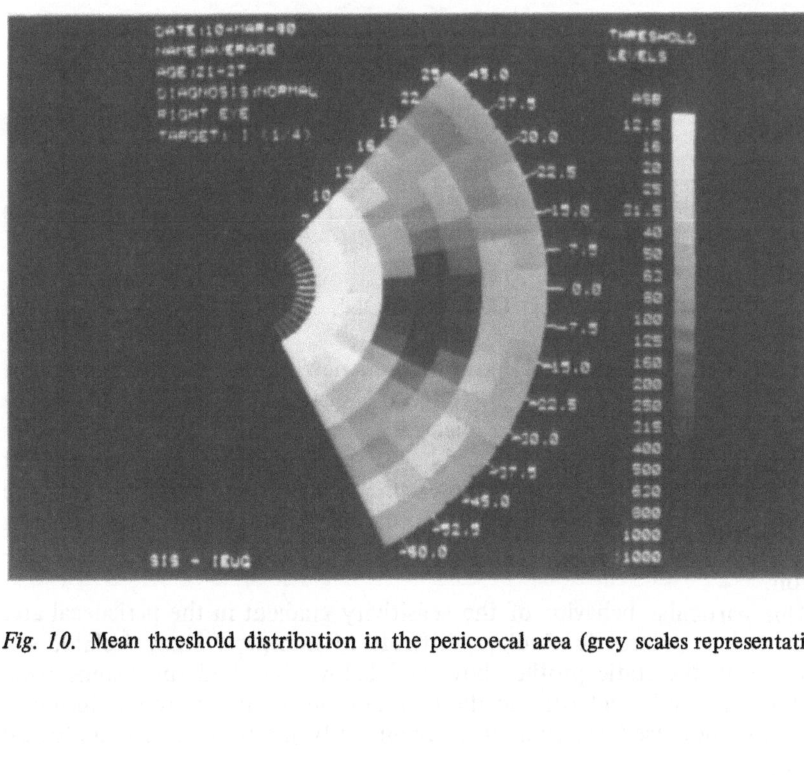

Fig. 10. Mean threshold distribution in the pericoecal area (grey scales representation).

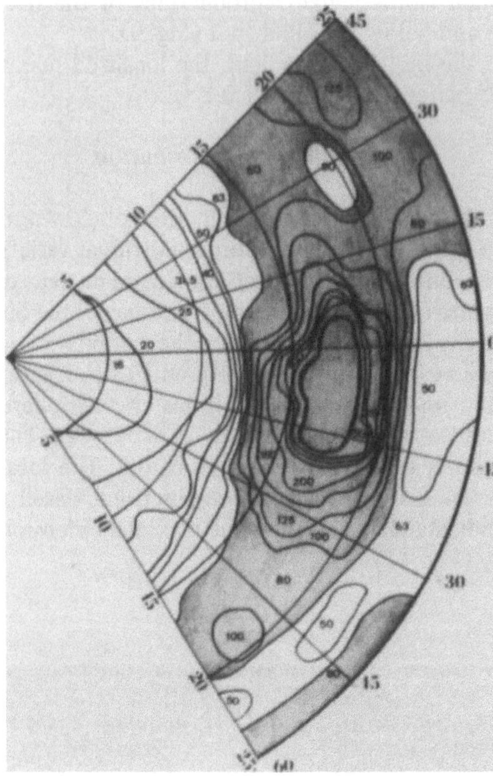

Fig. 11. Mean threshold distribution in the pericoecal area (isopteric-like representation).

CONCLUSIONS

The present investigation does not propose a new exploration method for the pericoecal area, but attempts to verify the distribution mode of sensitivity threshold in this area in normal subjects.

The reduced sensitivity above and below the blind spot is correlated to but not completely explained by the presence of angioscotomata. Probably the particular enlargement mode of the coecal funnel toward both the superior and inferior direction is another explanation for this irregular threshold distribution.

This particular behavior of the sensitivity gradient in the pericoecal area often makes perimetric findings difficult to interpret. Many isolated depressions in the static profile above and below the blind spot; some paracentral isopteric irregularities in the temporal quadrants and the exclusion of the blind spot itself are sometimes erroneously interpreted as pathological signs.

The only reliable element in these cases can arise from the quantitiative assessment of the sensitivity reductions.

On the basis of our investigation localized sensitivity reductions in the pericoecal area with a maximum density of 0.6 to 0.8 L.U. can be assumed to be still within physiological limits. The width of these low sensitivity areas is very large, until above 8° to 10° for slight sensitivity depressions (0.2 to 0.3 L.U.), being more restricted (from about 2° to 3°) if the sensitivity depression is deeper (0.6 to 0.8 L.U.),

These variations in width are still larger when the areas of reduced sensitivity extend along the parallels. Of course further experimental confirmation of these results is needed before definitive conclusions are drawn.

REFERENCES

1. Benjumeda, A. S. Rodriguez Rubio & J. D. Campos. Perimetria estatica circular seriada. Topografia normal de la mancha ciega. Arch. Soc. Esp. Oftal. 34: 635–644 (1974).
2. Greve, E. L. Single and multiple stimulus static perimetry; the two phases of perimetry. Doc. Ophth. 36: 147–155 (1971).
3. Ourgaud, A. G. & L. Aubert. Adaptométrie topographique circulaire chez le sujet normal. Bull. Soc. Opht. France 59: 528–532 (1959).

This study was supported by a grant from the Consiglio Nazionale delle Ricerche, Roma, Italy.

Authors' address:
University Eye Clinic
Viale Benedetto XV
16132 Genoa
Italy

AUTHORS INDEX